"A very complete compilation that I would recommend to anyone interested in going to the Big Sur area."

—*Ada Babine*
Chair of the Sierra Club's Santa Barbara group
& veteran Big Sur hiker

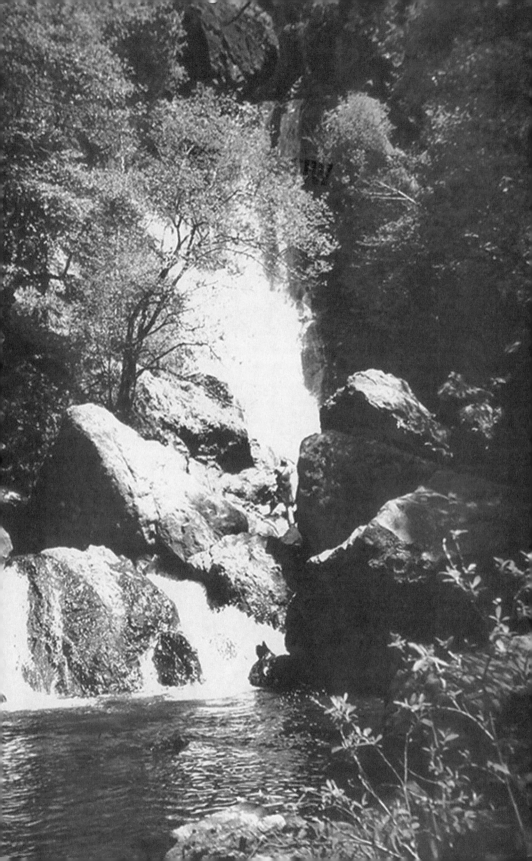

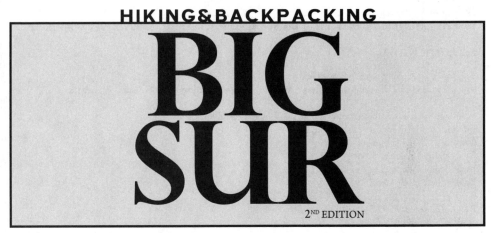

HIKING&BACKPACKING

BIG SUR

2ND EDITION

Your complete guide to the trails of Big Sur,
Ventana Wilderness, and Silver Peak Wilderness

Analise Elliot Heid

 WILDERNESS PRESS ... *on the trail since 1967*

Hiking & Backpacking Big Sur
Your complete guide to the trails of Big Sur, Ventana Wilderness, & Silver Peak Wilderness

2nd EDITION 2013

ISBN: 978-0-89997-727-0
eISBN: 978-0-89997-726-3

CATALOGING-IN-PUBLICATION DATA IS AVAILABLE FROM THE LIBRARY OF CONGRESS.

Manufactured in the United States of America

Published by: **Wilderness Press**
                Keen Communications
                P.O. Box 43673
                Birmingham, AL 35243
                (800) 443-7227; FAX (205) 326-1012
                info@wildernesspress.com
                www.wildernesspress.com

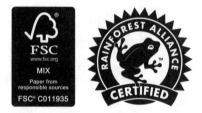

Visit our website for a complete listing of our books and for ordering information.

Distributed by Publishers Group West

SAFETY NOTICE: Although Wilderness Press and the author have made every attempt to ensure that the information in this book is accurate at press time, they are not responsible for any loss, damage, injury, or inconvenience that may occur to anyone while using this book. You are responsible for your own safety and health while in the wilderness. The fact that a trail is described in this book does not mean that it will be safe for you. Be aware that trail conditions can change from day to day. Always check local conditions and know your own limitations.

ACKNOWLEDGMENTS

■ ■ ■ ■ ■ ■ ■ ■ ■ ■ ■ ■ ■

FOREMOST, I would like to thank Jeff Schaffer, author of Wilderness Press's *Hiking the Big Sur Country*, which this book replaces. I drew upon his incredibly accurate mapping and trail descriptions in writing this book.

My parents are at the head of the list of acknowledgments. Their love and support has given me the confidence to live passionately and follow my dreams. To Craig, for making my first experiences in the backcountry filled with adventure and fun. To Heid, for countless hours spent listening and encouraging. To Matt, for guidance and inspiration to go for it. To Jannie, for your willingness to stand up for what you believe in. To Laurie and Chris, for your incredible generosity. To Briezer and Wickland, whom I can always count on for an adventure. To E, for many words of advice. To Trevor, for your friendship and flexibility. To my community of friends and avid adventurers: Heart & Lissin, Hammer, Aaron, Pogen, Thomas, Isabel, Bill, and Joanne for accompanying me on unknown and overgrown trails. To Michelle and Leah, for taking the path less traveled. To Jan and Sid, for opening your home and hearts.

I wish to thank Thomas and Caroline Winnett at Wilderness Press for the opportunity to pursue professionally what I love. Thank you to David Lauterborn, who read the manuscript, contributing his knowledge and art of good writing, and to Roslyn, for picking up the pieces and guiding me through the process to completion.

A special thank-you goes to the hundreds of volunteers who built, maintained, and continue to work on the trails of the Santa Lucia Mountains. Unfortunately, the USFS has said that budgetary constraints preclude them from restoring most of the trails in the wilderness in the foreseeable future. Without the grassroots volunteer efforts of the folks at the Ventana Chapter of the Sierra Club and the Ventana Wilderness Alliance, many of the remote trails that traverse the heart of Ventana would be lost. The dedication of these volunteers to protecting and restoring the wildlands of the Big Sur coast is vital to the preservation of the rugged wilderness and biodiversity of the Northern Santa Lucia Mountains for generations to come. Without their efforts, this book would not have been possible.

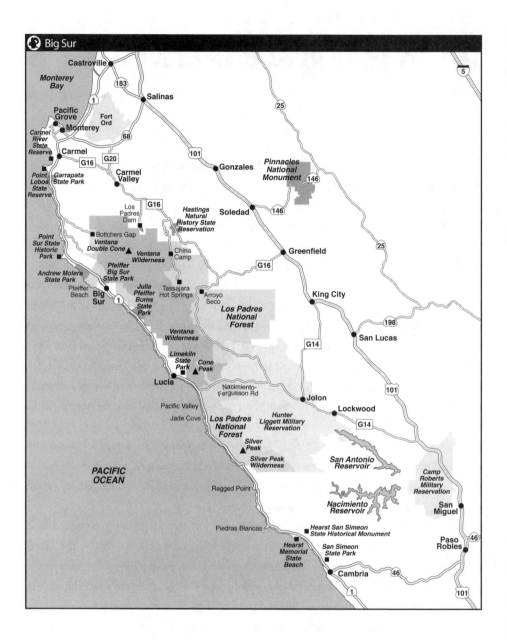

C O N T E N T S

PART II Ventana & Silver Peak Wildernesses

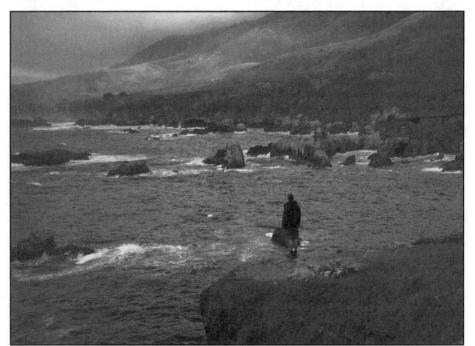

Solitude overlooking a vast ocean at the edge of our continent

CHAPTER one

Introducing Big Sur

■ ■ ■ ■ ■ ■ ■ ■ ■ ■ ■ ■ ■

BIG SUR. THE NAME EVOKES IMAGES of a wild and rugged coast. In the mid-1800s, a handful of independent and adventurous homesteaders, fur traders, ranchers, and entrepreneurs settled the area along steep, narrow wagon roads. But Big Sur would remain remote until Highway 1 was completed in 1938. Modern-day visitors are struck by the drama of this two-lane roller coaster, which twists and winds through blankets of fog along sheer cliffs hundreds of feet above the Pacific.

Just where Big Sur begins and ends has long been a matter of debate. Historically, early Spanish explorers named the vague unexplored wilderness south of Monterey *El Sur Grande* ("The Big South"). Today, the region encompasses a 90-mile coastal stretch between Carmel to the north and San Simeon to the south, flanked on one side by the high peaks of the Santa Lucia Range and on the other by the jagged coast and broad Pacific Ocean.

While Big Sur is widely renowned for its exceptional beauty, few people venture beyond Highway 1. In addition, few roads cross the Santa Lucia Range, making it one of the largest roadless areas along the continental US coast. The result? A vast, remote wilderness waits to be explored.

About This Book

IN THIS BOOK, trips in Big Sur country are described in two parts: Part I, State & Federal Lands of the Big Sur Coast, and Part II, Ventana & Silver Peak Wildernesses.

Trips in Part I list day hikes only, as state and federal lands are limited to day use. While some state parks offer campgrounds, backcountry camping is forbidden. In contrast, the wilderness areas described in Part II offer more than 300 miles of trails and restricted roads to explore on either day hikes or extended backpacking treks. Each part is subdivided into chapters that list trips in geographic order from north to south.

Each trip includes summary information and the hike description itself.

Summary

Summary information for each trip includes:

TITLE The highlighted destination(s) along the route.

LENGTH AND TYPE The overall length of the hike and whether the route is out-and-back, point-to-point, or a loop. Distances to specific waypoints are listed in each hike description.

RATING This book rates each trip according to physical effort and ease of access. Ratings are as follows:

> *Easy:* Typically a short hike on level terrain with less than 500 feet of total elevation gain.
>
> *Moderate:* Hikes with a consistent medium grade with roughly 500–1000 feet of total elevation gain.
>
> *Strenuous:* Typically longer hikes with approximately 1000–2000 feet of elevation gain.
>
> *Challenging:* A very strenuous hike with roughly 2000–3000 feet of total elevation gain over many miles of steep, rugged trails in often remote regions. Wilderness experience and ethics required.

TRAIL CONDITION Many routes within the wilderness areas are ill maintained, suffering from landslides, encroaching brush, and vanishing tread. The five-level rating system described below summarizes the general navigability of the trail. This section also advises whether the trail is good for kids, and whether you're likely to encounter poison oak.

> *Well maintained:* Typically heavily used and regularly maintained.
>
> *Clear:* A well-defined trail with no major obstructions.
>
> *Passable:* The trail is evident with some encroaching brush and/or downed debris. Lightly traveled and not regularly maintained.
>
> *Difficult:* The trail is faint with waist-high or above brush and/or fallen debris.
>
> *Impassable:* The trail is unrecognizable with major trail obstructions, including encroaching brush, landslides, and/or much fallen debris.

HIGHLIGHTS The natural feature(s) that distinguish each hike.

TO REACH THE TRAILHEAD Concise directions to the start of the trail. Where necessary, information is provided regarding facilities, water, entrance fees, and parking fees.

TRIP SUMMARY A basic description of the route, including any day hike or extended overnight options. Includes information on potential difficulties/hazards, as well as advice on the best time of year to visit.

Maps

Each trip is shown on a map, which is placed adjacent to the trip itself or adjacent to a nearby trip. Please see the map legend for details about the maps.

Map Legend

Trail Maps

——	Trail	▲	Mountain
- - - -	Alternate Trail	⊞	Picnic Area
T	Trailhead		National Park
P	Parking		National Monument; Wilderness Area
⚠	Camp		National Forest
🏠	Ranger Station	(5)	Interstate
?	Information	(395)	US Highway
S	Fee Collection Gate	(41)	State Highway

Trip Description

Each trip description offers a thorough breakdown of the route, including trail conditions, seasonal considerations, water sources, historical notes, geology, plant and animal life, etc. Directions include all trail and spur junctions, camps, natural landmarks, and other notable features. Camps, junctions, and certain key features are listed in bold type followed by a parenthetical notation of the distance from the trailhead in miles and elevation in feet—for example, **Hiding Canyon Camp** (5.5 miles, 2500').

In certain instances, trail descriptions may overlap from one trip to the next. In such cases, the reader might be directed to a previous description for the route up to a certain point—for example, "See TRIP 49 Pine Valley (page 199) for the first 5.3 miles of this route to **Pine Valley**."

If a spur leads to a notable feature (e.g., a camp, swimming hole, etc.), the trip description may include a Side Trip that elaborates on that feature. You'll also find sidebars throughout the text that offer more detail about natural features, historical anecdotes, and the like.

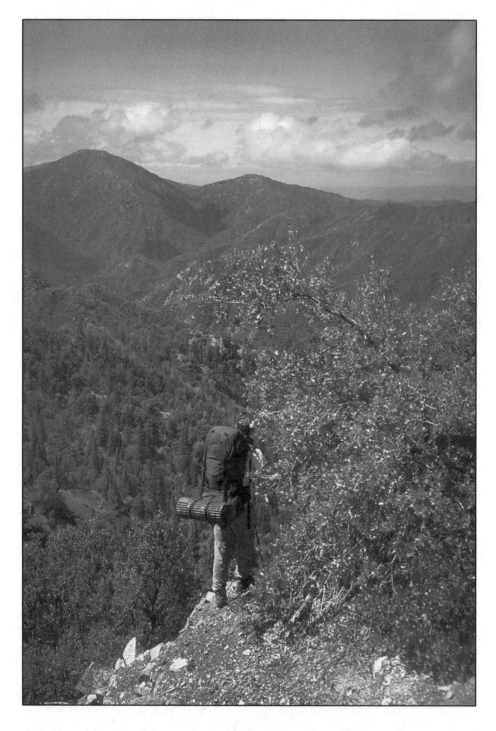

Tectonic activity created the prominent peaks and ridges of the Santa Lucia Range.

CHAPTER two

Natural History

■ ■ ■ ■ ■ ■ ■ ■ ■ ■ ■ ■ ■

Geology

BIG SUR'S RUGGED LANDSCAPE speaks to a tumultuous past, when ocean and rock collided in a dramatic convergence. It is a geologically youthful region. In just 5 million years, Big Sur has been smashed between colliding tectonic plates, compressed by massive faults, and rammed upward to form the jagged peaks, steep ridges, and deep gorges of the Santa Lucia Range.

While the mountains themselves may be relative toddlers, many of the rocks bear ancient origins, tens of millions of years old. The convoluted topography means that rock types formed under radically different conditions lie confusingly side by side. Ancient mountain ranges, seafloors, stream sediments, and molten rock form a jumbled matrix that continues to baffle geologists.

The story for most of these rocks begins 130 million years ago, amid sediments from an ancient mountain range 1800 miles southeast in present-day Mexico. In that era, North America's western shoreline lay about where the Sierra Nevada stands today, everything west was submerged beneath the ocean, and the Santa Lucia Range did not exist. In the following millennia, westbound rivers deposited the sediments along the coast, where these layers eventually solidified into sandstone, siltstone, and limestone.

Over subsequent millions of years, a massive oceanic plate slid slowly beneath the continental plate. The increasing depth and pressure melted the sandstone, siltstone, and limestone, which slowly cooled and solidified underground as various types of granite, marble, schist, and gneiss. The cooling process formed large crystals that lend these rocks a salt-and-pepper appearance in the sunlight. Geologists believe that rock types along the Big Sur coast and Santa Lucia Range share traits with granites of the Sierra Nevada, comprising a group called the Salinian block.

The hard, crystalline rocks of the Salinian block comprise many of the prominent high peaks of the range, such as Ventana Double Cone and Pico Blanco, as well as many of the rugged coves, cliffs, and promontories along the Big Sur coastline, particularly at Garrapata, Julia Pfeiffer, and Partington Cove. These durable, erosion-resistant granitic rocks hold up well in the pounding surf, producing little sediment to cloud the waters. Any sediment is coarse-grained and quickly sinks to the bottom, unlike finer sediments that cloud coastal waters elsewhere in California.

These rocks are readily identified when exposed. Limestone and marble outcrops are vivid white with a sugary texture. Granitic rocks in the surf zone appear coarse with reflective faces, while rocks higher on the bluffs weather a rusty orange. Collectively, the Salinian block rocks form the basement layers in the north half of the Santa Lucia Range.

As the denser oceanic plate dove under the lighter continental plate, mas-

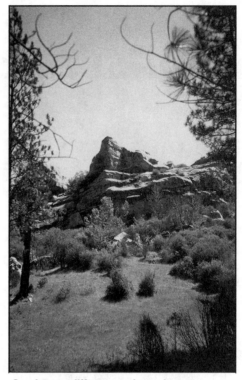

Sandstone cliffs tower above the open grasslands and pine-studded meadows of Ventana Wilderness.

sive accumulations of sand, mud, and the skeletons of microscopic sea creatures scraped off and slipped into a deep undersea trench. The resulting jumble appears along the Big Sur coast in the Franciscan formation, part of the Nacimiento block, which forms the underlying rock in the south half of the Santa Lucia Range.

The exposed cliffs at Andrew Molera State Park include excellent examples of Franciscan rocks. Formed from silica-rich sea creature skeletons, chert features jagged layering and an erosion-resistant glasslike texture. Sandstone is characterized by its tan color, rough surfaces, and fine sand grains. Comprising hardened, compressed mud, shale is gray-black in color with microscopic grains.

Serpentine, California's state rock, forms in layers that solidify above molten rock. These layers are scraped off and jumbled near the surface, where they react with groundwater to form this slippery green stone. You'll find dramatic serpentine outcrops in the Silver Peak Wilderness amid the Salmon Creek and San Carpoforo drainages.

Other younger rocks formed in the vicinity of the Santa Lucia Range before a single peak rose above the surface. A few million years ago, this area was a drainage basin that collected sediments in the form of sand, silt, and boulders. In time these solidified into sandstone, siltstone, and conglomerate. Conglomerate is least common, although at Point Lobos it is the dominant sedimentary rock and forms dramatic outcrops and cobblestone promontories.

While these theories may explain how the rocks formed, they don't explain how the rocks traveled hundreds of miles and rose to form the Santa Lucia Range. That story begins along the San Andreas Fault system some 30 million years ago. Once again, tectonic forces brought oceanic and continental plates together. This time, the North American plate and the Pacific plate met and began to grind past one another, marking the San Andreas Fault boundary.

Two massive chunks of Earth's crust, the Nacimiento and Salinian blocks, were ripped from their moorings along the North American plate and pushed northward along the numerous major faults associated with the San Andreas system. These faults generally run northwest-southeast, paralleling the coastline and general trend of the coastal mountains. A prime example is the Sur-Nacimiento Fault, which separates the Salinian and Nacimiento blocks, relieving pressure along the San Andreas Fault. As the tectonic plates collided, compressed, and fractured along these major fault lines, the land buckled in on itself like folds in a loose carpet, giving rise to the peaks, ridges, and gorges of the Santa Lucia Range.

Stream courses mark many of these otherwise indiscernible faults. The lower Big Sur River from the gorge to Andrew Molera State Park offers startling proof of how fault movement can alter a watercourse. Along this section, the river flows straight down the Sur Thrust Fault until it is forced into a conspicuous 90-degree turn out to Molera Beach.

Coastal bluffs, or marine terraces, offer evidence that the Santa Lucia Range continues its abrupt rise above sea level. These bluffs form as waves carve into the bedrock and deposit coarse sand and sediments. As land west of the San Andreas Fault buckles, these platforms rise above sea level, exposing the layered sand and cobblestones. Prominent marine terraces stretch from Point Sur to Andrew Molera State Park, while broader terraces form the flat terrain at Pacific Valley.

Erosion serves as a counteracting force to the recent uplifted Santa Lucia Range. As mountain flanks rise ever steeper, streams cut deep, fast channels through the rock, carrying away thousands of tons of sediment. A clear creek in summer can become a muddy torrent during heavy winter rains or after wildfires remove anchoring vegetation. Landslides are a common phenomenon in Big Sur. Of course, the Pacific Ocean also accounts for its fair share of erosion.

Geologists believe the recent uplift has thus far outstripped these erosive forces. If the uplift slows or stops, however, the tables will turn and gradually return the region to a rumpled landscape of low, rolling hills and plains.

Climate

CLIMATOLOGISTS HAVE LONG COMPARED California's climate to that of the Mediterranean coastline, with dry summers, wet winters, and moderate year-round temperatures. Big Sur's climate differs markedly, however, due primarily to consistent summer fog and the sheer topography of the Santa Lucia Range. Temperatures and humidity run the extremes along the fog-shrouded coast, atop 5000-foot mountain peaks, amid deep river canyons, and across the sun-drenched south-facing slopes.

An air circulation pattern known as the North Pacific High dominates regional weather patterns. From May through September, the sun most directly strikes the Northern Hemisphere. Surface air warms and rises into the upper atmosphere toward the North Pole. This heated air mass cools quickly in the upper atmosphere, subsequently sinking toward the surface as a large high-pressure cell. This massive high-pressure cell drives Big Sur's westerly winds and summer drought, as well as its summer fog, a very stable phenomenon off the California coast that is absent in the Mediterranean basin.

Thick fog forms when westerly winds brought by the North Pacific High push cold ocean water inland, forcing warmer surface water offshore. Rich in nutrients from nearshore submarine canyons, the cold water wells to the surface, sustaining abundant marine life along the Big Sur coast. With temperatures in the low 50s Fahrenheit, it also makes a swim here

In the wake of winter rains, fog retreats and grasslands and forests burst with new growth.

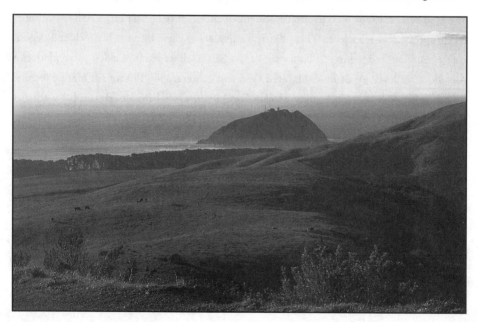

brisk at best, even in summer. The cold water chills the air directly above it. When this cold water comes in contact with warm, moist air along the coast, water vapor condenses into fog.

This pattern continues until late fall, when the sun strikes Earth farther south and the North Pacific High dissipates. No longer deflected by the high-pressure cell, the jet stream flows over California and brings with it strong winter storms. From November through April, California's wet season, these storms batter the coastal ranges until the sun's path again swings north to rebuild the North Pacific High.

Plant & Animal Communities

BIG SUR IS HOME TO A DIVERSE ARRAY of plant communities and associated wildlife. Botanists have long been fascinated by the proximity of northern and southern species living beside one another along the region's steep-sided ridges, narrow valleys, deep canyons, sun-drenched grasslands, and chaparral. Here, moisture-dependent redwoods may tower alongside drought-tolerant yuccas.

The story begins 5 million years ago, when the Santa Lucia Range was more of a low, rolling plain blessed with a moderate climate. Winters were warmer and summers wetter than today's more Mediterranean climate. The climate was likely too damp for chaparral species and too warm for redwoods and their shade-loving companions. Given the relatively uniform landscape and climate, botanists suggest the area supported fewer species than today's diverse topography permits.

Squeezed by tectonic plates and compressed by massive faults, the region rose and folded in on itself, creating the Santa Lucias' jagged peaks, steep ridges, and deep gorges. This topographic shift occurred in concert with climatic changes from the most recent Ice Age some 2.5 million years ago. These profound changes disrupted the uniform vegetation, paving the way for a major plant invasion.

The cool, damp climate allowed redwoods to take root in narrow, deep canyons along the coast. Fog encroached inland in dry months, supplying much-needed moisture to northern species. Thunderstorms became commonplace, as moist air rose abruptly to form thick cumulonimbus clouds, or thunderheads. These clouds arrived in summer, when temperatures were at a maximum and moisture at a minimum. Lightning sparked regular wildfires, and fire-adapted plant species thrived.

Drought-tolerant species also had an advantage. As the range continued to rise, coastal lands received the lion's share of precipitation, depriving eastern slopes of moisture. The steep topography also meant accelerated erosion, preventing mature soils from developing. The resulting shallow, primitive soils held considerably less ground water. But the hardy vegetation that populated these slopes shrugged at the arid conditions.

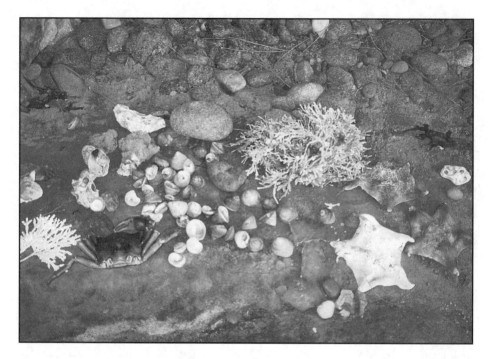

Low tide reveals diverse inter-tidal life.

Today, drought-tolerant plants still thrive on arid slopes, moisture-loving species grow along creeks and rivers, and shade-seeking plants retreat to the deep canyons and ravines. To categorize these patterns, botanists devised the concept of plant communities. A plant community is a group of species that grow together in a particular environment. Although it's possible to break these down into more detailed divisions, following is a basic breakdown of Big Sur's primary plant communities and their resident animals:

Coastal Scrub

Coastal scrub communities extend along the entire California coast and are divided into two major types: northern coastal scrub and southern coastal scrub. Although Point Sur is considered the loose boundary between the two types, northern and southern species intermingle along the Big Sur coast.

Common coastal shrubs include coyote brush (*Baccharis pilularis*), California lilac (*Ceanothus thyrsiflorus*), California coffeeberry (*Rhamnus californica*), and poison oak (*Toxicodendron diversilobum*). Headlands and bluffs feature such fragrant shrubs and herbs as California sagebrush (*Artemisia californica*), black sage (*Salvia mellifera*), hedge nettle (*Stachys bullata*), California mugwort (*Artemisia douglasiana*), and yerba buena (*Satureia douglasii*). Spring welcomes colorful purple, orange, and yellow blossoms from species such as silver and yellow bush lupine (*Lupinus albifrons* and *arboreus*), sticky monkeyflower (*Mimulus aurantiacus*), seaside daisy (*Erigeron glaucus*), and seaside wooly sunflower (*Eriophyllum staechadifolium*). Trees in this community are shrub-like, and few exceed 10 feet in height. California bay (*Umbellularia californica*) and coast live oak (*Quercus agrifolia*) nestle in ravines, while dense clusters of willows (mostly *Salix coulteri*) huddle near water.

The coastal bluffs and low rolling hillsides endure the constant assault of wind and salt spray, which sculpt and prune the plants to grow low and rounded. These species favor areas of heavy fog, average precipitation, abundant sunlight, and mild year-round temperatures. In Big Sur, northern plants thrive in moist locations, while southern species are more abundant in arid locations. When fire burns mature stands of coastal scrub, lush herbs and nutritious new growth thrive, providing prime foraging and nesting habitat to a greater number of animals.

Seeds, berries, roots, flowers, and young seedlings provide excellent food sources for herbivores, while woody plants provide nesting material. Omnivores and predators use the abundant scrub as cover from which to hunt, while prey species such as rodents, snakes, and small birds use it to hide from the former. Resident species include:

MAMMALS Mule deer, coyote, bobcat, gray fox, brush rabbit, black-tailed hare, California ground squirrel, Botta's pocket gopher, California meadow mouse, brush mouse, pinyon mouse, Merriam's chipmunk, long-tailed weasel, striped skunk, and dusky-footed woodrat.

BIRDS California condor, red-tailed hawk, white-tailed kite, California quail, western scrub jay, wrentit, California thrasher, song sparrow, white-crowned sparrow, bushtits, rufous-sided and California towhees, Anna's hummingbird, and western meadowlark.

REPTILES Western fence lizard, alligator lizard, western skink, gopher snake, California mountain king snake, western terrestrial garter snake, and western rattlesnake.

New growth of this native pine appears purple as new cones form the next generation of Monterey pines.

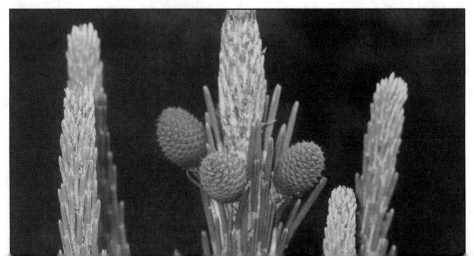

Chaparral

Comprising dense thickets of hardwood shrubs with stiff evergreen leaves, chaparral is unquestionably the dominant plant community in Big Sur, particularly in the Ventana and Silver Peak Wildernesses.

The predominant species of this fire-loving vegetation type is chamise, or greasewood (*Adenostoma fasciculatum*). This member of the rose family features a tough, woody stem, wiry branches, and bundles of needlelike evergreen leaves. It is named for its oily wood, which emits a pungent odor when brushed against. This brush species is a favorite perch for ticks, which wait to hitchhike on unsuspecting passersby.

The majority of chaparral in the Santa Lucias can be divided into two types: chamise chaparral and mixed chaparral. Chamise can grow in pure stands, while other plants grow in association with chamise to form mixed chaparral, where species such as ceanothus and manzanita dominate. The community includes manzanita species (*Arctostaphylos spp.*), buck brush (*Ceanothus cuneatus*), wartleaf (*Ceanothus papillosus*), California coffeeberry (*Rhamnus californica*), monkeyflower (*Mimulus bifidus*), California yerba santa (*Eriodictyon californicum*), poison oak (*Toxicodendron diversilobum*), and Our Lord's candle (*Yucca whipplei*).

Chaparral carpets the hottest, driest slopes, where summer temperatures can soar above 100°F. When lightning strikes, fire spreads quickly through mature chaparral stands. The volatile oils in some chaparral shrubs make this one of the most fire-adapted plant communities in the world. Historically, in the Santa Lucia Range, fire ravages chaparral slopes once every 10 to 40 years. The community provides critical stabilizing cover on steep, rocky slopes. When fire rips through, the slopes are left barren and unstable, resulting in massive floods and landslides when heavy winter storms strike.

Resident animal species include:

MAMMALS Mountain lion, coyote, gray fox, bobcat, mule deer, spotted skunk, ringtail, brush rabbit, California ground squirrel, Santa Cruz kangaroo rat, desert woodrat, California mice, deer mice, brush mice, Merriam's chipmunk, pallid bat, and Brazilian free-tailed bat.

BIRDS Turkey vulture, golden eagle, red-tailed hawk, Cooper's hawk, sharp-shinned hawk, California quail, mountain quail, Anna's hummingbird, wrentit, California thrasher, rufous-sided and California towhee, blue-gray gnatcatcher, Bewick's wren, bushtit, black swifts, white-throated swifts, and barn, violet-green, and cliff swallows.

REPTILES Western fence lizard, sagebrush lizard, western whiptail, coast horned lizard, garter snake, gopher snake, striped racer, western rattlesnake, and common kingsnake.

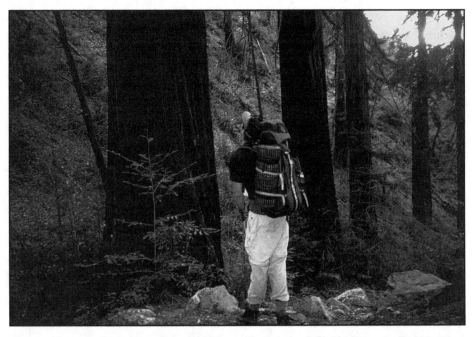

Coast redwoods show signs of vigorous regrowth after the 1999 Kirk Complex Fires in the narrow ravines of Hare Creek Canyon.

Redwood Forests

California is blessed with Earth's largest, oldest, and tallest living organisms. The largest tree in volume, the giant sequoia (*Sequoiadendron giganteum*), lords over the western slopes of the Sierra Nevada. The world's oldest tree, the bristlecone pine (*Pinus aristata*), perches along the flanks of the White Mountains. The tallest living organism, the coast redwood (*Sequoia sempervirens*), grows along the California coast, making its southern home in the Santa Lucia Range.

Redwood forests form a narrow belt along the coast from central California to southern Oregon. They are prized for their longevity (1000 years or more) and height (stretching some 250 to 300 feet above the forest floor). The tallest trees and healthiest groves rise farther north at Redwood National Park. Big Sur represents the redwood's southern stronghold, which peters out near Salmon Creek in southern Big Sur, close to the coastal California fog belt. As redwoods approach their southern limit, the trees are noticeably diminished in size.

In its warmer, drier southern range, this moisture-loving species is restricted to cool, damp valleys, canyons, ravines, and gullies. The fossil record proves that 50 million years ago redwoods were widespread throughout the Northern Hemisphere, including Greenland, Asia, and Europe. As the climate changed, so did the species' range.

Although redwoods can live for thousands of years, the desire for lumber makes the fast-growing, massive trees commercially valuable. At the turn of the century, the Big Sur region sustained massive logging operations that cleared much of the ancient stands. Remaining old-growth redwood forests are confined to a few coastal drainages, including the Little Sur, Big Sur, Partington, McWay, Big Creek, and Palo Colorado Canyons.

A number of other moisture-loving trees, shrubs, and herbs grow in association with redwoods. Common neighboring trees include tanoak (*Lithocarpus densiflorus*), California bay (*Umbellularia californica*), western sycamore (*Platanus racemosa*), white alder (*Alnus rhombifolia*), and bigleaf maple (*Acer macrophyllum*). Although redwood canopies all but blot out the sun, a surprisingly dense understory of ferns, herbs, and shrubs obtain enough sunlight to carpet stream corridors and steep slopes along the forest floor. Understory plants include western sword fern (*Polystichum munitum*), bracken fern (*Pteridium aqulinum*), giant chain fern (*Woodwardia fimbriata*), American maidenhair fern (*Adiantum pedatum*), California maidenhair fern (*Adiantum jordani*), coastal wood fern (*Dryopteris arguta*), fairy lantern (*Calochortus alkus*), western hound's-tongue (*Cynoglossum grande*), fairy bells (*Disporum hookeri*), western starflower (*Trientalis latifolia*), poison oak (*Toxicodendron diversilobum*), evergreen huckleberry (*Vaccinium ovatum*), and redwood sorrel (*Oxalis oregana*).

The lush forest seems surprisingly void of wildlife. The understory supports few seed-bearing plants to attract herbivores and their predators. One of the most common plants, redwood sorrel, is even toxic to herbivores. Regardless, a few animals do thrive here. One notable and highly visible resident is the banana slug, a bright yellow gastropod that grazes on understory plants and fungi. Its bright coloration is a defense mechanism, signaling predators that the slug is extremely distasteful. Other common species include:

MAMMALS Trowbridge shrew and broad-handed mole.

BIRDS Steller's jay, winter wren, brown creeper, Pacific slope flycatcher, dark-eyed junco, hermit thrush, varied thrush, American robins, chestnut-backed chickadee, common flickers, great horned owl, northern pygmy owl, and golden-crowned kinglet.

REPTILES & AMPHIBIANS Coast Range newt, red salamander, slender salamander, alligator lizard, western fence lizard, and sharp-tailed snake.

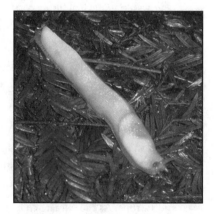

The ubiquitous banana slug

Riparian Woodland

By definition, riparian (riverside) woodlands follow clear water in Big Sur country. Characterized by moisture-loving trees, this community nestles alongside creeks, streams, and rivers in
the heart of the wilderness. The most
common trees are the deciduous western sycamore (*Platanus racemosa*), bigleaf maple (*Acer macrophyllum*), red alder
(*Alnus rubra*), white alder (*Alnus rhombifolia*), and several species of willow
(*Salix spp.*). In fall the major drainages of
the Santa Lucia Range, notably the Carmel and Big Sur Rivers and Arroyo Seco,
boast vibrant hues as autumn leaves catch
the slightest canyon breezes. In spring
the forest flaunts such delicate moisture-
loving flowers as leopard lily (*Lilium par-
dalinum*), giant stream orchid (*Epipactus
gigantean*), scarlet monkeyflower (*Mimulus

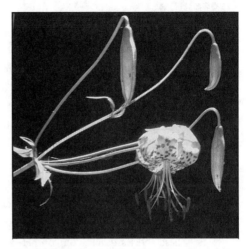

*During spring tiger lilies adorn the banks of
riparian corridors.*

cardinalis*), red columbine (*Aquilegia formosa*), and thimbleberry (*Rubus parviflorus*).

This is one of the best areas to view wildlife. Butterflies, dragonflies, amphibians, reptiles, fish, birds, and mammals all gather here to drink, hunt, forage, and mate. Resident
species include:

MAMMALS Mule deer, mountain lion, bobcat, coyote, raccoon, gray fox, striped skunk,
opossum, Pacific shrew, ornate shrew, western harvest mouse, deer mouse, dusky-footed
woodrat, big brown bat, silver-haired bat, red bat, and hoary bat.

BIRDS American dipper, belted kingfisher, red-shouldered hawk, Cooper's hawk, western
screech owl, long-eared owl, downy woodpecker, white-headed woodpecker, black phoebe,
willow flycatcher, violet-green swallow, tree swallow, plain titmouse, white-breasted nuthatch, Bewick's wren, Swainson's thrush, warbling vireo, yellow warbler, Wilson's warbler,
American goldfinch, lesser goldfinch, and song sparrow.

REPTILES Western pond turtle, western terrestrial garter snake, sharp-tailed snake, ringneck
snake, rubber boa, California mountain kingsnake, western rattlesnake, western fence lizard,
and alligator lizard.

FISH & AMPHIBIANS Pacific tree frog, steelhead trout, brown trout, rainbow trout, lamprey, arboreal salamander, red salamander, slender salamander, Coast Range newt, tiger salamander, bullfrog, and crayfish.

Grassland

Grasslands usually mix with coastal scrub along the slopes of the Santa Lucia Range. In the drier interior, they grow alongside arid thickets of chaparral on oak- and pine-studded hillsides. Grasslands also thrive along marine terraces and coastal bluffs, including El Sur Ranch north of Andrew Molera State Park, where cattle continually graze.

Those who believe the central coast to be void of seasonal changes have not taken a stroll through the grasslands of Big Sur. Following winter rains, vibrant green grasses sprout from the damp earth. This annual growth cycle may end before summer if little rain falls in spring. By late May, the rolling hills turn golden as the grasslands fade and lay dormant until the following winter's rains.

Most grasses responsible for these seasonal bursts of color are exotic species to the California landscape. In the mid 19th century, settlers brought in invasive annual grasses to feed livestock. These species quickly outcompeted native perennial grasses and thrived in areas ravaged by grazing, fire, or landslides.

Though grasses are the dominant species, forbs and herbs also thrive here, weaving colorful tapestries along the open slopes of the Coast Range. Among the most recognized are the blue, purple, and orange hues of sky lupines (*Lupinus nanus*) and California poppies (*Eschscholzia californica*). Other fragile, ornate flowers include the padres shooting star

Seasonal changes are most dramatic within the grassland ecosystem, where vibrant new growth carpets the landscape.

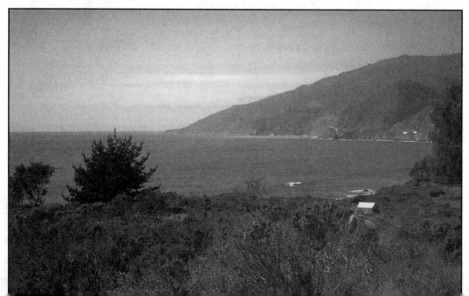

(*Dodecatheon clevelandii*), California buttercup (*Ranunculus californicus*), Johnny-jump-up (*Viola pedunculata*), and blue dicks (*Dichelostemma pulchella*).

Many animals forage and hunt in the grasslands, though few find safe refuge to nest and breed. Common species include:

MAMMALS Coyote, mule deer, bobcat, gray fox, pocket gopher, California ground squirrel, and long-tail weasel.

BIRDS Western meadowlark, grasshopper sparrow, savannah sparrow, lark sparrow, burrowing owl, horned lark, white-tailed kite, red-tailed hawk, red-shouldered hawk, American kestrel, golden eagle, barn owl, great horned owl, California quail, mourning dove, swallows, swifts, and finches.

REPTILES Gopher snake, western rattlesnake, yellow-bellied racer, ringneck snake, alligator lizard, and western fence lizard.

Oak Woodland

Majestic oak woodlands form some of Big Sur's most picturesque, enchanting forests. The southern region shelters centuries-old blue and valley oaks, while coastal slopes are studded with sprawling coast live oaks draped with lacy lichens. The most common trees are coast live oak (*Quercus agrifolia*), blue oak (*Quercus douglasii*), California black oak (*Quercus kelloggii*), valley oak (*Quercus lobata*), and canyon live oak (*Quercus chrysolepis*). Oak woodlands vary from dense forests to grassy savannas, and plants from neighboring communities often occupy the understory.

Unfortunately, tens of thousands of tanoaks, coast live oaks, and black oaks between Big Sur and the Oregon border are dying from sudden oak death. Researchers have isolated a previously unknown fungal species they believe causes the disease. This pathogen is a member of the genus *Phytophthora* (Latin for plant destroyer) and is related to species blamed for such agricultural plagues as the Irish potato famine. Scientists are conducting far-ranging research to determine how the fungus spreads and how it can be stopped. It's critical to slow the spread of the fungus by preventing the movement of infected leaves, wood, and soil. Visitors to Big Sur's oak woodlands should clean their tires, shoes, and animals' feet thoroughly before leaving the area.

Acorns are the most important food item for animals living in or around oak woodlands. In fall, as acorns ripen and fall, the forest chatters with excitement as birds and mammals flock to harvest the nutritious nuts. Resident species include:

MAMMALS Mule deer, bobcat, mountain lion, gray fox, coyote, striped skunk, wild boar (introduced from Europe), California mouse, western gray squirrel, pocket gopher, Audubon cottontail, lump-nosed bat, big brown bat, silver-haired bat, red bat, and hoary bat.

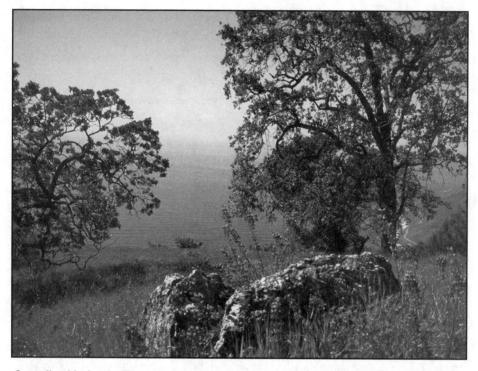

Sprawling black oaks filter views northwest toward the ocean along the Buckeye Trail.

BIRDS Western bluebird; chestnut-backed chickadee; northern flicker; acorn, Lewis', and Nuttall's woodpeckers; violet-green and tree swallows; scrub jay; common raven; plain titmouse; bushtit; white-breasted nuthatch; orange-crowned and Townsend's warblers; Hutton's vireo; black-headed grosbeak; band-tailed pigeon; mourning dove; western screech and great horned owls; Cooper's, red-tailed, and red-shouldered hawks; and American kestrel.

REPTILES Western fence lizard, alligator lizard, western skink, gopher snake, common kingsnake, and western rattlesnake.

AMPHIBIANS Arboreal salamander, California newt, and western toad.

Mixed Evergreen Forest

The mixed evergreen forest is an extremely varied community, in which endemic, rare, isolated, or disjunct coniferous species grow amid a diverse array of hardwood trees. Member species include the Santa Lucia fir, Coulter pine, ponderosa pine, sugar pine, gray pine, Monterey pine, Douglas fir, and incense cedar.

Nestled along deep, dark canyon floors and atop the Santa Lucias' dry, rocky slopes and summits lives the rarest, most distinct, and narrowly distributed of all fir species, the endemic Santa Lucia fir. They are easily identified by droopy, densely foliated crowns that extend from the base of the tree with lower branches that nearly touch the ground. The tree's differing habitats share one characteristic: each is relatively fire resistant. Although the range is subject to periodic wildfires, the Santa Lucia fir is not fire adapted and cannot survive in areas susceptible to burning.

Fossil evidence from the Miocene period (22 million to 6 million years ago) proves the Santa Lucia fir was once widely distributed throughout western North America. During the Miocene, the climate was much warmer and wetter than today, including regular summer rainfall. During the Pliocene period (5.2 to 1.6 million years ago), the climate cooled, leading to the ice ages of the Pleistocene (1.6 million to 11,000 years ago). The Santa Lucia fir could not withstand these colder, drier conditions and thus retreated to milder coastal climates.

Botanist Thomas Coulter first described the Coulter pine in 1832 near Cone Peak. Its enormous, sharp-spurred cones are the heaviest of any pine species. The tree grows in association with canyon live oaks, tanoaks, California bays, and madrones. On the flanks of Junipero Serra Peak, Coulter pines grow alongside stately sugar pines.

A Scottish botanist first described sugar pines in 1831 while climbing Cone Peak. These largest of all pines boast enormous cones that are longer and more slender than the Coulter pine's cones. Distinct from their Sierra Nevada and Southern California cousins, Big

Climate change millions of years ago isolated this stand of Santa Lucia fir to the milder coastal climate of Big Sur.

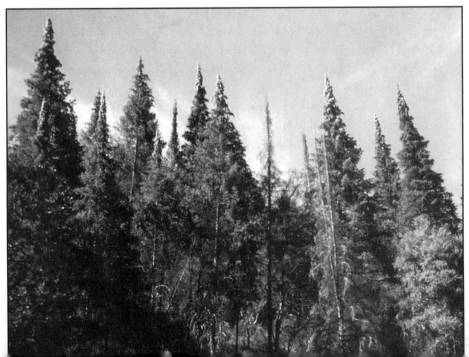

Sur's sugar pines are restricted to isolated peaks and higher elevation slopes atop Cone and Junipero Serra Peaks.

The incense cedar is another disjunct tree removed from its Sierra Nevada population. When crushed, its flat, scaled foliage emits a pungent aroma. Botanists speculate that this tree was also once widespread, but as the climate warmed over the past 10,000 years and wildfires became more commonplace, its range shrank drastically.

The mixed evergreen plant community shares many of the plant and animal species commonly seen in Big Sur's oak woodlands. Consult that wildlife list for representative species.

BIG SUR SEASONS ■ ■ ■ ■ ■ ■ ■ ■ ■ ■ ■ ■ ■ ■ ■ ■ ■ ■ ■

Big Sur's steep, rugged topography and proximity to the ocean lead to a diverse array of regional microclimates. Deep, narrow canyons remain shady and cool even in sweltering summer heat. High, barren peaks regularly freeze and receive snow in winter. Cool onshore breezes sweep coastal terraces, while the sun beats down on arid south-facing slopes. Though visitors may complain about a lack of defined seasons along the coast, locals know Big Sur is markedly different and beautiful each season.

Summer

In summer, inland temperatures along the Santa Lucia Range often soar into the 90s Fahrenheit during the day and drop to the 40s Fahrenheit by night both in the valleys and at high elevation. This contrasts dramatically with stable, cool temperatures along the coast, which generally range from the low 50s to mid 60s Fahrenheit.

Separated from the ocean by 2000-foot Pfeiffer Ridge, the Big Sur River gorge is much warmer than the fog-shrouded beaches to the west. Campers and hikers flock to deep swimming holes within the gorge for bracing dips. Occasionally, the fog encroaches inland and is drawn up-canyon, bringing gray and overcast conditions even to high ridges.

Although rain is unlikely in summer, tropical low-pressure systems occasionally approach the coast in the form of puffy cumulus clouds. As this warm, humid air moves in, thunderheads may develop, spawning lightning and rain. During periodic summer droughts, wildfires are a real threat, so residents are watchful for any signs of lightning or smoke. Lightning sparked the 180,000-acre Marble–Cone Fire (1977), the 60,000-acre Rat Creek Fire (1985), the 90,000-acre Kirk Complex Fires (1999), and the 160,000-acre Basin Complex Fire (2008).

Fall

Indian summer brings warmer temperatures to the coast in fall. As the North Pacific High dissipates, nearshore cold-water upwelling stops, lowering humidity and driving fog well offshore. Views from high mountain peaks are outstanding in the crisp, clear air. Northwesterly winds diminish, and coastal waters become flat, calm, and warm (upper 50s instead of low 50s Fahrenheit). Deep within the riparian woodlands, deciduous trees change color and shed their kaleidoscopic leaves on the canyon floors.

Winter

Winter storms generally approach the central California coast from the northwest or southwest. Forming in the cold regions of the North Pacific and Bering Sea, northern fronts bring cold air masses and moderate rainfall. Forming over warm water in the South Pacific, southern storms typically bring extensive rainfall.

Arriving on the Big Sur coast, the moisture-laden air lashes the steep terrain and is forced upward. As the air rises, it cools and condenses, releasing moisture as rain or snow. When the North Pacific High lingers into winter, it prevents storms from reaching the coast and often leads to severe winter droughts.

Precipitation varies dramatically from year to year. Rainfall along the coast averages about 40 inches annually, while some 90 inches fall near the crests and ridges. In winter the high peaks are dusted in snow, which may remain on the ground for weeks or even months above 3500 feet.

A rain shadow effect occurs along eastern slopes, similar to that seen along the eastern slopes of the Sierra. Moisture-laden air deposits its precipitation along the rising western slopes and ridges, leaving eastern slopes drier on average, as the air warms and descends into the Salinas Valley. King City averages only about 11 inches annually.

Spring

Spring is glorious along the Big Sur coast. Plants and animals awake from dormancy, and the sights and sounds of life abound. In the wake of winter rains, grasslands and forests burst forth with new growth. Colorful, fragrant wildflowers carpet the grasslands and ridges, while oak and riparian woodlands bud in vibrant green hues. Views are spectacular on cold, crisp days.

The arrival of spring varies with the timing of winter rains. If rains continue until May, expect incredible wildflower displays through summer, while an end to rains in March turns the hillsides gold as dry season descends on Big Sur. Expect encroaching fog by late spring as the North Pacific High returns offshore, spawning cold-water upwelling.

Big Sur Cultural History & Lore

I MAGINE A LAND OF STUNNING BEAUTY with a wealth of resources, where thousands of steelhead swim upstream along crystal clear creeks and rivers. Grizzly bears, wolves, and mountain lions roam sheer mountains that jut toward the heavens. Sea otters, seals, and whales forage in nearshore waters. Condors, falcons, and eagles soar overhead. Acorns, wild berries, nutritious herbs, and medicinal plants flourish amid valleys and hillsides. This vision is perhaps what early Europeans saw as they explored the vast wilderness inhabited by the American Indians of Big Sur.

American Indians

ARCHAEOLOGICAL EVIDENCE PROVES that people have lived along the rugged Big Sur coast for some 8000 years. When Spanish explorers of the 16th and 17th centuries arrived in Big Sur, the native population numbered nearly 5000 people among three separate coastal tribes: the Ohlone (from Point Sur north to San Francisco), the Esselen (from Point Sur south to Big Creek and inland to the upper Carmel River and Arroyo Seco watersheds), and the Salinian (from Big Creek south to San Carpoforo Creek and inland from Junipero Serra Peak north up the Salinas River valley). These groups differed dramatically from one another, adopting different languages, religious beliefs, customs, and dress.

The American Indians were hunter-gatherers, harvesting a variety of food sources throughout the year rather than farming. In fall they moved inland to bountiful oak woodlands to collect acorns, in spring to the valleys and grasslands to harvest nutritious herbs, and in winter to the Pacific to fish and hunt along the rich coastal waters.

Ancient middens speak to this variety in their diet. Lying amid former Indian villages and encampments, middens are essentially trash heaps, offering a stratified record of animal bones, shellfish remains, stone tools, weapons, and ornamental artifacts. Coastal middens largely contain the remains of mussels, abalone, chitons, barnacles, seabirds, marine mammals, and fish, while inland middens feature the bones of deer, skunks, raccoons, coyotes, foxes, rabbits, squirrels, mice, and gophers.

Aside from the middens and written records from Spanish explorers, missionaries, and anthropologists, we know little about these people and how they lived. Tragically, their culture vanished soon after contact with the Europeans. Within a few decades, thousands succumbed to European diseases for which they had no immunity. Many of those who survived such diseases as whooping cough and measles were driven from their lands, converted to Christianity, and put to work raising cattle within the mission system.

Spanish Exploration & the Mission Period

In 1542, Spain hired Portuguese navigator Juan Rodríguez Cabrillo to sail the California coast in search of riches and a water route between the Pacific and Atlantic Oceans. The first European to see Big Sur and the Santa Lucia Range, Cabrillo remarked, "There are mountains which seem to reach the heavens, and the sea beats on them; sailing along close to land, it appears as though they would fall on the ships." He also encountered Monterey Bay, naming it Bahia de los Pinos (Bay of Pines).

In 1602, 60 years after Cabrillo's expedition and nearly 20 years before pilgrims landed at Plymouth Rock, Spanish explorer Sebastian Vizcaíno sailed coastal California. His expedition spent two weeks surveying Monterey and Carmel Bays, proclaiming both to be excellent safe harbors. Vizcaíno named the coast Monte-Rey after Spain's new viceroy, the count of

In 1542, Cabrillo described the California coastline aptly: "There are mountains which seem to reach the heavens and the sea beats on them."

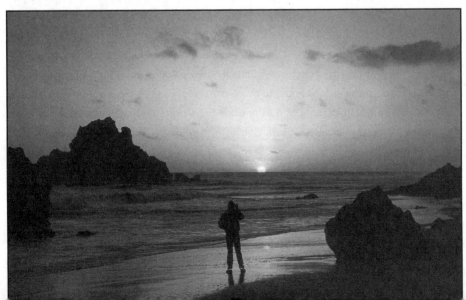

Monte-Rey. Vizcaíno's glowing reports and fears that Russian explorers were encroaching south along the coast from Alaska prompted Spain to claim Monterey Bay as its own.

In 1769, Gaspar de Portolá led an inland expedition north from Baja California near present-day San Diego. When the expedition reached the daunting coastal cliffs near Ragged Point, it turned inland. Protected by its sheer topography, Big Sur was left unexplored. After Portolá reached the San Francisco Bay, the expedition returned south, bypassing entirely Monterey, Carmel, and environs. Although disheartened, Portolá persevered and planned another trip.

In 1770, Portolá departed on another land expedition accompanied by Father Junipero Serra, who sailed north with the intent to establish Catholic outposts in the unknown territory. Serra established Mission San Carlos at present-day Carmel River State Beach and two other missions east of the Santa Lucia Range in the San Antonio River Valley and at Soledad in the Salinas Valley. Again, Big Sur was left unexplored.

The missionaries' arrival drastically altered native life in the Big Sur region. The newcomers claimed the land and brought Ohlone, Esselen, and Salinian natives into the missions. Some welcomed the priests, while others were lured by exotic gifts of glass beads, colored fabric, metal tools, and livestock. Forced conversion and de facto enslavement was not mission policy prior to 1800, but when natives resisted, more coercive methods were used. Missionaries justified their enslavement of "heathens" as acceptable if the natives ultimately converted to Christianity and found salvation.

In 1821, Mexico declared independence from Spanish rule, and in 1834 the vast mission lands were secularized and divided into livestock "ranchos." Any law-abiding Mexican Catholic was now eligible to receive land grants. California's ranching era had begun.

VISITING THE SAN CARLOS BORROMEO DE CARMELO MISSION ■ ■ ■

Step back in time and enter Father Junipero Serra's chosen home and final resting place, founded near the mouth of the Carmel River on August 24, 1771. Serra wished to build a permanent stone house of worship that required skilled masons to cut and dress the stones in the style of missions that Serra had erected in Mexico. With no skilled masons available in California, many of the missions never progressed past the humble adobe style, and the Carmel Mission we see today was delayed until years after Serra's death.

The construction of the stone church began in 1795 and was basically complete by 1797, when it was dedicated for worship on Christmas Day of that year. When the church was originally constructed, the sandstone walls were quarried from the Santa Lucia Mountains, but most of the exterior is different today. Inside, the statue of the

Virgin Mary in the side chapel of Our Lady Bethlehem is the same one that Father Serra carried back from Mexico in 1769.

Carmel Mission served both as headquarters for the mission's agricultural holdings in the Carmel Valley and as command center for the statewide California mission system. Today, the mission serves as a parish church, school, and basilica. Its distinction as a basilica is the highest honorary rank for a church and implies great historical and artistic importance. Pope John XXIII honored Carmel Mission's church with the rank of basilica in 1961 in recognition of Serra's work in the establishment of Christianity on the western coast of the United States, as well as the unique architectural features of the structure such as the Moorish dome and the parabolic ceiling. Since that designation, Carmel Mission Basilica was honored with a visit by Pope John Paul II, who visited the church to lay a wreath at the foot of the grave of Father Serra, who is buried beneath the floor of the sanctuary (near the altar).

Carmel Mission is open to the public Monday–Saturday 9:30 a.m.–5 p.m. and Sunday 10:30 a.m.–5 p.m. The admission fee to visit the mission grounds, basilica, and museums is $6.50 for adults, $4 for seniors (age 65 and up), and $2 for children age 7 and up (children under 6 are admitted free). These funds are used to support the continued maintenance and restoration of Carmel Mission. To get there, turn west from Highway 1 onto Rio Road and drive 0.7 mile to the corner of Lausen Drive. For more information, call (831) 624-1271 or visit **carmelmission.org**.

Ranching & Homesteading

As MEXICO REDISTRIBUTED the vast mission holdings as land grants, homesteaders claimed several outlying areas of Big Sur. Monterey soon developed into an important Pacific trading port, and the United States began to set its sights on California. Tensions arose between land-owning *Californios*, as they called themselves, and American pioneers immigrating through the treacherous passes of the Sierra Nevada. Conflict erupted at the outset of the Mexican War in 1846. In 1848, Mexico ceded California to the United States. The following year, gold was discovered in the foothills of the Sierra, and statehood was declared in 1850.

Pioneers and prospectors headed to California in droves. By this time, many outlying areas, including the Carmel, Nacimiento, and San Antonio River Valleys, were already privately owned. Two land grants spanned Big Sur: the 8984-acre Rancho El Sur, owned by Juan Bautista Alvarado, covering most of Point Sur, and the 8876-acre Rancho San Jose y Sur Chiquito, from the Carmel River to Palo Colorado Canyon.

Would-be homesteaders found the remaining steep, rocky terrain ill suited for farming, difficult to cross, and isolated from the world. Nonetheless, by the late 1800s a small community of determined pioneers had settled in Big Sur. These strong-willed folks survived by hunting, fishing, foraging, raising livestock, planting orchards, and tending gardens amid the lush canyons and steep ridges. Today, much of the land is named for these early pioneer families, including the Pfeiffers, Posts, Plasketts, Prewitts, and Partingtons.

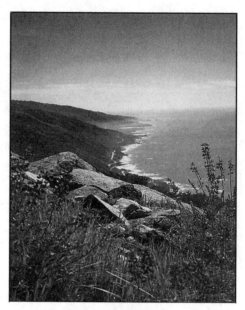

Highway 1 Construction & Recent Settlement

The sheer coastal topography has kept the Big Sur coastline rugged and largely uninhabited even to the present day.

UNTIL 1938, early settlers could only dream of a safe, fast route down the coast from Monterey to Big Sur. Even a simple supply trip to Monterey required a three-day trek up steep ridges and across creeks and deep canyons. In 1919, after lobbying pressure from a local politician, the federal government began construction of a road along the central California coast. The construction project pitted settlers who wanted to preserve their privacy against those who sought to profit from California's growing tourist trade.

Built by convicts and local labor, Highway 1 would become one of America's most popular roadways, revealing a gorgeous natural landscape. Artists and writers, social activists, scientists, philosophers, and other visionaries flocked to the area for inspiration, forming small artists' colonies and Bohemian sanctuaries. In the 1940s and '50s, playwright Henry Miller lived and worked in Big Sur. Other famous people who spent time here include Robert Louis Stevenson, Ansel Adams, Jack Kerouac, Mary Austin, Jack London, Sinclair Lewis, John Steinbeck, Robinson Jeffers, Lillian Ross, and Edward Weston.

Today, millions of annual visitors drive the Big Sur coast in appreciation of its unparalleled natural beauty. While the road literally paved the way for so many of us to access this wild, remote coast, it has also spurred government agencies, conservation groups, and local activists to preserve its exquisite beauty.

Big Sur Lore

WITHIN THE JAGGED cliffs and narrow valleys live generations of mysteries: tales of buried treasures, haunted beings, and supernatural speculation. The awe-inducing beauty and eerie isolation experienced by many who venture to Big Sur, whether to call it home or a place of refuge, gave birth to many interesting and irksome stories. In my countless days in the backcountry, I have yet to experience any evidence that these tales shed light on life within the Santa Lucia Mountains, yet they still remain an alluring part of Big Sur's cultural heritage, and I do not intend to endorse or debunk them.

The Dark Watchers

The sighting of the Dark Watchers originates from the Chumash Indians. They first spoke of these dark humanlike beings inhabiting the forests and high country of Big Sur in legends and their cave paintings. More recently, legendary author John Steinbeck described them in his story, "Flight":

"Pepe looked up to the top of the next dry withered ridge. He saw a dark form against the sky, a man's figure standing on top of a rock, and he glanced away quickly not to appear curious. When a moment later he looked up again, the figure was gone."

In 1937, the poet Robinson Jeffers mentioned them in his poem "Such Counsels You Gave to Me" as "forms that look human . . . but certainly are not human." If Jeffers or Steinbeck ever actually saw one of the Dark Watchers is unknown, but the local legend has been around since long before they wrote about it. Longtime Big Sur resident Rosalind Sharpe Wall claims to have seen the Dark Watchers near Bixby Bridge. If you happen to come across a Dark Watcher, the prevailing wisdom warns against looking at them.

The Ventana

The Ventana Wilderness is named for a unique notch called "The Window" on a granite ridge between Ventana Double Cone and Peak. According to local legend, this notch was once a natural stone arch that created a natural "window," which is supposedly what inspired the Spanish explorers gazing up toward the peaks to call it Ventana. The Ventana, or "The Slot" as local rock climbers call it, is the 200-foot-deep gap in the ridge. Geologists have yet to find rubble of a collapsed arch to support the legend, but nonetheless there are many arches and small complete "windows" in rock formations in the Santa Lucias. You can view the notch by looking west from Ventana Double Cone or along Coast Ridge Road with views north and looking northeast from Post Ranch Inn.

Supernatural Stories of Point Lobos

During the mission period, the Ohlone Indian neophytes at Carmel Mission would go out on foggy evenings to "cheer up" their lonely and forlorn fog spirits. The mission fathers strictly forbade any such pagan activity, and one night they followed them out into the fog and performed an exorcism. The fog spirits flew off angry and offended, departing with howls and causing sadness among the Indians. Some believe poetic justice prevailed, when the priest who performed the exorcism went mad, jumped off a cliff into the sea at Point Lobos, and was drowned.

A Goddess and a Hidden Gold Mine on Pico Blanco

With the discovery of gold and silver in Big Sur in the late 19th century, miners began searching for the precious metals along the flanks and valleys of the Santa Lucias. Today, the Pico Blanco area is littered with the rusting remnants of mining operations.

More than tales of fortunes found, historians have uncovered a curious tale that was circulated in response to the miners' arrival. According to local legend, an American Indian goddess zealously protected Pico Blanco. Historians recorded these accounts by miners claiming to have encountered the goddess, who cursed them with madness for pursuing gold.

During this same gold exploration period in Big Sur, a seemingly illiterate prospector named Al Clark became Pico Blanco's best-known resident. For decades he wandered the area around the mountain and told local ranchers stories of the goddess and a vast subterranean cavern filled with ancient pictographs that matched the descriptions of saber-toothed tigers and mastodons. In an effort to hide the cave, Clark said he used dynamite to destroy its entrance. Clark was an eccentric Columbia University graduate who posed as an illiterate. Rumors swarmed that he also found a hidden gold mine, but since he had no use for money, he left it alone and concealed the mine's location. Clark's hoard of gold still remains a mystery.

Driving & Destinations Along Highway 1

■ ■ ■ ■ ■ ■ ■ ■ ■ ■ ■ ■

MORE THAN 3 MILLION VISITORS a year travel Highway 1, so it's no surprise that sightseers and vacationers have a myriad of services and attractions from which to choose—from resorts, spas, hotels, campgrounds, and retreats to galleries, hot springs, and coastal coffeehouses. The following attractions and businesses are listed in order from north to south under specific categories. While not comprehensive, the listings include many of the Hotels & Motels, Campgrounds & RV Parks, Restaurants & Cafés, Art Galleries, Automotive Services, and Events along Highway 1 between Carmel and San Simeon.

Hotels & Motels

LAMP LIGHTER INN SE corner of Ocean Avenue at Camino Real, Carmel-by-the-Sea, (831) 624-7372, carmellamplighter.com ($185–450/night). Just west of Highway 1, this is one of the most photographed inns in the country, offering rooms and cottages a short stroll from the beach and village.

CARMEL RIVER INN At Carmel River Bridge, (831) 624-1575 or (800) 882-8142, carmel riverinn.com ($165–450/night). Just past Carmel River State Beach, this inn is widely considered the best lodging bargain in Carmel.

PARK HYATT CARMEL, HIGHLANDS INN 120 Highlands Drive, Carmel, (831) 624-3801 or (800) 682-4811, highlandsinn.hyatt.com ($440–675/night). Ocean-view rooms with fireplaces and spa baths, as well as wine tasting and a fantastic restaurant.

RIVERSIDE CAMPGROUND & CABINS 22 miles south of Carmel, (831) 667-2414, river sidecampground.com ($90–200/night). Cabins on the Big Sur River.

BIG SUR RIVER INN 24 miles south of Carmel, (831) 667-2700 or (800) 548-3610, bigsur riverinn.com ($125–225/night). Balconies overlook the Big Sur River. Includes heated pool, restaurant, general store, and live entertainment in the bar on weekends.

GLEN OAKS BIG SUR 25 miles south of Carmel, (831) 667-2105 ($195–450/night). Standard rooms, as well as four separate cottages for rent in the redwoods, offering both river and forest views.

BIG SUR CAMPGROUND & CABINS 26 miles south of Carmel, (831) 667-2322 ($95–450/night). Tent cabins and A-frame cabins with kitchens, fireplaces, and redwood decks overlooking the river.

FERNWOOD RESORT 26 miles south of Carmel, (831) 667-2422 ($45–195/night). One of the least expensive spots above the Big Sur River, offering 66 campsites, 10 cabins, and 13 motel-style units.

BIG SUR LODGE 26 miles south of Carmel, (831) 667-3100, bigsurlodge.com ($159–364/night). Within Pfeiffer Big Sur State Park, this lodge offers simple cottages, a restaurant, gift shop, grocery, laundry, and a heated pool in summer.

RIPPLEWOOD RESORT 27 miles south of Carmel, (831) 667-2242, ripplewoodresort.com ($105–225/night). Another affordable option above the Big Sur River, with a convenience store, gas station, and café.

VENTANA INN 28 miles south of Carmel, (831) 667-2331 or (800) 628-6500, ventanainn .com ($440–1,500/night). Nestled on a hillside, this inn offers elegant cottages and luxury suites with ocean or mountain views, as well as a restaurant and spa services.

POST RANCH 28 miles south of Carmel, (831) 667-2200 or (800) 527-2200, postranchinn .com ($675–2,485/night). This cliffside ranch offers rustic yet elegant rooms with awe-inspiring ocean views. Voted one of the best hotels in North America. Award-winning Sierra Mar Restaurant serves world-class cuisine.

DEETJEN'S BIG SUR INN 28 miles south of Carmel, (831) 667-2377, deetjens.com ($105–260/night). Rustic, funky rooms offer an offbeat hideaway in a shady redwood canyon.

ESALEN INSTITUTE 8 miles south of Big Sur, (831) 667-3005, esalen.org ($140–220/night). Offering natural hot springs and workshops that emphasize the potentialities of human existence.

LUCIA LODGE 22 miles south of Big Sur and 38 miles north of San Simeon, (831) 667-2391, lucialodge.com ($150–275/night). These cabins are set along a 300-foot cliff above the Pacific, offering ocean views from the dining deck.

TREEBONES RESORT 37 miles south of Big Sur and 23 miles north of San Simeon, (877) 424-4787, treebonesresort.com (campsite: $90/night; yurt: $215–400/night). There are 16 canvas-covered yurts, along with ocean-view campsites and the Wild Coast Restaurant and Sushi Bar, which focuses on sustainably harvested local food. No children under age 6 allowed.

GORDA SPRINGS COTTAGES 42 miles south of Big Sur and 25 miles north of San Simeon, (805) 927-4600 or (805) 927-3918, gordaspringsresort.com ($150–300/night). Cottages feature a private patio overlooking the ocean; some have hot tubs, fireplaces, and ocean views. General store, restaurant, gift shop, and excellent whale-watching. Pet the resident llamas.

RAGGED POINT INN 50 miles south of Big Sur and 15 miles north of San Simeon, (805) 927-4502, raggedpointinn.net ($159–309/night). You'll find 21 rooms with coastal views, as well as a conference/wedding pavilion, restaurant, snack bar, gallery and gift shop, espresso stand, convenience store, gas station, and gardens.

Campgrounds & RV Parks

ANDREW MOLERA STATE PARK 21 miles south of Carmel and 70 miles north of San Simeon, (831) 667-2315 (24 sites, $25/night). A walk-in campground about 0.3 mile from the parking area. No dogs allowed. Sites are granted on a first-come, first-serve basis.

RIVERSIDE CAMPGROUND & CABINS 22 miles south of Carmel, (831) 667-2414, riversidecampground.com (45 sites, $40/night for tent site and $50/night for RV site). Perched along the Big Sur River in the shade of redwoods, this campground offers swimming and fishing in season.

BIG SUR CAMPGROUND & CABINS 24 miles south of Carmel, (831) 667-2322 (tent: $45–60/night for 2 people; $5 for each additional person up to 5; cabin: $180–535/night). Offers full-hookup campsites along the Big Sur River, as well as tent cabins and A-frame cabins.

FERNWOOD RESORT CAMPGROUND 25 miles south of Carmel, (831) 667-2422 (tent: $30–50/night for 2 people; $5 for each additional person up to 6; RV: $35–50/night). This campground offers 60 sites, showers, a restaurant, bar, and general store.

PFEIFFER BIG SUR STATE PARK 26 miles south of Carmel, (800) 444-7275, parks.ca.gov (218 sites, $35/standard site, $45/river site, $150/group site; reservations recommended). Along the Big Sur River, this 1006-acre park offers showers, Wi-Fi, and swimming.

VENTANA CAMPGROUND 30 miles south of Carmel, (831) 667-2712, ventanacampground.com (80 sites, $27–55/night prior to closure in 2008; will reopen summer 2013). Nestled in a redwood grove in Post Canyon, this rustic campground provides electricity and showers.

JULIA PFEIFFER BURNS STATE PARK 37 miles south of Carmel, (800) 444-7275, parks.ca.gov (2 tent-only sites, $30/night; reservations highly recommended). Near the trail to 100-foot McWay Falls, these primitive hike-in campsites are in high demand. Restrooms and water at the parking lot.

KIRK CREEK CAMPGROUND 54 miles south of Carmel and 40 miles north of San Simeon, (805) 434-1996, campone.com/campsites/kirk-creek (34 sites, $22/night; reservations recommended). This campground offers magnificent views of the Big Sur coast and a short trail to the beach.

LIMEKILN STATE PARK 56 miles south of Carmel, (831) 667-2403, parks.ca.gov (33 sites, $35/night; reservations recommended in summer and on holidays). At the mouth of Limekiln Creek, this campground amid the redwoods offers developed sites with picnic tables and fire rings. Some sites accommodate RVs and trailers. There are showers, picnic areas, and flush toilets.

PLASKETT CREEK CAMPGROUND 59 miles south of Carmel and 35 miles north of San Simeon, (805) 434-1996, recreation.gov (41 sites, $22/night; 3 group sites, $80/night; reservations recommended spring–fall and on holidays). This campground offers a parklike setting under the canopy of large pines and cypress a short walk from Sand Dollar Beach and Jade Cove.

TREEBONES RESORT 37 miles south of Big Sur and 23 miles north of San Simeon, (877) 424-4787, treebonesresort.com (campsite: $90/night; yurt: $215–400/night). There are 16 canvas-covered yurts, along with ocean-view campsites and the Wild Coast Restaurant and Sushi Bar, which focuses on sustainably harvested local food. No children under age 6 allowed.

SAN SIMEON CREEK CAMPGROUND Within San Simeon State Park, 5 miles south of San Simeon, (800) 444-7275, parks.ca.gov (134 sites, $35/night; reservations recommended in summer; first come, first served October 1–March 14). On a plateau overlooking the Pacific, this campground includes showers and RV sites (no hookups).

WASHBURN CAMPGROUND Within San Simeon State Park, 5 miles south of San Simeon, (800) 444-7275, parks.ca.gov (68 sites, $22/night; reservations recommended in summer; no showers). This campground lies a mile inland on a plateau overlooking the Santa Lucia Range.

Restaurants & Cafés

ROCKY POINT RESTAURANT 10 miles south of Carmel, (831) 624-2933, rockypoint restaurant.com. Promises spectacular coastal views from all tables.

BIG SUR RIVER INN 24 miles south of Carmel, (831) 667-2700 or (800) 548-3610, bigsur riverinn.com. Offers patio and indoor dining on the banks of the Big Sur River. Live entertainment on Sunday afternoons.

BIG SUR VILLAGE PUB 24 miles south of Carmel, (831) 667-2355. In the Village Shops, the pub features specialty beers and a pub-style menu.

REDWOOD GRILL 25 miles south of Carmel, (831) 667-2129, fernwoodbigsur.com. Serving buffalo burgers, salmon burgers, hamburgers, and veggie burgers in the shade of redwoods.

BIG SUR LODGE RESTAURANT & ESPRESSO HOUSE 26 miles south of Carmel, (831) 667-3100, bigsurlodge.com. Indoor and patio dining beneath the redwoods along the Big Sur River.

BIG SUR DELI 27 miles south of Carmel, (831) 667-2225, bigsurdeli.com. Known for reasonable prices, Big Sur Deli offers sandwiches, tacos, salads, and desserts at the deli, as well as groceries, camping supplies, and a gift shop.

BIG SUR BAKERY & RESTAURANT 28 miles south of Carmel, (831) 667-0520, bigsurbakery .com. Fresh pastries, breads, and pizza baked daily in a wood-fire oven, with sweeping views of the Big Sur River gorge.

CIELO 28 miles south of Carmel, (831) 667-2331 or (800) 628-6500, ventanainn.com. At Ventana Inn, this restaurant offers elegant dining, seasonal ingredients, and 50-mile vistas from the outdoor terrace.

SIERRA MAR RESTAURANT 28 miles south of Carmel, (831) 667-2800, postranchinn.com. At Post Ranch, this restaurant offers gourmet and eclectic California cuisine with a spectacular ocean view. Reservations required.

NEPENTHE 29 miles south of Carmel, (831) 667-2345, nepenthebigsur.com. Elegant dining in a rustic setting that overlooks 40 miles of incredibly scenic coastline.

CAFÉ KEVAH 29 miles south of Carmel, (831) 667-2344, nepenthebigsur.com. Just below Nepenthe, this café offers brunch and lunch on an outdoor terrace.

WILD COAST RESTAURANT AND SUSHI BAR At Treebones Resort, 37 miles south of Big Sur and 23 miles north of San Simeon, (831) 877) 424-4787, treebonesresort.com. Along with yurts and campsites, Treebones Resort features the Wild Coast Restaurant and Sushi Bar, which focuses on sustainably harvested local food.

WHALE WATCHER CAFE 25 miles north of Hearst Castle and 69 miles south of Carmel, (805) 927-1590, gordaspringsresort.com. At Gorda Springs Resort, this restaurant offers California cuisine and delicious homemade desserts, with spectacular ocean views.

RAGGED POINT RESTAURANT 14 miles north of Hearst Castle and 80 miles south of Carmel, (805) 927-5708, raggedpointinn.net. California cuisine, with ocean and mountain views.

Art Galleries

HEARTBEAT GIFT GALLERY 24 miles south of Carmel, (831) 667-2557, heartbeatbigsur .com. Adjacent to the Big Sur River Inn, this gallery offers art, jewelry, and collectibles from local artists and from around the world.

LOCAL COLOR 24 miles south of Carmel, (831) 667-0481, bigsurlocalcolor.com. Home to the Central Coast Artisan Gallery, where talented local artists display handmade goods.

STUDIO ONE 24 miles south of Carmel, (831) 667-1530. Owned by the Big Sur Arts Initiative, a local nonprofit arts enrichment organization. In addition to the gallery, the initiative provides teaching space for art classes, workshops, and seminars.

THE GARDEN GALLERY 27 miles south of Carmel, (831) 667-2000. The gallery offers local art, crafts, jewelry, clothing, and herbal products.

HAWTHORNE GALLERY 28 miles south of Carmel, (831) 667-3200, hawthornegallery.com. Represents local artists, featuring painting and sculpture in granite, wood, steel, bronze, glass, and ceramics.

THE PHOENIX SHOP 29 miles south of Carmel, (831) 667-2347, nepenthebigsur.com. At Nepenthe, this shop offers a collection of gifts, books, jewelry, and clothing.

HENRY MILLER LIBRARY 30 miles south of Carmel, (831) 667-2574, henrymiller.org. A nonprofit organization dedicated to the works of the American author, artist, and Big Sur resident Henry Miller. The gallery offers a wide assortment of art and fine and rare books.

COAST GALLERY BIG SUR 33 miles south of Carmel, (831) 667-2301, coastgalleries.com. A historic showplace for local artists and coastal craftsmen, featuring an art gallery, candle studio, and boutique.

Automotive Services

CHEVRON 3645 Rio Road, Carmel, (831) 624-7764. Open 6 a.m.–midnight; gas only.

CHEVRON CARMEL TOWING & GARAGE 4th Avenue and Junipero Avenue, Carmel, (831) 624-3827, carmeltow@redshift.com. Offers 24-hour towing and full-service repairs. Open 8 a.m.– 6 p.m.

BIG SUR GARAGE & TOWING 24 miles south of Carmel, (831) 667-2181. Offers 24-hour services: towing, tires, auto repair, and lockouts.

GORDA SPRINGS RESORT, RESTAURANT, STORE & GAS STATION 25 miles north of Hearst Castle and 69 miles south of Carmel, (805) 927-3918, gordaspringsresort.com. Open 8 a.m.–8 p.m.

RAGGED POINT INN RESORT & GAS STATION 14 miles north of Hearst Castle and 80 miles south of Carmel, (805) 927-4502, raggedpointinn.com. Open 8 a.m.–9 p.m.; gas only.

CAMBRIA TOWING 4363 Bridge Street, Cambria, (805) 927-4357. Offers 24-hour services: lockouts and tires.

Events

BIG SUR INTERNATIONAL MARATHON (831) 625-6226, bsim.org. Last Sunday in April. Voted best marathon in North America.

BIG SUR JAZZFEST (831) 667-1530. Spring. Three days of jazz at various Big Sur venues.

BIG SUR RIVER RUN (831) 624-4112, bigsurriverrun.org. Late October. Referred to as "the most beautiful run in the world," through redwoods along the Big Sur River.

HENRY MILLER LIBRARY (831) 667-2574, henrymiller.org. Summer calendar of international music, circus events, family entertainment, and community open mic.

HIDDEN GARDENS TOUR (831) 667-1530. Late June. One-day tour of various private Big Sur gardens, featuring presenters, artists, and musicians.

JADE FESTIVAL (831) 394-8315, surcoast.com/jfest.html. Early October. Jade, gems, wood, stone, barbecue, and live music in Pacific Valley.

Highway 1 Mileage Log: From Carmel River or Cambria

DESTINATION	Miles from Carmel River (*heading south*)	Miles from Cambria (*heading north*)
Carmel River Bridge	0	97.5
Carmel Meadows (Ribera Road)	0.6	96.9
Missionary Beach	1	96.5
Point Lobos State Reserve	1.9	95.6
Carmel Highlands general store	2.7	94.8
Malpaso Creek Bridge	4.5	93
Garrapata State Park (GSP north boundary)	5.2	92.3
GSP: Soberanes Canyon Trailhead	6.6	90.9
GSP: Whaleback Peak Trailhead	6.9	90.6
California Department of Fish and Game	7.8	89.7
Granite Creek Bridge	8	89.5
Garrapata Creek Bridge	9.4	88.1
Rocky Point Restaurant (turnoff west)	10.4	87.1
Palo Colorado Road (turnoff east)	11	86.5
Rocky Creek Bridge	12.5	85
Old Coast Road (turnoff east)	13	84.5
Bixby Bridge	13.1	84.4
Hurricane Point (viewpoint)	14.4	83.2

DESTINATION	Miles from Carmel River (*heading south*)	Miles from Cambria (*heading north*)
Little Sur River	16.4	81.1
Point Sur Historical Park & Lighthouse (turnoff west)	18.5	79
Point Sur Naval Facility (west gate)	18.9	78.6
Old Coast Road (turnoff east)	21.5	76
Andrew Molera State Park (west entrance)	21.5	76
River Inn Resort	24	73.5
Big Sur Center Village Shops (west)	24	73.5
Big Sur Campground & Cabins (west)	24.3	73.2
Riverside Campground & Cabins (west)	24.4	73.1
Ripplewood Resort, Gas Station, Store, Café	24.7	73.1
Glen Oaks (lodging & restaurant)	24.7	72.8
St. Francis of the Redwoods Catholic Church (west)	25.1	72.4
Fernwood Park Resort (west)	25.3	72.2
Pfeiffer Big Sur State Park (east)	26	71.5
Big Sur Lodge	26	71.5
Big Sur River Bridge	26.2	71.3
Big Sur Station (multi-agency facility; east)	26.4	71.1
Ripplewood Resort (west)	27	72.8
Sycamore Canyon Road (Pfeiffer Beach; turnoff west)	27.2	70.3
Big Sur Post Office & Store (east)	27.7	69.8
Big Sur Deli (gas station, store, bakery; turnoff west)	27.8	69.7
Ventana Inn turnoff (Old Post Ranch; east)	28.3	69.2
Post Ranch Inn & Cielo Restaurant (turnoff west)	28.3	69.2
Coastlands (residential neighborhood; turnoff west)	28.4	69.1
Nepenthe, Café Kevah, & the Phoenix Gift Shop (west)	29	68.5
Henry Miller Library (Graves Canyon; turnoff east)	29.3	68.2
Deetjen's (Castro Canyon; turnoff east)	29.7	67.8
Coast Gallery (turnoff east)	32.1	65.4
Torre Canyon Bridge	33.2	64.3
DeAngulo Trailhead (east)	34	63.5
Partington Ridge Road (residential; turnoff east)	34.3	63.1
Partington Cove & Tanbark Trailheads	35.1	62.4
Fire Road Trail to Tin House (turnoff east)	36	61.5
Large Vista Point (turnoff west)	36	61.5

DESTINATION	Miles from Carmel River (*heading south*)	Miles from Cambria (*heading north*)
Pfeiffer Burns State Park & McWay Creek Waterfall (turnoff east)	37.1	60.4
Anderson Creek Bridge	37.6	59.9
Burns Creek Bridge	38.7	58.8
Buck Creek Bridge	39.3	58.2
Esalen Institute (turnoff west)	40.3	57.2
Lime Creek Bridge	40.7	56.8
Dolan Creek Bridge	41.8	55.7
Rat Creek Bridge	42.9	54.6
Big Creek Bridge	45	52.5
Gamboa Point (west)	46.8	50.7
Vicente Creek Bridge	47.3	50.2
Lucia	50.1	47.4
New Camaldoli Monastery (east entrance)	50.6	46.9
Limekiln State Park	52.2	45.3
Vicente Flat Trailhead (east)	54.1	43.4
Kirk Creek Campground (turnoff west)	54.1	43.4
Nacimiento-Fergusson Road (turnoff east)	54.2	43.3
Mill Creek Bridge	54.5	43
Prewitt Loop Trailhead (north end turnoff east)	57.9	39.6
Pacific Valley Ranger Station & Prewitt Loop Trailhead (south end turnoff east)	58.5	39
Sand Dollar Beach parking & picnic area (turnoff west)	59.4	38.1
Plaskett Creek Campground; Pacific Valley School (turnoff east)	59.5	38
Plaskett Ridge Road (turnoff east)	59.6	37.9
Jade Cove turnout (west)	60	37.5
Willow Creek Bridge & Beach	61.5	36
Willow Creek Road & Treebones Resort (east turnoff)	62.1	35.4
Gorda (gas, lodging, store, restaurant)	63	34.5
Alder Creek Bridge	65.5	32
Villa Creek Bridge	66.2	31.3
Cruikshank Trailhead (east)	66.8	30.7
Soda Springs Trail (east)	69.5	28
Buckeye Trail (just past old ranger station on northeast side of highway)	71	26.5
Salmon Creek Bridge & Trailhead (east)	71.1	26.4

DESTINATION	Miles from Carmel River (*heading south*)	Miles from Cambria (*heading north*)
Monterey–San Luis Obispo county line	73.6	23.9
Ragged Point Inn (gas, lodging, restaurant; turnoff west)	75	22.5
San Carpoforo Creek Bridge	76.4	21.1
Arroyo de la Cruz Bridge	80.8	16.7
Piedras Blancas Lightstation (turnoff west)	84.1	13.4
Elephant Seal Vista Point (west)	85.1	12.4
Elephant Seal Vista Point (west)	85.4	12.1
Elephant Seal Vista Point (west)	86.4	11.1
Arroyo Laguna Bridge	87.5	10
W. R. Hearst Memorial Beach (turnoff west)	90.2	7.3
Hearst Castle entrance (turnoff east)	90.2	7.3
San Simeon Acres (lodging, restaurants; turnoff west)	93.3–93.7	4.2–3.8
San Simeon Creek Road to San Simeon State Park (turnoff east)	94.8	2.7
San Simeon Creek Bridge	95.1	2.4
Washburn Day Use Area & San Simeon State Beach	95.3	2.2
Moonstone Beach Road (north end; turnoff west)	95.7	1.8
Main Street, Cambria (turnoff east)	97.5	0

CHAPTER five

Driving & Destinations Along Big Sur Back Roads

■ ■ ■ ■ ■ ■ ■ ■ ■ ■ ■ ■ ■

IF YOU ARE LOOKING TO ESCAPE the tourism and development of Highway 1, consider venturing east and turning along some of the back roads that gain access into the remote wildlands of Big Sur County.

With this remoteness comes ruggedness. Often county road departments and the US Forest Service close these back roads during storm events and keep them closed until the wet season dissipates in the spring. Maintenance is not high priority along these relatively unused roads, so expect to find ruts and debris (boulders, rocks, trees, and limbs) if you choose a more adventurous route.

Be prepared and note that most unpaved back roads are not suitable for low clearance vehicles, trailers, and RVs. Fortunately, there are a few paved roads that are suitable for your average two-wheel drive vehicle, but you should still expect a steep, windy, and, at times, single-lane ride. Regardless of the route you choose (paved or unpaved), inquire locally about road conditions before you head out, respect private property, fill up your tank, and make sure your vehicle is in good running condition with everything you might need to repair a spare or wait for some time for assistance.

If you plan to enter Fort Hunter Liggett, note the special rules at the three public-access points (Jolon Road, Nacimiento-Fergusson Road, and the northern end of Milpitas Road). All passengers will need to show photo identification to the sentry, and drivers will need to show car registration and proof of insurance. Entry may be denied due to security alerts or military training. Biking, hiking, camping, picnicking, and swimming are prohibited except to anglers and hunters who obtained the required permits from the Outdoor Recreation Office.

For information on road closures contact the following offices:

Fort Hunter Liggett: Call (831) 386-2503 or (831) 386-2310 for military road closures.

Los Padres National Forest: Call the King City office at (831) 385-5434 or visit www.fs.fed.us for seasonal or permanent closures of forest service roads.

Big Sur Station: Call (831) 667-2315 for information on state park and forest service roads.

Cal Trans: Call (888) 836-0866 for information about traffic and road conditions on Highway 1 from Carmel to Cambria.

Back Road Camping

IF YOU ARE TURNED OFF by the high price of camping along Highway 1, consider the primitive and remote camping that exists along Big Sur's back roads. The plus side is that many of these camps provide free camping (simply unheard of along the coast). With the exception of Arroyo Seco Campground and the developed sites at Nacimiento and San Antonio Reservoirs, these primitive, rarely maintained camps provide few to no amenities, so expect to bring in water and/or purifying systems and everything else you might need to be comfortable and safe.

Alder Creek Camp

DIRECTIONS: Located 8 miles from Highway 1 on Willow Creek Road (23S01).

CAMPSITES: 2 | **COST:** Free

WATER: On the creek; no potable water

COMMENTS: For more information contact the Los Padres National Forest Service at (831) 385-5434 or **www.fs.fed.us**.

Arroyo Seco Campground

DIRECTIONS: Coming from the south on Highway 101 to Greenfield, take the Arroyo Seco exit into town. Turn left on Elm Street. Go west to Arroyo Seco Road and turn left; campground is at the end of Arroyo Seco Road.

Coming from the north on Highway 101 just pass Soledad. Go west to Arroyo Seco Road and turn left; campground is at the end of Arroyo Seco Road.

CAMPSITES: 50 | **COST:** $15–30 (primitive sites), $20–40 (with showers and flush toilets), $75 (group site)

COMMENTS: For more information contact Rocky Mountain Recreation at (831) 674-5726.

Bottchers Gap Campground

DIRECTIONS: Located 8 miles inland, off Highway 1 on Palo Colorado Road (18S05), 15 miles north of Big Sur and 11 miles south of Carmel.

CAMPSITES: 11 | **COST:** $12/night, $5/day use

COMMENTS: For more information contact Parks Management Co. at (805) 434-1996, (805) 434-9199, or **campone.com**.

China Camp

DIRECTIONS: From Highway 101 north, exit at Arroyo Seco Road near the city of Greenfield. Proceed 16.2 miles to the junction of Carmel Valley Road and Arroyo Seco Road and bear right. Take Carmel Valley Road 17.2 miles to the junction with Tassajara Road and turn left. Go 11 miles to China Camp.

From Highway 101 south, exit at Arroyo Seco Road and make an immediate left at Elm Avenue. (If you get to the ENTERING GREENFIELD sign, you have passed the left turn.) Follow Elm Avenue for 6 miles and turn left at the T onto Arroyo Seco Road. Proceed 6.5 miles along Arroyo Seco Road to the junction with Carmel Valley Road and bear right. Take Carmel Valley Road 17.2 miles to the junction with Tassajara Road and turn left. Go 11 miles to China Camp.

CAMPSITES: 6 | **COST:** Free

COMMENTS: No water; vault toilets. For more information contact the Los Padres National Forest Service at (831) 385-5434 or **www.fs.fed.us**.

Escondido Campground

DIRECTIONS: Take Highway 101 to Jolon Road, turn onto Mission Road, to Del Venture Road. Travel 12 miles to the campground. Last 3 miles is unsurfaced.

CAMPSITES: 9 | **COST:** Free

COMMENTS: Closed during the winter and periodically during the wet season (November–March). No water, but the Arroyo Seco River is nearby (bring a water purification system); vault toilets. For more information contact the Los Padres National Forest Service at (831) 385-5434 or **www.fs.fed.us**.

Nacimiento Campground

DIRECTIONS: From the north, take Highway 101 south and take the Ft. Hunter Liggett exit. Then go 17.5 miles to the junction with Mission Road. From the south, take Highway 101 south to Exit 252. Drive 21.7 miles on County Road G18 to the junction at Mission Road. From the junction travel 3.2 miles on Mission Road to Nacimiento-Ferguson Road and turn left. It is 13 miles to Nacimiento CG from this point.

CAMPSITES: 8 | **COST:** $10/night

COMMENTS: No water; vault toilets. For more information contact Parks Management Co. at (805) 434-1996, (805) 434-9199, or **campone.com**.

Ponderosa Campground

DIRECTIONS: From Salinas take Highway 101 south and take the Ft. Hunter Liggett exit. Then go 17.5 miles to the junction with Mission Road. From Highway 101 south, take Exit 252. Drive 21.7 miles on County Road G18 to the junction at Mission Road. From the junction travel 3.2 miles on Mission Road to Nacimiento-Ferguson Road and turn left. It is 12 miles to Ponderosa CG from this point.

CAMPSITES: 23 | **COST:** $15/night

COMMENTS: No water (April–October); vault toilets. For more information contact Parks Management Co. at (805) 434-1996, (805) 434-9199, or **campone.com**.

CHAPTER six

Safety & Conservation

■ ■ ■ ■ ■ ■ ■ ■ ■ ■ ■ ■ ■

HUNDREDS OF MILES OF TRAILS AND ROADS crisscross Big Sur's state parks, the Ventana Wilderness, and the Silver Peak Wilderness. Plan carefully before you venture into the backcountry. This chapter describes potential hazards and offers gear suggestions to help you prepare for your hike.

The fact that a trail is described in this book does not mean it's safe for everyone. Trails vary greatly in difficulty and condition. Some sections are choked with poison oak, encroaching brush, fallen trees, and debris. The sheer landscape is also subject to floods and landslides. Conditions can change rapidly. A riverside trail that's safe on a dry day may be impassable during heavy rains, even for the fittest hiker.

It is essential that you tell someone where you're hiking and when you expect to return so rescue groups know where to look if you're overdue. Always respect your limits and avoid hiking alone. Stay on the trail, both to limit erosion and avoid injury.

Following the preparation tips is a partial list of regulations and advice on how to preserve this beautiful landscape for fellow hikers. If you'd like to volunteer your time, refer to the list of conservation organizations on page 50.

Wildlife Hazards

Ticks

Particularly in the Ventana and Silver Peak Wildernesses, trails are often overgrown with brush. This encroaching brush, in turn, harbors ticks. Tick numbers boom following winter's first major rains and don't drop again till early summer. They're most prevalent amid dense thickets of chamise, Big Sur's most widespread plant.

Once one of these blood-sucking arachnids latches on, it climbs till it reaches an exposed patch of skin. Deer ticks start out the size of a comma on a printed page, while wood ticks are only about twice that size. The tiny hitchhikers often go unnoticed until they swell with blood.

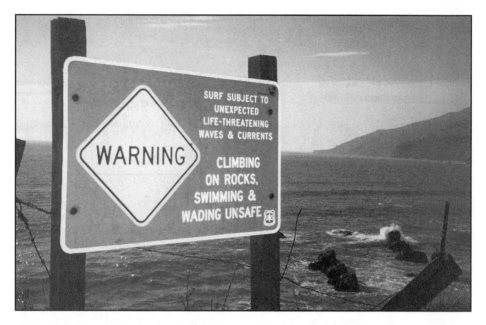

Along the coast, enjoy the coarse sand between your toes, but beware of cold water and dangerous currents.

Ticks usually take an hour or more to burrow into your skin, though in heavily infested areas you should check for them every few minutes. Wear long, light-colored clothing to make it easier to spot ticks. Consider wearing breathable rain gear, as the slow-moving insects have difficulty latching onto the synthetic material.

If you do find a tick burrowed into your skin, take a pair of tweezers, grip the tick as close to the skin as possible, and pull it straight out. Avoid squeezing the tick, as it may emit bacteria into the skin. While tick-borne Lyme disease remains rare in the northern Santa Lucia Range, that risk could change in the future. A tick must be attached for at least 24 hours to transmit the disease, which is very treatable if diagnosed early. If you develop a bull's-eye rash, pain, fever, headache, or muscle ache after a tick bite, see your doctor immediately.

Flies

How can such a small insect be so vexing? A number of fly species thrive when temperatures rise above 70°F. Though certain types can deliver a painful bite, these are typically slow and easy to swat. Much more of a nuisance are persistent nonbiting gnats, which continually buzz around your face. You may encounter flies on a warm winter day, but populations increase markedly between April and October. Dense oak woodlands are their favorite habitat in summer.

Rattlesnakes

Found throughout the Santa Lucia Range, these venomous snakes like to bask on warm rocks or sunny patches of dirt. They are most common in spring when their food supply (mostly rodents) also peaks. Rattlesnakes usually flee when startled and will only strike if threatened.

To avoid being bitten, stay on paths, always give snakes the right of way, wear high-sided hiking boots, and carry a walking stick. When climbing, watch where you place your hands and feet.

If someone is bitten, keep the person as calm and still as possible, gently wash the area with soap and water, apply a clean bandage, and seek immediate medical attention. Do not apply a tourniquet or pack the bite area in ice, as either method will only block circulation. Do not use your mouth to suck out venom, as that may lead to a complicating infection. Following treatment, most snakebite symptoms resolve within a few days.

Giardia lamblia

People often return from camping trips suffering from giardiasis, an infection of the small intestine that can cause nausea, diarrhea, loose or watery stool, and stomach cramps. A single-celled parasite, *Giardia lamblia* is passed in the stool of an infected person or animal or through contaminated food or water. Symptoms generally begin one to two weeks after being infected and may last two to six weeks.

Purify all water taken from springs, lakes, creeks, and rivers with a portable filter, chemical treatment, or by boiling it for one to three minutes.

Raccoons & Skunks

These night visitors are drawn by food left out by campers. Never leave your food unattended and always store it somewhere safe at night, preferably in a food canister hung from a tree. Avoid feeding wildlife. Raccoons and skunks are known carriers of rabies and are also infested with disease-carrying fleas, ticks, lice, and mites.

Mountain Lions

While mountain lions do roam throughout the Santa Lucia Range, they are extremely elusive and pose a minimal threat. Don't hike alone, and keep children within arm's length. If you encounter a lion, neither approach nor run from it. Do all you can to appear larger, and fight back if attacked.

Wild Boars

Hunters introduced these destructive, nonnative animals to the Santa Lucia Range as game in the 1920s, and their population has since exploded. Boar hunting is permitted within the

Ventana and Silver Peak Wildernesses, but regulations govern how far hunters must keep from trails and roads. For more information, contact the Los Padres National Forest Headquarters: (805) 968-6640 or www.fs.usda.gov/lpnf.

Plant Hazards

Poison Oak

Poison oak is a common trailside companion in Big Sur country. It grows as a low-lying bush, shrub, or vine along stream banks, rocky canyons, mountain flanks, and coastal bluffs from sea level to below 5000 feet (it's only absent on the highest rocky summits). Learning to identify this toxic plant is the first step toward avoiding a painful, annoying rash.

Poison oak leaves are clustered in threes. Shiny when young, the leaflets usually range from half an inch to 2 inches long. In fall the leaves turn a brilliant red, while branches are bare in winter. Unfortunately, all parts of the plant (the leaves, flowers, stem, roots, and fruit) are toxic year-round.

Since many trails are overgrown, particularly within the Ventana and Silver Peak Wildernesses, it's likely you'll brush up against poison oak at some point. It's best to wear long pants while hiking, regardless of temperature. If you're extremely susceptible, bring extra pants and long-sleeved shirts, and place each day's clothes in a plastic bag upon reaching camp. Wash your skin thoroughly with products designed to remove the plant's toxic oil, such as Tecnu.

Poison oak's oily resin contains the toxin urushiol. Contact can cause painful blistering, weeping soars, and maddening itching. The rash may appear in a few hours or days, depending on the extent of exposure and your degree of sensitivity. Most exposures are through direct contact with the plant. Other sources include smoke and secondary exposure from pets, soiled clothing, and gear. If your symptoms are severe, see a physician for treatment with strong corticosteroids.

Stinging Nettle

Another unpleasant plant you may encounter on the trail is the stinging nettle, which grows in clusters along the banks of creeks and rivers. Nettle leaves bear raised prickly hairs that stick in your skin, instantly delivering a painful sting and burning sensation. You'll know once you've walked through stinging nettles—the key is to recognize them in advance.

Growing in slender stalks up to 6 feet tall, nettles sport dense, drooping clusters of flowers where the leaves join the stalk. Leaves are heart-shaped, finely toothed, and grow on opposite sides of the stem. When you brush against the plant, the tiny hollow hairs break off and release an acid. Symptoms are usually gone within 24 hours.

You can neutralize the acid by mixing it with a base, such as baking soda. Bring a packet of baking soda with you, and apply it to your skin as soon as possible to soothe the burn. If baking soda is unavailable, try your own spit, which is somewhat basic and will help neutralize the acid.

Gear

Survival Essentials

You should always carry:

Water

Many wilderness trails are dry for several miles, and small seasonal creeks are not always reliable. Carry at least 1–2 liters of water and some means of purifying backcountry sources (filter or chemical treatment such as iodine).

Food

An energy bar, nuts, or trail mix may be critical if you're out longer than you planned to be.

First-Aid Kit

Accidents and injuries can happen to anyone. Properly preparing for these instances can save you from a backcountry disaster. Prepackaged first-aid kits are readily available at outdoor equipment stores. A basic kit should include at least the following:

- Ace bandages
- Advil or other anti-inflammatory medicine
- alcohol pads
- antibiotic ointment
- Band-Aids and moleskin
- cotton balls or swabs
- gauze pads and bandages
- hydrogen peroxide
- medical tape
- poison oak soap (Tecnu)
- space blanket
- tweezers (for removing ticks)
- Tylenol (fever and pain reduction)
- waterproof matches (for emergency fire)

Knife

Pocketknives and all-in-one tools can be invaluable in the event of a mishap.

Map & Compass

Some of the more remote trails are heavily overgrown with brush and easily lost to slides and fallen debris. A map and compass may help you find your way home.

Important Hiking Gear

Backpack

The ideal daypack should have enough room to carry survival essentials (see the previous page), ideally somewhere between 1000 and 2000 cubic inches of volume. Overnight packs should provide between 3000 and 4000 cubic inches.

Flashlight

Whenever possible, avoid hiking in the dark, as trails are steep, slippery, and lined with poison oak in places. However, if you're delayed or tire unexpectedly, you may end up hiking in the dark. Be prepared and always carry a flashlight. Hands-free headlamps are preferred over handheld flashlights.

Essential Overnight Gear

Sleeping Bag

Temperatures can drop dramatically at higher elevations along the Santa Lucia Range. Choose a sleeping bag with a temperature rating of 20°F or lower to ensure a warm and restful night's sleep. Be prepared for temperatures to occasionally drop below freezing from late fall through early spring.

Sleeping Pad

Inflatable and foam sleeping pads keep you off the cold, hard ground. They also provide spots to sit and lounge at camp.

Tent

Too often hikers leave tents at home, particularly in summer when rainfall is unlikely. However, fog creeps inland and can saturate a sleeping bag with condensation by morning.

The Kitchen Sink

Be sure to pack plenty of food, spices, cooking supplies, and utensils. There's nothing like eating gourmet in the backcountry. Don't forget the chocolate and warm drinks.

Camp Wear

Backcountry hiking can be a sweaty slog. When you arrive at camp, it's wonderful to hang out beneath the stars in a set of comfortable camp clothes (e.g., long underwear, comfortable fleece pants, and slip-on shoes). Again, those extremely sensitive to poison oak should store the previous day's clothes in a plastic bag.

Other Necessities

Don't forget a wide-brimmed hat, polarizing sunglasses, sunscreen, a towel, toiletries, a warm knit cap, waterproof backpack cover, duct tape, and trowel.

If there's still room in your pack, bring a camera, binoculars, a Frisbee, cards, and small travel games.

The Wilderness Ethic

TREATING BIG SUR'S PUBLIC LANDS as a precious resource will ensure they remain unspoiled for future generations. Please refer to the following commonsense guidelines:

Group Size

Visit in small groups. Although US Forest Service guidelines allow groups of up to 25 individuals at backcountry camps, most backcountry camps only have room for up to 10. You'll find designated group camping at Pfeiffer Big Sur State Park, Kirk Creek Campground, and Arroyo Seco Campground.

Camping

Camp at an established site. Keep your camp clean and never leave food out. Scout the area to be sure you leave nothing behind.

Fire Safety

Careless campfire use has sparked devastating blazes. Where fire use is authorized, please observe the following measures:

Campfires are permitted only in established fire rings and must be kept small, using as little wood as possible. Use only dead and downed wood. Always make sure your fire is completely extinguished before you break camp.

Regardless of the time of year, a fire permit is required for backcountry camping. The permits allow full campfires during the wet season (November through April) or the use of camp stoves the rest of the year. East side campers should contact the Los Padres National Forest Headquarters in Goleta at (805) 968-6640. West side campers can obtain a permit either at Big Sur Station, a half mile south of Pfeiffer Big Sur State Park, or at Pacific Valley Station, 5 miles north of Gorda.

Noise Pollution

Respect the natural peace, fellow hikers, and neighboring campers by keeping all trail and camp chatter down. Raucous behavior may also spook wildlife.

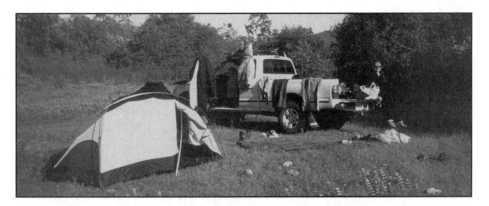

Camp at established sites to minimize your impact and "leave no trace."

Sanitation

Keep soap and detergent away from all natural water sources. If you're susceptible to poison oak and need to wash with medicated soap, do not bathe in the streams. Such products contain toxic chemicals that pollute water. Wash with water from a pot, and rinse at least 100 feet from any water source.

Also refrain from washing dishes or clothing in natural water sources. Wash using minimal water and dispose of wastewater at least 100 feet from any water source.

If a pit toilet is unavailable, dig a hole at least 6 inches deep, make your deposit, and cover it with the soil you removed. Do not bury toilet paper or trash, as an animal may dig it up.

Garbage

If you pack it in, you must pack it out. Before leaving camp, clean up and pack out any trash left by inconsiderate campers. Leave the site looking as lightly used as possible.

Pack Stock & Horses

Hikers must yield right-of-way to all pack and saddle animals. Forage is often scarce, so be sure to pack plenty of food for your animals. Such animals can severely damage trails and camps if not properly handled. Avoid tying animals to trees, as they may dig up roots and strip bark.

Wildlife

Do not feed wild animals. They will associate humans with food and may become aggressive pests. Juvenile animals may never learn normal foraging behavior, instead becoming dependent on handouts that are not part of their natural diets. Wild animals may also congregate in unnaturally high numbers, which might increase chances of disease transmission.

Conservation

WITH LITTLE MONEY ALLOCATED for maintenance, the US Forest Service is unable to devote much attention to trails within the Ventana and Silver Peak Wildernesses. Fortunately, groups of dedicated volunteers have taken responsibility for rebuilding trail networks and caring for this backcountry that belongs to us all. Many of these volunteers work for the following listed conservation groups, grass-roots organizations dedicated to protecting, preserving, enhancing, and restoring public lands within the Santa Lucia Range.

> *Let us leave a splendid legacy for our children . . . let us turn to them and say, "This you inherit: Guard it well, for it is far more precious than money . . . and once destroyed, nature's beauty cannot be repurchased at any price."*

> *Ansel Adams, American photographer, 1902–1984*

We owe a debt of gratitude to such volunteers. The trails would not be passable and this book would not be possible without them. Be sure to do your part to leave Big Sur's natural spaces as pristine as you found them.

Conservation Organizations

The Big Sur wilderness hangs in fragile balance between humans and nature. Were it not for the foresight and efforts of grass-roots conservationists, much of the region's untamed splendor might be lost to development. Please contact the following groups if you'd like to get involved:

Big Sur Land Trust
PO Box 221864
Carmel, CA 93922
(831) 625-5523; **bigsurlandtrust.org**

Ventana Wilderness Alliance
PO Box 506
Santa Cruz, CA 95061
(831) 423-3191; **ventanawild.org**

Sierra Club, Ventana Chapter
PO Box 5667
Carmel, CA 93921
(831) 624-8032; **ventana.sierraclub.org**

Ventana Wilderness Society
19045 Portola Dr., Suite F-1
Salinas, CA 93908
(831) 455-9514; **ventanaws.org**

PART ONE

■ ■ ■ ■ ■ ■ ■ ■ ■ ■ ■ ■ ■ ■

State & Federal Lands of the Big Sur Coast

THIS SECTION COVERS the 90-mile stretch of coast from Carmel River State Beach south to San Simeon State Beach. All lands are accessible from Highway 1, which winds past golden hillsides, redwood-lined ravines, ancient oak forests, and sheer granite cliffs. Lying primarily west of the highway, the region comprises six state parks (Garrapata, Andrew Molera, Pfeiffer Big Sur, Julia Pfeiffer Burns, Limekiln, and San Simeon), seven beaches (Carmel River, Pfeiffer, San Simeon, Hearst Memorial, Piedras Blancas, Jade Cove, and Sand Dollar), one reserve (Point Lobos), and one historic park (Point Sur). These public spaces are relatively small, thus trails are short and for day use only.

Due to its proximity to the ocean, the region is fertile in both terrestrial and marine life. Northern and southern biogeographical regions converge here in a kind of suture zone that supports a wide range of vegetation. Fog shrouds the coast in summer, nurturing moisture-loving plants in deep ravines, while the sheer, exposed slopes host such drought-tolerant species as yuccas. Cold-water upwellings from deep marine canyons bring nutrient-rich waters to the surface, luring fish, seals, birds, whales, and sharks close to shore.

Recreational opportunities are equally diverse. Visitors can dive the waters off Point Lobos or Jade Cove, summit granite peaks, marvel at 5,000-pound male elephant seals, plunge into swimming holes along the Big Sur River, explore Hearst Castle, surf the rollers at Andrew Molera, learn about maritime history at Point Sur Lighthouse, or simply take a barefoot stroll on the beach. Whatever you choose, you're bound to return.

CHAPTER seven

Carmel River State Beach & Point Lobos State Reserve

Carmel River State Beach

THIS PARK ACTUALLY comprises two beaches: Carmel River State Beach at the river mouth and San Jose Creek Beach (aka Monastery Beach) farther south. Together they form a mile-long crescent of coarse sand backed by bluffs that offer spectacular views. Visitors can go for a stroll, build a sandcastle, picnic, or watch wildlife on the sheltered inland side of the beach at Carmel River Lagoon.

While the turquoise Pacific may look inviting, neither beach is safe for swimming or wading. A deep underwater canyon just offshore contributes to hazardous surf conditions. Even on calm days, unpredictable "sleeper waves" have risen up to surprise waders, sometimes dragging them in. Year-round strong currents and water temperatures that linger in the mid-50s Fahrenheit make submersion a real danger, though experienced, properly trained surfers and scuba divers do brave these waters.

DIRECTIONS: From Carmel, drive south on Highway 1 and turn right at the Rio Road signal light. In a half mile you'll pass Carmel Mission (Mission San Carlos Borromeo de Carmelo) on the left. One block past the mission, turn left on Santa Lucia Avenue. Drive 0.4 mile west on Santa Lucia to Carmelo Street and turn left. Within a half mile Carmelo dead-ends at the beach's north parking lot.

VISITOR CENTER: Point Lobos State Reserve, off Highway 1, 2.2 miles south of the Rio Road intersection. Open daily 9 a.m.–7 p.m. in summer, 9 a.m.–5 p.m. in winter.

NEAREST CAMPGROUND: See Chapter 10: Pfeiffer Big Sur State Park (page 98) for coastal campgrounds or Chapter 14: Bottchers Gap (page 148) for inland options.

INFORMATION: Open 7 a.m.–10 p.m. Dogs must be on a leash.

WEBSITE: parks.ca.gov

PHONE: (831) 649-2836

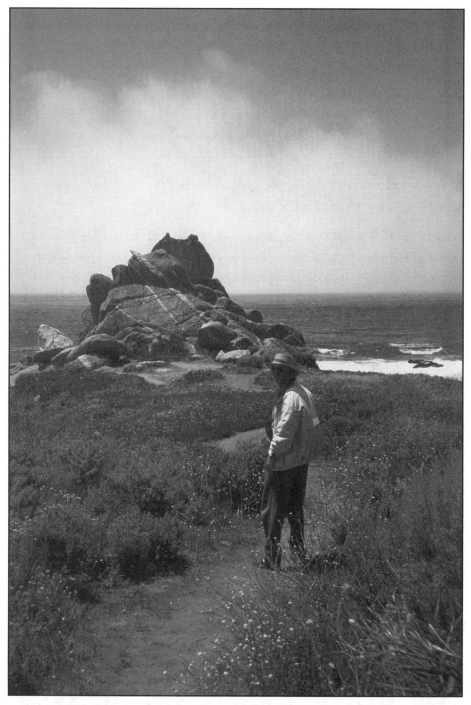

Short spur trails lead to stunning views from rocky granite outcrops along Carmel River State Beach.

CARMEL RIVER STATE BEACH

LENGTH AND TYPE: 2-mile out-and-back

RATING: Easy

TRAIL CONDITION: Well maintained, poison oak, good for kids

HIGHLIGHTS: A wildlife haven amid the Carmel River lagoon and estuary, featuring a mile-long crescent of coarse white sand and views of the open ocean

TO REACH THE TRAILHEAD: This hike begins at Carmel River State Beach, where you'll find a phone, restrooms, and water at the free parking lot.

TRIP SUMMARY: Carmel River State Beach actually comprises two beaches: Carmel River State Beach, at the river mouth, and Monastery Beach (aka San Jose Creek Beach), just south of the river. The trail saunters along these wave-washed beaches and atop the adjacent bluffs. The first 0.2 mile of the route crosses soft sands deposited by the Carmel River and pounded into fine powder by the often-heavy surf. The bluffs overlook granite pinnacles, wind-sculpted Monterey cypress, and a marsh and estuary that teem with life.

Trip Description

From the north end of **Carmel River State Beach,** the hike strikes out across sand and heads southwest toward the river mouth. Sand bridges the river mouth in summer, but expect a wet crossing after winter rains. If you prefer to keep your feet dry, park at Monastery Beach and hike north, following this trail description in reverse. Parking stretches for 0.2 mile along

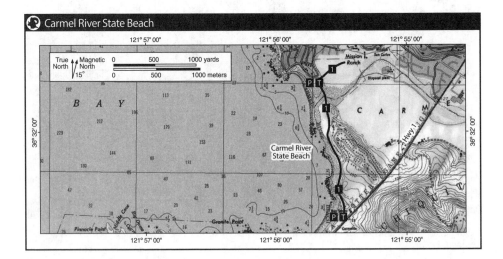

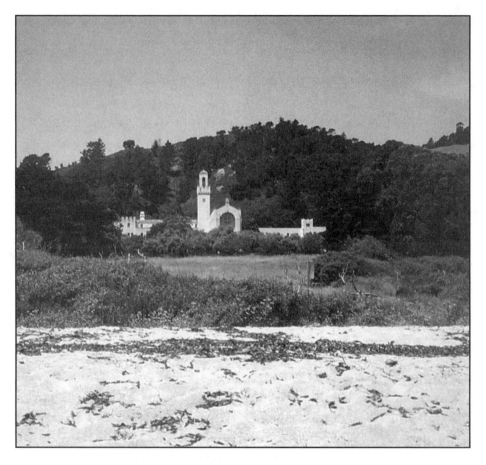

Monastery Beach offers views inland that give rise to its name.

Highway 1 at Monastery. Just south of the lagoon you can either continue along the shoreline or climb atop the bluffs for sweeping views of Carmel Bay, the lagoon, and the marsh.

The bluff trail leads up a half dozen stairs to a fork (0.2 mile, 25'). The left spur traverses the east edge of the bluff for views of the marsh and lagoon. This spur then turns south through thickets of coyote brush, sagebrush, and lupine, ascending a small knoll capped by a large **wooden cross** (0.3 mile, 35'). A plaque explains its significance. In 1769 the Portolá-Crespi expedition traveled overland from Mexico. After waiting in vain for the long-overdue supply ship *San Jose*, they erected a cross here to signal their early return to San Diego. From here the spur veers west and rejoins the main bluff trail.

The direct route to the south end of the beach leads from atop the stairs along the west edge of the bluff, blanketed in fragrant coastal chaparral. A half mile south, the trail passes very large, striking homes in the **Carmel Meadows** subdivision. Farther along you'll encounter another short, narrow spur that leads down to prominent boulders pounded by surf. Beyond this spur, the main trail curls southeast to emerge at **Monastery Beach** (0.9 mile).

WHERE RIVER & SEA COLLIDE ■ ■ ■ ■ ■ ■ ■ ■ ■ ■ ■ ■ ■ ■ ■

The opposing forces of the Carmel River and Pacific Ocean form a unique ecosystem at Carmel River State Beach. Longshore currents deposit sand on the beach at the river mouth, forming sandbars that periodically dam its flow. The water that accumulates in the lagoon and surrounding marsh is a mix of freshwater and saltwater, creating a rare habitat. In the 160 miles between San Francisco Bay and Morro Bay, coastal salt marshes occur only at Elkhorn Slough, Pescadero Marsh, and here. It takes heavy rainfall to flood the river and once again break through the sandbars, allowing the lagoon to drain into the ocean.

Among Monterey County's prime birding locations, the lagoon and marsh shelter a wide variety of waterfowl and songbirds during their migration along the Pacific Flyway. Pelicans, seagulls, and several duck species bathe in the brackish water, while great blue herons, egrets, sandpipers, and plovers work the shallows for food. Red-winged blackbirds enact courtship displays atop tule reeds at the edge of the marsh. In the evenings, cliff swallows swoop down from nests south of the lagoon to nab flying insects. Also watch for the occasional northern harrier, black-shouldered kite, or red-tailed hawk, which soar over the wetlands in search of prey.

The river also hosts the southernmost major steelhead trout run in North America. Native steelhead return annually from the ocean to spawn. Strict rules protect this population, as the run dwindled to just a handful of fish in the early 1990s. As of 2002, the Carmel River averaged 123 juvenile steelhead per hundred feet of stream—numbers reflective of well-stocked streams, though this group and other California steelhead populations remain threatened species under the federal Endangered Species Act. Contact the California Department of Fish & Game for current fishing regulations: (831) 649-2870.

■ ■

Dramatically different rock formations anchor either end of the beach. On the north end, the trail passes large granitic outcrops laced with veins of blocky white crystals—excellent examples of Hobnail granite. Over the past 65 million years, the Pacific plate carried these ancient rocks hundreds of miles north from their origin in Mexico. In contrast, the south end features a narrow ridge of russet and tan conglomerate, composed of well-cemented stream sediments from a flood plain that was later supplanted by the Santa Lucia Range.

Monastery Beach is a popular launching spot for divers exploring the nearshore kelp forests. Cold upwelling in the Carmel Submarine Canyon brings nutrient-rich water to the surface, supplying food to abundant marine life. The canyon extends 3.5 miles west before deepening and turning northwest for 12 miles along an active fault to join the Monterey Submarine Canyon, the West Coast's largest submarine canyon.

Enjoy the coarse sand between your toes before returning the way you came.

Point Lobos State Reserve

THIS EXCEPTIONAL STRETCH of the Big Sur coast has been dubbed "the crown jewel of the California state park system." Seven hundred of the reserve's 1250 acres lie underwater, encompassing rocky coves, shallow tide pools, and broad kelp beds. The remaining 550 acres take in 14 trails that crisscross through wind-sculpted pines, across jagged rocky headlands, and along white sand beaches beside cobalt waters. Strolling this dynamic, diverse landscape, you'll find plenty of opportunities to sightsee, take photos, paint, picnic, and study nature, while water lovers can scuba dive or snorkel.

In addition to harboring incredibly diverse flora and fauna, unique geology, rare plant life, and spectacular scenery, Point Lobos is also rich in human history. At one time or another over the past 200 years, the point has been home to American Indians, Chinese fishermen, Japanese abalone harvesters, and Portuguese whalers. Throughout the park, historic relics and endangered archaeological sites offer visitors insight into the varied occupations that once thrived here.

Whether you walk the windswept coastline or head inland through Monterey pine groves and meadows, you'll hear the raucous barking of sea lions from their nearshore colonies—an enduring reminder of the earlier Spanish name for the reserve: *Punta de los Lobos Marinos* (Point of the Sea Wolves).

DIRECTIONS: The reserve entrance is off Highway 1, 2.2 miles south of the Rio Road intersection in Carmel and 1.2 miles north of the Highlands Inn entrance road (Highlands Drive) in Carmel Highlands.

VISITOR CENTER: An information kiosk at the entrance offers books, maps, and interpretive displays about the zoology, geology, and botany of Point Lobos.

NEAREST CAMPGROUNDS: See Chapter 10: Pfeiffer Big Sur State Park (page 98) for coastal campgrounds or Chapter 14: Bottchers Gap (page 148) for inland options.

INFORMATION: Open daily 9 a.m.–7 p.m. in summer, 9 a.m.–5 p.m. in winter. There's an $10-per-vehicle entrance fee (discounts offered to seniors and the disabled). Entry is limited to 450 visitors at any one time. Bicycles are restricted to paved

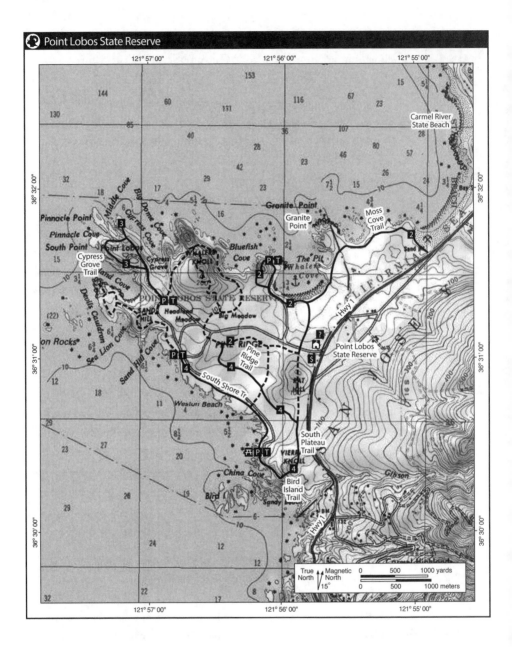

roads. Fires and the use of stoves are prohibited. Fishing, Frisbee, kite flying, and other games are prohibited. Pets are not allowed in the reserve, though guide dogs for the blind and certified service dogs are permitted. Diving is restricted to Bluefish and Whalers Coves with advance permits and proof of dive certification.

WEBSITE: pointlobos.org

PHONE: (831) 624-4909

Trip 2

CARMELO MEADOW, GRANITE POINT, & MOSS COVE TRAILS

LENGTH AND TYPE: 4.4-mile out-and-back

RATING: Easy

TRAIL CONDITION: Well maintained, good for kids

HIGHLIGHTS: Visit the Whaling Station Museum and adjacent Whalers Cabin Museum to learn about the area's cultural history.

TO REACH THE TRAILHEAD: Once at Point Lobos, park in the lot just past the entrance kiosk. If that lot is full (often the case on weekends), bear right at the first fork and head north 0.3 mile to Whalers Cove. Follow the trail description from Whalers Cove, bypassing the 0.2-mile Carmelo Meadow Trail description.

TRIP SUMMARY: This hike begins amid colorful coastal wildflowers in Carmelo Meadow and leads to Whalers Cove, the former site of a prosperous whaling station. A short stroll up the road leads to the Whalers Cabin Museum and Whaling Station Museum, each of which display historical artifacts, diagrams, and photographs. The **Granite Point Trail** leads through dense Monterey pines to Coal Chute Point, which overlooks the surging surf and thick floating kelp mats. Keep a close watch for harbor seals and sea otters amid the kelp.

Trails at Point Lobos lead to jagged, rocky headlands, turquoise waters, and wind-sculpted pine forests.

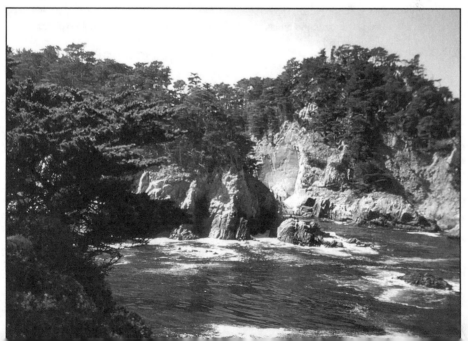

Trip Description

The **Carmelo Meadow Trail** leads from the entrance road north to Whalers Cove or south toward Gibson Beach and Bird Island. Head north through **Carmelo Meadow**. In spring, grasses and herbacious plants give way to a spectrum of wildflowers. At 0.2 mile the Carmelo Meadow Trail ends at **Whalers Cove** and a junction with the Granite Point Trail. Turn left onto the **Granite Point Trail** and stroll 0.1 mile to the **Whaling Station Museum** and **Whalers Cabin Museum** (0.3 mile, 30').

WHALE TALES ■

In the 1850s, Chinese fishermen sailed to California in 30-foot junks in order to harvest abalone along these rocky shores. Their settlement at Whalers Cove consisted of about a dozen structures, one of which now houses the Whalers Cabin Museum. Artifacts and memorabilia span several time periods in the cultural history of the cove.

Portuguese whalers arrived at Point Lobos in 1862 and established the Carmel Bay Whaling Company, one of 16 whaling stations on the California coast. The men hunted gray whales, which still roam these waters from mid-December through May during their migration from Baja to Alaska. The station closed in 1879, but the Whaling Station Museum offers a historical perspective of the industry alongside equipment, photographs, and drawings that depict the lives of whalers and their families. Docents are often on hand to answer questions.

After killing a whale, the whalers towed it into the cove and sliced its blubber into strips. They then cut the blubber into smaller pieces and melted it down in large iron cauldrons called try pots. The reduced blubber was used primarily as lamp oil. Two try pots are on display next to the museum alongside an enormous finback whale skeleton.

■ ■

Just past the museums, the trail leads to a small parking lot where an abalone cannery and a granite quarry once operated. At the height of abalone harvesting, the cannery supplied 75% of the abalone sold in California, while granite from the quarry was used to build the U.S. Mint in San Francisco. From here return to the junction with the Carmelo Meadow Trail.

Past this junction the Granite Point Trail leads through dense stands of Monterey pine and climbs toward **Coal Chute Point**, the first spur on your left (0.4 mile, 30'). At this site in the mid-1870s, coal was dumped from ore carts down a coal chute to the cove below, where deep water enabled coastal steamships close access to shore. The 200-foot spur loops back to Granite Point Trail.

The trail continues through dense, fragrant coastal scrub, descends to the edge of a former pasture, then reaches a junction with the spur toward **Granite Point**. Turn left and climb 0.1 mile to the point (1.6 miles, 30'), where spectacular views abound. Carmel Bay lies to the north, boasting wave-washed beaches and rocky promontories. Abundant life teems in the kelp forests, which rise and fall with the tides. Herons and egrets often "surf" atop these floating mats. The spur loops around to join the **Moss Cove Trail.**

This trail follows the road once used to transport coal from the hills above Point Lobos to Coal Chute Point. It also leads to the newest addition to the reserve, a pasture that once supported grazing cattle. Today small mammals such as mice, voles, and rabbits scurry in the underbrush, while hawks, kestrels, and kites soar overhead, taking advantage of the open hunting grounds. The trail emerges at the south end of **Monastery Beach** (2.2 miles, 20'). Return the way you came.

Trip 3

CYPRESS GROVE TRAIL

LENGTH AND TYPE: 0.8-mile loop

RATING: Easy

TRAIL CONDITION: Well maintained, good for kids

HIGHLIGHTS: Stroll past gnarled Monterey cypress trees in one of only two remaining native groves of this species.

TO REACH THE TRAILHEAD: From the entrance station of the park, drive 0.8 mile to the Sea Lion Point parking area. The trailhead is on the north side of the lot, just past the restrooms and information kiosk. Water is available at the trailhead.

TREES THAT INSPIRED A RESERVE ■ ■ ■ ■ ■ ■ ■ ■ ■ ■ ■ ■

Monterey cypress trees bear distinct twisted branches, shallow exposed roots, and dense flattened canopies. Their contorted appearance attests to the harsh environment of salt spray, rocky granite soil, and gale-force winds the trees must endure. Protection of the celebrated cypress prompted the acquisition of Point Lobos as a state reserve in 1933.

The Monterey cypress trees along North and South Point stand as a memorial to Mr. and Mrs. A.M. Allan, former owners of Point Lobos. In 1888 several land claimants banded together to develop a portion of the headland as residential lots. Fortunately, A.M. Allan, in conjunction with the Save-the-Redwoods League, had the foresight to buy back the residential lots, limit access, and seek public support to make Point Lobos part of the new state park system.

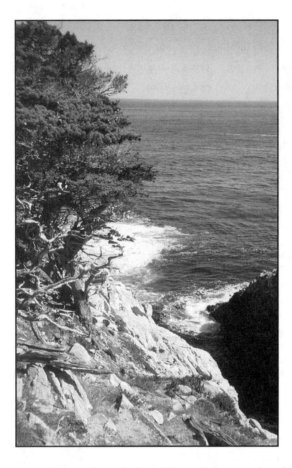

The Monterey cypress clings its bare roots to the sheer granite cliffs of Point Lobos.

TRIP SUMMARY: This short, easy trail leads to overlooks of near-shore islands and rocky coves, where sea otters, harbor seals, and sea lions frolic amid multicolored kelp beds.

Trip Description

From the information kiosk, the trail leads north and soon forks. The **North Shore Trail** heads off to the right, while the **Cypress Grove Trail** veers left 0.1 mile, then splits again into a loop trail through the **Allan Memorial Grove.** Taking the loop in either direction will lead you back to this junction.

Along the northwest fork, the trail offers views into **Headland Cove,** where with any luck you'll see all three species of resident marine mammals: California sea lions, sea otters, and harbor seals. If thick summer fog obscures your view, listen for the boisterous barking of sea lions from nearshore rocks.

Strolling past Headland Cove, you soon enter the grove, one of only two naturally growing stands of Monterey cypress in the world (the other grove is at Cypress Point on the north end of Carmel Bay). In the colder, wetter climate of the Pleistocene epoch some 15,000 years ago, these wind-sculpted trees extended over a much wider range. As the climate slowly turned hotter and drier, the cypress trees withdrew to the cool, fog-shrouded coast. Closely inspect the branches and buttressed trunks to spot a deep orange velvety encrustation. This plush substance is lichen that coexists with the tree, using its branches merely as a roost rather than obtaining nourishment at the tree's expense.

The trail soon veers right, offering dramatic views of secluded coves and granite pinnacles stretching north to Cypress Point. At **North Point** a spur climbs 50 feet to a rocky ledge. Clinging to crevices along the granite walls are such coastal plants as *Dudleya,* or bluff lettuce, featuring succulent silver leaves arranged in a spiral. In summer and fall especially, be sure to bring binoculars, as humpback and gray whales pass within sight of shore along their migratory route from Alaska to the Sea of Cortez, in Baja, Mexico.

Farther along the main trail, a long staircase leads down toward the blue-green waters of **Cypress Cove,** where you may distinguish the heads of several sea otters, resting on their backs atop an underwater forest of 70-foot giant bull kelp. Ascend the steps and continue along the main trail 0.1 mile to complete your loop around the peninsula. From here retrace your steps to the parking area.

Trip 4

SOUTH SHORE, BIRD ISLAND, SOUTH PLATEAU, & PINE RIDGE TRAILS

LENGTH AND TYPE: 2.6-mile loop

RATING: Easy

TRAIL CONDITION: Well maintained, good for kids

HIGHLIGHTS: Explore cliffside gardens, pebbly beaches, blue-green waters, wave-sculpted archways and coves, and forests of majestic Monterey pines.

TO REACH THE TRAILHEAD: From the entrance station of the park, drive 0.8 mile to the Sea Lion Point parking area, bear left, and follow the road another 0.3 mile toward Little Mound Meadow. A parking area on the right leads to the South Shore Trail. If this lot is full, turn left and drive 100 yards farther to the Piney Woods parking and picnic area. You'll find picnic tables, water, and restrooms at the trailhead.

TRIP SUMMARY: This scenic loop takes in an array of habitats, from cliffside gardens, coarse pebbly beaches, and wave-sculpted archways and coves to Monterey pine forests and golden grasslands. Watch egrets walk atop dense rafts of floating kelp, listen for barking sea lions, and smell the salt spray. You may spot the fluke of a passing gray whale or surprise grazing black-tailed deer in a wildflower-strewn meadow.

Trip Description

From the parking area, the **South Shore Trail** leads west toward the typically gentle surf along this rocky shoreline, protected by its southern orientation and wave-thwarting offshore rocks. Low tide exposes pools teeming with unfamiliar life. Pause a moment to peer into a pool. At first you may only notice a few rocks and plants, but the longer you wait, the more alive the pool becomes. Blue-handed hermit crabs scurry nervously along the bottom, while camouflaged sculpin fish dart across the pool to new hiding places. Do be careful where you step—the exposed rocks are covered with slippery seaweed, not to mention tiny tide pool creatures. Check at the information kiosk for daily tide charts.

EBB & FLOOD ■

Ocean tides have perplexed humans throughout history. One ancient theory stated that a water god swallowed seawater and a few hours later released it, thus creating the tides. Science has since explained the phenomenon. High (or flood) tide is when the water level is at its maximum and the beach is covered. During low (or ebb) tide, the water recedes and the beach is exposed.

The tides are generated when the combined gravitational forces of the moon and sun tug on the planet's surface against the force of gravity pulling inward toward Earth's core. Both the sun and moon draw ocean water to positions directly beneath them. High tides are actually bulges that form as water flows toward two regions on the surface—one facing the moon, where gravitational pull is strongest, and the other facing directly away, where gravitational pull is weakest. Low tides represent the corresponding withdrawal of water from regions midway between these bulges. The tides shift as Earth's daily rotation moves the surface closer or farther from these gravitational pulls.

■ ■

Onward, the trail turns southeast toward a junction with the **Mound Meadow Trail** (0.3 mile, 15'), on the left heading northwest. You could take this to the Pine Ridge Trail for a short half-mile loop back to **Piney Woods**. For a richer visit, continue on the South Shore Trail along the reserve's exquisite southern boundary, encompassing some of the state's most beautiful coves and inlets.

The trail meanders within sight of the shore and colorful kelp beds off **Weston Beach**. These rocky promontories are typical of the Carmelo formation, a mix of water-sculpted rocks, fine sediment, and debris deposited by ancient avalanches that occurred in a narrow underwater canyon. Wave action, erosion, and uplift over the past 39 million years have exposed the formation, leaving a complex pattern of graded beds and pebbly beaches.

Leaving Weston Beach, you may want to duck off the trail and descend a few feet to **Hidden Beach** (0.4 mile). Look amid the intertidal rocks for feeding shorebirds such as the black oystercatcher, which boasts a red bill and loud whistled yelps.

Past Hidden Beach the South Shore Trail emerges at the southern parking area, where the **Bird Island Trail** begins (0.6 mile, 25'). If you're short on time, you could park here and explore China Cove and Bird Island, favorite destinations in the reserve.

The short detour to **China Cove** leads up a set of stairs to the headland, where another long, steep set of stairs descends to the white sand beach and sparkling waters. This calm, protected cove is a safe place to wade or explore nearby arches. Year-round water temperatures hover in the 50s Fahrenheit, so you may only want to get your feet wet.

Bird Island Trail heads west to a 0.4-mile loop around **Pelican Point,** passing brittle granite cliffs that do battle with the pounding Pacific. Over time these cliffs crack and fault, forming caves and archways that eventually collapse, leaving spires like **Bird Island**. Bring your binoculars to scan the thousands of migratory and residential seabirds and shorebirds. In spring and summer the island is a nesting site for hundreds of cormorants, known for their sleek black torsos and snakelike necks. Also keep watch for sea otters floating atop the kelp forests and great blue herons surfing on the thick nearshore kelp rafts. Eventually retrace your steps to the junction with the **South Plateau Trail.**

As you turn inland along the South Plateau Trail, you'll soon pass a short spur to **Gibson Beach,** one of the few wide, protected sandy beaches at Point Lobos. The South Plateau Trail is a nature trail, where numbered markers correspond to a pamphlet in a box at the trailhead near the entrance kiosk. When the trail forks (1.9 miles, 50'), turn left onto the **Pine Ridge Trail.**

Farther from the sea breeze and salt spray, the Pine Ridge Trail winds through a tall shady grove of Monterey pines—one of only three remaining natural groves on Earth. Similar to the cypress, Monterey pines require heat or fire to release seeds from their cones. Hiking on a carpet of pine needles, you may notice charcoal or basal fire scars on the pines, evidence of controlled burns. In general, natural processes at the reserve are left undisturbed.

Pristine pocket beaches are nestled under stands of Monterey pine.

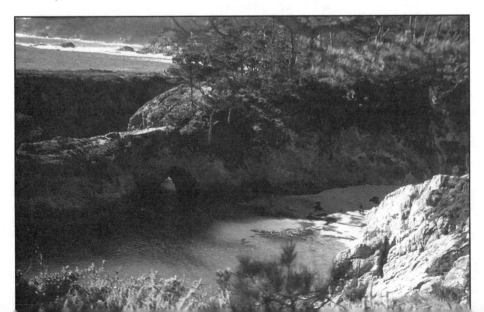

However, rangers do use fire to promote healthy pine regeneration and to limit wood debris and understory regrowth. Black-tailed deer, white-rumped northern flicker woodpeckers, and western gray squirrels may remind you of the Sierra Nevada. But the ever-present noisy barks of California sea lions carry deep into the grove, a reminder that you're but a short walk from the fresh, fragrant sea air, salty spray, and soothing waves.

As you begin a shady moderate climb, you'll cross several small plank bridges conveniently placed along the trail over seasonal wet areas. Half a mile later the trail gently descends 0.2 mile to a Y junction. Turn left toward Piney Woods on a level walk, catching ocean glimpses beyond the towering pines. You'll soon emerge at the parking area. Restrooms, water, and picnic tables are 50 feet farther on your left. If you're parked along the shore adjacent to the South Shore Trail, continue 100 feet along the paved road.

C H A P T E R **eight**

Garrapata State Park & Point Sur State Historic Park

■ ■ ■ ■ ■ ■ ■ ■ ■ ■ ■ ■ ■

Garrapata State Park

GARRAPATA STATE PARK offers a scenic slice of the beauty and ruggedness we associate with Big Sur, where redwoods burrow deep within the folds of steep mountains that abruptly rise above a rocky shoreline and wave-washed sandy beaches. On the northern edge of the Big Sur coast, the park features 4 miles of coastline and spans 2879 acres between Andrew Molera State Park to the south and Point Lobos to the north. Created in 1983, Garrapata is one of the more recent additions to the state park system along the central California coast. Coastal and inland access and miles of hiking trails promise numerous recreational opportunities.

Do heed tick warnings. In 1830, Spanish explorers were so exasperated by these blood-sucking arachnids, they named the canyon and creek *Garrapata* (Spanish for "tick"). Despite its unappealing name, the park shelters rich and diverse plant and animal life. The terrain encompasses five vegetation zones: coastal scrub, chaparral, redwood forest, riparian wood-land, and mixed evergreen forest. From late December through January and March through April, gray whales migrate along the coast—south for the winter to Baja, then back north to arctic waters in spring, marking the longest migratory route of any mammal in the world. Near the park's south end, Soberanes Point offers a good vantage point for whale sightings.

As with the other state lands along the Big Sur coast, Garrapata limits trail and road access to day use only, so if you're planning a visit, arrive early. There is no main entrance or entrance fee. Access is via Highway 1 turnouts, which are often crowded by midday in summer and on weekends. The climate is moderate year-round, with average temperatures between 50°F and 65°F. Weather varies from cool, damp fog to strong onshore winds and

67

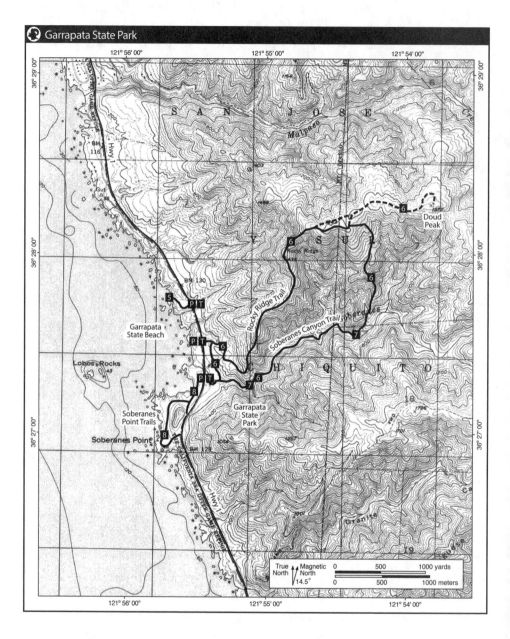

Garrapata State Park

the occasional warm, glorious day. Wear layered clothing and be prepared for changing conditions. Fall promises more consistent, warm fogless days, while summer days are often cool, as fog shrouds the coast. After winter rains the bluffs and hillsides sprout verdant plant life that by spring blankets the headlands, valleys, and hillsides amid decadent orange, purple, yellow, and red wildflower blooms.

DIRECTIONS: Garrapata State Park lies 7 miles south of Carmel and 18 miles north of Big Sur. There is no official park entrance. Parking and trail access is via 19 turnouts along Highway 1, the first on the Monterey County line at Mile 67.2 and the last at Mile 65.3. The turnouts correspond to numbered gates. Gates 17, 17A, 18, and 19 lead to Garrapata State Beach, while gates 8, 9, and 10 lead to the Soberanes Point trails.

VISITOR CENTER: Big Sur Station: (831) 667-2315. The station is on Highway 1, 18 miles south of Garrapata State Park. Open daily 8 a.m.–6 p.m. Memorial Day through Labor Day, 8 a.m.–4:30 p.m. the rest of the year.

NEAREST CAMPGROUNDS: The nearest developed state campground is at Pfeiffer Big Sur State Park (see page 98 for details). The nearest walk-in campground is at Andrew Molera State Park (see page 82 for details).

INFORMATION: Park closes at sunset. Camping and fires are not permitted. Dogs are only allowed on Garrapata Beach (not on trails) and must be kept on a leash at all times (6-foot maximum). Bicycles are permitted only on Rocky Ridge Trail. Do not remove plants, minerals, or other natural features.

WEBSITE: parks.ca.gov

PHONE: (831) 624-4909

Enjoy the journey along the many short spur trails that lead to dramatic vistas and sheltered coves within Garrapata.

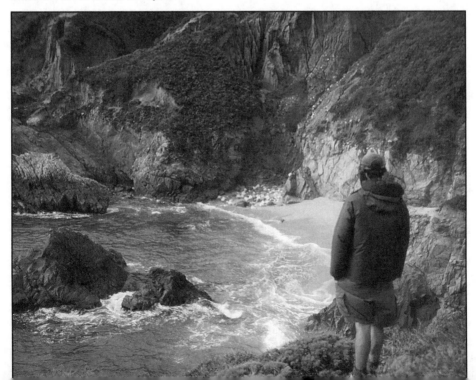

Trip 5

COASTAL ACCESS TRAILS

LENGTH AND TYPE: 2-mile out-and-back

RATING: Easy

TRAIL CONDITION: Well maintained, poison oak, good for kids

HIGHLIGHTS: Rugged rocky shores, wave-washed beaches, and isolated coves

TO REACH THE TRAILHEAD: This hike description begins from turnout 17 along Highway 1.

TRIP SUMMARY: The hike stretches about a mile to the south end of the park via the headlands or the beach.

EARLY BEACHCOMBERS ■ ■ ■ ■ ■ ■ ■ ■ ■ ■ ■ ■ ■ ■ ■ ■

Between dense thickets of coastal brush, shellfish remains and the bones of seals, otters, and land mammals such as deer and rabbits poke up from the bare sand, marking ancient middens, or human garbage heaps. The middens in Garrapata State Park date to coastal tribes that roamed the coast centuries before Spanish missionaries arrived. One shell bead dated from 100 to 300 A.D., while archaeologists traced obsidian flakes to the Borax Lake region of the Coast Range, nearly 200 miles north of Big Sur.

Garrapata's natives were likely members of the Rumsen subgroup of Ohlone Indians. Through extensive trade, the Ohlone were able to obtain items from both neighboring and distant tribes. The tribe relied on hunting and gathering along the coast in mild summer months, moving inland for the winter. They ate primarily mussels and other shellfish.

Before the arrival of Spanish missionaries, an estimated 10,000 Ohlone lived in an area stretching from San Francisco Bay south to Big Sur and east to the Central Valley. By the late 1700s, the Spanish had claimed much of the land and missionaries' conversionary zeal had all but erased native culture. Within a few short decades, exposure to deadly European diseases reduced Ohlone's numbers to some 2500 people. Today, descendants of the Ohlone still live in the area and preserve their ancestors' native traditions.

■ ■

Trip Description

From 17, the northernmost turnout, a short spur leads a few yards west to a bench atop a scenic overlook, an ideal spot to watch migrating whales in winter and spring. April and

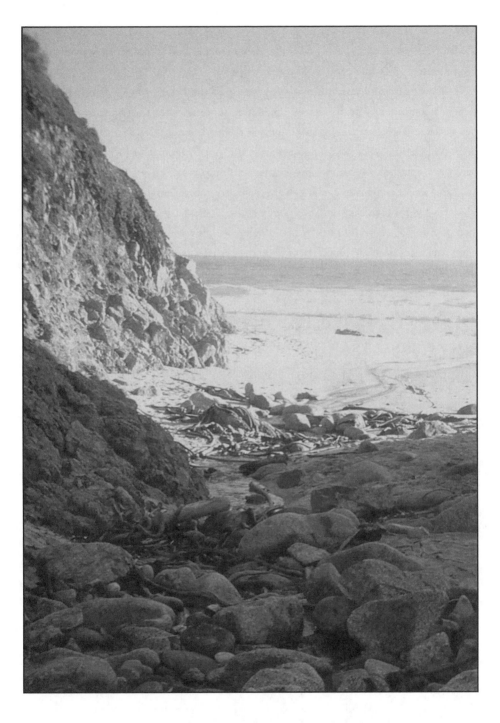

A natural symphony of seals barking, creeks gurgling, and waves pounding is common along the 4 miles of rocky shoreline and wave-washed sandy coves in Garrapata State Park.

May are the best months, as mothers steer their calves closer to shore for safety from such predators as great white sharks and orcas. Park naturalists often lead whale-watching hikes on spring weekends (call the park for specific dates).

The trail meanders south and then west past dramatic views of a rocky shoreline pounded continuously by foamy surf. You'll soon turn east past a small isolated cove and an overlook south to Garrapata Beach. A spur veers left to **turnout 17A** (0.3 mile, 40'), while the main trail continues south past another spur, this one to **turnout 18** (0.5 mile, 40'). From here you'll descend to a narrow canyon carved by **Doud Creek** (0.6 mile, 10'). Cross the creek and head south, either farther along the headlands or across **Garrapata State Beach.**

Beyond the creek, the bluff trail climbs and curls east a few paces to the spur for **turnout 19** (0.8 mile, 30'). Past this spur, the main trail descends west to emerge on the south end of Garrapata State Beach (1 mile). Pause to appreciate its timeless beauty before heading back the way you came.

Trip 6

ROCKY RIDGE TRAIL

LENGTH AND TYPE: 6-mile out-and-back or 4.6-mile loop

RATING: Strenuous

TRAIL CONDITION: Well maintained, poison oak

HIGHLIGHTS: Breathtaking views from mountains that rise dramatically beside a craggy coast

TO REACH THE TRAILHEAD: Both the Rocky Ridge and Soberanes Canyon Trails start from turnout 8, amid a strip of Monterey cypress on the east side of Highway 1, 7.1 miles south of Carmel Valley Road (County Road G16) and 14 miles north of Andrew Molera State Park. The trailheads lie beyond the numbered gate adjacent to a dilapidated barn. There are no facilities or water at the trailhead.

TRIP SUMMARY: You can approach this hike either as a 6-mile out-and-back along the Rocky Ridge Trail or as a 4.6-mile loop trip through Soberanes Canyon via the Soberanes Canyon Trail. Both routes are strenuous. The Rocky Ridge Trail drops abruptly from a 1435-foot ridge to 400-foot Soberanes Creek. Although the loop is 1.4 miles shorter, it's along a steeper, more strenuous grade, plunging 1000 feet to the canyon bottom in less than 0.7 mile.

The 3-mile Rocky Ridge Trail climbs past creekside willows and fragrant coastal scrub along a ridge of arid, boulder-strewn golden grasslands to a promontory more than 1600 feet above the sea. You'll enjoy 360-degree views, stretching from Point Sur to the Monterey Peninsula and the Santa Cruz Mountains to the Pacific. The topography is so sheer that despite a long climb, you'll still hear barking sea lions less than a mile away. Its difficulty keeps crowds at bay, though hikers, joggers, and bicyclists do flock here in summer. The best time to visit is in spring when coastal scrub is in bloom, migrating gray whales pass just offshore, and fog rarely encroaches inland.

Trip Description

From turnout 8, the trail begins a gentle climb up a closed road past the barn, soon crossing **Soberanes Creek.** Thirty yards beyond the creek, the trail meets the Soberanes Canyon Trail junction (0.1 mile, 120'), which branches right. Keep left and head north. Fifty yards farther, the trail passes a spur on the left, which descends some 130 yards to **turnout 12** (parking here would shave 0.2 mile off your hike). A minute farther north, the trail leaves the canyon and passes the first sign for the Rocky Ridge Trail (0.3 mile, 180').

Onward, the trail climbs 0.3 mile southeast up to a ridgetop (410') that boasts views of Garrapata's inland mountains and valleys. Pause for a breather, as your easy walk is over. The trail climbs more than 1200 feet in the next 1.5 miles, crests a knoll, then contours along a prominent saddle, nearly topping another ridge marked with a U.S. Geological Survey benchmark (1435'). Hints of even more spectacular views will draw you up the final 250 feet.

Farther up the main trail, look east for glimpses of the lush redwood groves that line Soberanes Creek, in stark contrast to the surrounding arid slopes of coastal scrub and grasslands. The trail heads northeast across a saddle, then north to its terminus atop a ridge (3 miles, 1680'), 1600 feet above Highway 1.

From this point, you have three options: (1) retrace your steps along the Rocky Ridge Trail, 3 miles to the trailhead, (2) hike a mile farther, climbing the **Peak Trail** up 1977-foot **Doud Peak,** or (3) descend into **Soberanes Canyon** along the upper Rocky Ridge Trail to the **Soberanes Canyon Trail.** The latter two routes continue east along a north-facing ridge 0.3 mile to a fork—the right branch descends into Soberanes Canyon, while the left branch leads to Doud Peak. The remaining 0.7 mile along the Peak Trail offers sweeping views of the untamed central coast as far north as **Fremont Peak,** at the north end of the **Gabilan Range.** On exceptionally clear days, you may even spot **Pacheco Peak,** about 50 miles northeast.

If you're taking the 4.6-mile loop, head southeast, where an extremely steep passage leads down the Rocky Ridge Trail to the upper end of the Soberanes Canyon Trail. In just under a mile the trail plunges 1200 feet down loose gravel and sand. You'll find steps in sections where the grade exceeds 30%, but be sure to pace yourself. The trail eventually emerges from the coastal scrub to enter the shady, damp redwood forest. A final few steep, short switchbacks lead you down to the gurgling creek and the junction with the westbound Soberanes Canyon Trail.

See TRIP 7 Soberanes Canyon Trail (on the following page) for that trail description.

Trip 7

SOBERANES CANYON TRAIL

LENGTH AND TYPE: 2.2-mile out-and-back or 4.6-mile loop

RATING: Easy to strenuous

TRAIL CONDITION: Well maintained, poison oak

HIGHLIGHTS: A canyon that shelters primeval groves of the world's tallest living organism, *Sequoia sempervirens*

TO REACH THE TRAILHEAD: Both the Soberanes Canyon and Rocky Ridge Trails start from turnout 8, on the east side of Highway 1, 7.1 miles south of Carmel Valley Road (County Road G16) and 14 miles north of Andrew Molera State Park. The trailhead lies beyond the numbered gate adjacent to a dilapidated barn. There are no facilities or water at the trailhead.

TRIP SUMMARY: Depending on your time and fitness level, you can approach this as either an easy 2.2-mile out-and-back hike or a strenuous 4.6-mile loop. In this direction the 4.6-mile loop features a particularly grueling climb—instead, consider beginning with the Rocky Ridge Trail and returning along the Soberanes Creek Trail (see TRIP 6 Rocky Ridge Trail, page 72, for details).

The trail meanders upstream along Soberanes Creek. Where the canyon narrows, a dense redwood canopy shelters a myriad of shade- and moisture-loving plants.

Trip Description

From turnout 8, the trail climbs a closed road past the barn, soon crossing **Soberanes Creek.** Thirty yards beyond the creek you'll reach the **Soberanes Canyon Trail junction** (0.1 mile, 120'), which branches to the right. The left branch heads north along the Rocky Ridge Trail (see page 72 for description).

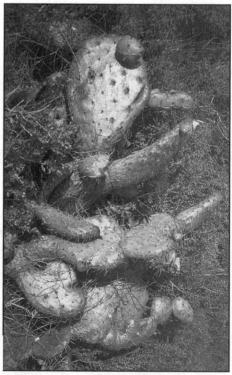

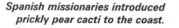

Spanish missionaries introduced prickly pear cacti to the coast.

Head east along the creek past clusters of coastal prickly pear cacti. Though not a native species, the plant thrives here. Spanish missionaries likely brought the plant north from Mexico as early as 1769. Beyond, the trail bends northeast past stunted, wind-sculpted redwoods (0.4 mile, 50') that are continually battered by salty onshore winds. As you hike farther up the canyon away from the surf, you'll find much healthier redwoods nestled along the canyon bottom. Farther inland, the trail enters a forest of mature redwoods that harbor a lush understory of ferns, mosses, and other creekside plants.

At 0.8 mile, the trail again crosses Soberanes Creek, then crosses it three more times over the next 0.3 mile. Just past the final crossing, a conspicuous spur branches off along the south bank. The main trail continues briefly along the north bank, ascends and descends several small, steep slopes, then descends a series of short switchbacks to the creek, where it meets the **Rocky Ridge Trail junction**. Over the years, high winds and flash floods have knocked down several large redwoods, providing excellent creekside seating, an ideal spot to rest and picnic. When ready, head back the way you came to complete the 2.2-mile round-trip.

The Rocky Ridge Trail continues up a few short, steep switchbacks, climbing above the cool redwood forest to exposed slopes of coastal scrub (see TRIP 6 Rocky Ridge Trail, page 72, for details).

Trip 8

SOBERANES POINT TRAILS

LENGTH AND TYPE: 2-mile loop

RATING: Easy

TRAIL CONDITION: Clear, poison oak, good for kids

HIGHLIGHTS: Roam the bluffs along one of California's most dramatic coastlines.

TO REACH THE TRAILHEAD: The Soberanes Point Trails are accessible via Highway 1 turn-outs 7 through 11. The trail description that follows starts on the west side of the highway at turnout 7.

TRIP SUMMARY: From turnout 7, the trail meanders south past uninhabited coves toward Soberanes Point. Along the way, watch pelicans skim wave crests in formation, peer down as surf surges into narrow inlets and coves, and maybe spot migrating whales. Some spurs lead to spectacular overlooks, while others descend to the beach for a barefoot stroll.

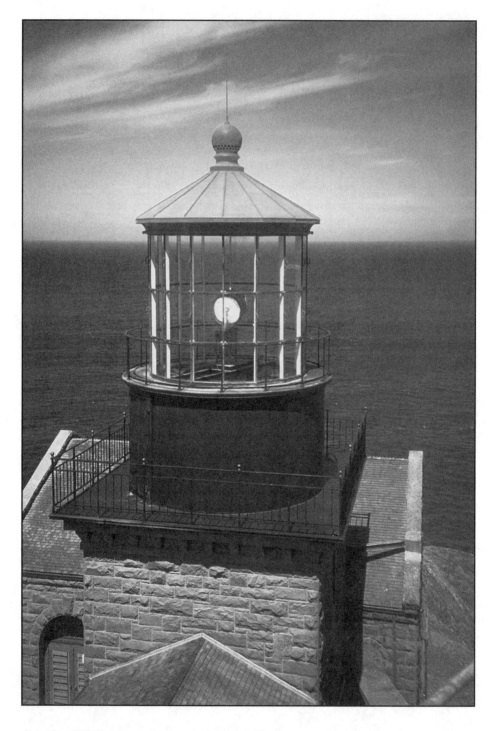

Point Sur Lighthouse stands as a sentinel of the bygone era of dangerous marine travel.

Trip Description

From turnout 7, the trail quickly reaches **Soberanes Creek** and a junction with a short spur down to the water's edge. Veer left across the creek through a dense stand of Monterey cypress between turnouts 8 and 9, where you'll find a portable toilet. If you parked at the Rocky Ridge and Soberanes Canyon Trailhead (turnout 8), your hike will begin here.

A few steps south of the cypress grove, you'll pass a junction with a trail to the left that skirts Highway 1. Those taking the 2-mile loop will return along this trail. Stay right and you'll soon reach a fork. Veer right to explore the dramatic shoreline that leads to rocky **Soberanes Point**. The route crosses bluffs covered with California sagebrush, bush lupine, coyote brush, coffeeberry, and other coastal scrub plants.

Beyond the point, the trail curls east and then north past the western flanks of **Whale Peak** to the junction between gates 8 and 9. If you parked at turnout 7, retrace your steps north across Soberanes Creek.

BIG SUR ROCKS ▨

Big Sur's coastal topography is a stunning blend of clear, cobalt water and the rugged granitic rocks of the Santa Lucia Range. Geologists believe these rocks originated in the southern Sierra in present-day Mexico and moved northwest hundreds of miles along the San Andreas Fault. These hard, crystalline rocks of the Salinian block also comprise many of the prominent high peaks of the range, such as Ventana Double Cone and Pico Blanco.

Deep underground, the molten rock slowly cooled, forming large crystals that glisten in the sun, lending the stone a grayish, salt-and-pepper appearance in the surf zone and a weathered rusty orange farther up the bluffs. As they slowly erode in the pounding surf, these durable rocks produce coarse-grained particles that sink quickly to the bottom, leaving little sediment to cloud the water.

▪ ▪

Point Sur State Historic Park

THE CENTERPIECE OF THIS historic park is Point Sur Lighthouse, perched 270 feet atop an isolated volcanic rock at the mouth of the Little Sur River. Built in 1889, the light provided invaluable warning to thousands of ships that plied this treacherous coast. Life for keepers and their families was lonely and isolated until the completion of Highway 1 in 1937. Then, in the 1960s, the U.S. Coast Guard began automating lighthouses. The last keeper left Point Sur in 1974. Year-round guided walking tours feature the lighthouse and supporting structures.

DIRECTIONS: The park is on the west side of Highway 1, 19 miles south of Carmel and a quarter mile north of the Point Sur Naval Facility.

VISITOR CENTER: Big Sur Station: (831) 667-2315. The station is on Highway 1, 18 miles south of Garrapata State Park and just south of Pfeiffer Big Sur State Park. Open daily 8 a.m.–6 p.m. Memorial Day through Labor Day, 8 a.m.–4:30 p.m. the rest of the year.

NEAREST CAMPGROUND: The nearest developed state campground is at Pfeiffer Big Sur State Park (see page 98 for details). The nearest walk-in campground is at Andrew Molera State Park (see page 82 for details).

INFORMATION: Closed to public except by guided tour. Docents lead three-hour tours year-round: Saturdays and Sundays at 10 a.m., Wednesdays at 1 p.m. The summer schedule includes Wednesday tours at 10 a.m. and 2 p.m. (April through October) and Thursday tours at 10 a.m. (July and August). Moonlight tours vary. Arrive early, as tickets are first come, first served. Admission: adults $12; ages 6–17, $5; children age 5 and under, free. Groups of 10 or more must call in advance. Groups of up to 40 people may also arrange private tours (minimum $200 charge). Visitors with disabilities should contact the park in advance to discuss access. No pets (even if left in car), picnicking, RVs or campers, strollers or baby carriages, beach access, or smoking.

PHONE: (831) 625-4419 or (831) 667-0528 (disabled access)

WEBSITES: pointsur.org or parks.ca.gov

Trip 9

POINT SUR STATE HISTORIC PARK

LENGTH AND TYPE: 0.4-mile out-and-back

RATING: Easy

TRAIL CONDITION: Well maintained, good for kids

HIGHLIGHTS: Experience life at a remote lighthouse perched on the edge of the Pacific.

TO REACH THE TRAILHEAD: At the park, meet at the farm gate along the west side of Highway 1 at the scheduled tour time. Arrive early, as tours occasionally fill up and reservations are not accepted. A docent or state park ranger will open the gate and direct you where to park. You'll drive less than a mile along a narrow paved road to the base of massive Point Sur. From here the three-hour tour begins.

TRIP SUMMARY: Point Sur Lighthouse is a lonely sentinel perched atop a massive rock formation at the mouth of the Little Sur River. The beacon reminds visitors of a bygone era,

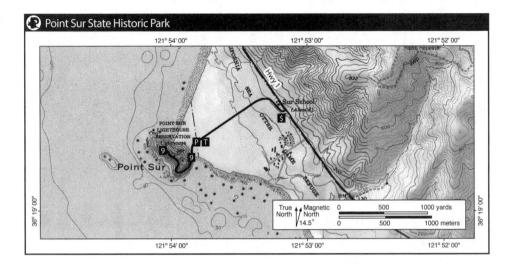

when mariners sailed blindly along the fogbound coast, often unaware of their proximity to the rocky shoreline. Swept by strong winds and big Pacific swells, the surroundings here remain largely unchanged.

Staffed from 1889 until 1974, Point Sur was home to families who stoically endured long months of isolation and solitude. Today, the lighthouse is automated and only traces of the keepers' stories remain in empty buildings, workshops, and barns.

Trip Description

From the parking area, you'll climb a steep paved road and two stairways to **Point Sur**. Count on plenty of rest stops along the way as your guide shares dramatic tales of life at this remote lighthouse.

Wildlife abounds on and around the point. Migrating gray whales pass within sight of shore. Pelicans fly by in formation, while cormorants vanish underwater and oystercatchers clamber across the rocks. Sea otters and seals swim beyond the surf line, feasting amid the kelp forests below. Also keep watch for golden eagles, peregrine falcons, and California condors, which soar overhead in search of prey or carrion.

Point Sur is a complete turn-of-the-century **lighthouse**. Your guide will lead you up the circular stairwell for a look at the lens and to stroll the catwalk. Weighing 4330 pounds, the first-order Fresnel lens is nearly 8 feet high and more than 6 feet in diameter. Its 16 panels of prisms bend light into a single focused beam visible for 23 nautical miles. Pause at this exposed point, taking in the fog, wind, sun, salt spray, and other raw elements.

Andrew Molera State Park

■ ■

THE LARGEST STATE PARK on the Big Sur coast, Andrew Molera is also one of the few places you can actually get your feet wet rather than just enjoying ocean viewpoints. This is an excellent place for beachcombers, surfers, and anglers, as well as hikers, joggers, bicyclists, and equestrians. Its 7.4 square miles boast more than 20 miles of trails, offering hikers passage across driftwood-strewn beaches, beside rivers lined with redwoods, and atop high ridges that overlook the Santa Lucia Range and broad Pacific. The wild and scenic Big Sur River winds amid the park's mountains, meadows, and a walk-in campground on its way down to the sea.

Diverse ecosystems shelter a broad range of plant and animal communities. Birders know the park well. In 1992 the nonprofit Ventana Wilderness Society established a research and education center and bird observatory here. The Big Sur Ornithology Lab has documented more than 380 migratory, resident, and transitory birds. Researchers point to multiple factors, including biotic diversity, the mild climate, a healthy lagoon and estuary, and a nearby lighthouse that may attract nocturnal migrants.

DISCOVERY CENTER ■ ■ ■ ■ ■ ■ ■ ■ ■ ■ ■ ■ ■ ■ ■ ■ ■ ■ ■

Don't miss the Discovery Center in Big Sur, located at Andrew Molera State Park. At the Discovery Center, you can see and interact with the exhibit Bringing the Condors Home and learn about the recovery efforts to bring the condors back to the wild. Enjoy a picnic or sign up for tours with on-site biologists and naturalists. Best of all, the Discovery Center is open to the public and free of charge.

■ ■

But this park isn't just for the birds. Keep watch for sea otters, seals, and sea lions amid the kelp beds and migrating gray whales just offshore. At dusk and dawn, deer graze in the Creamery Meadow as steelhead rise to feed on insects in the Big Sur River. Catch-and-release

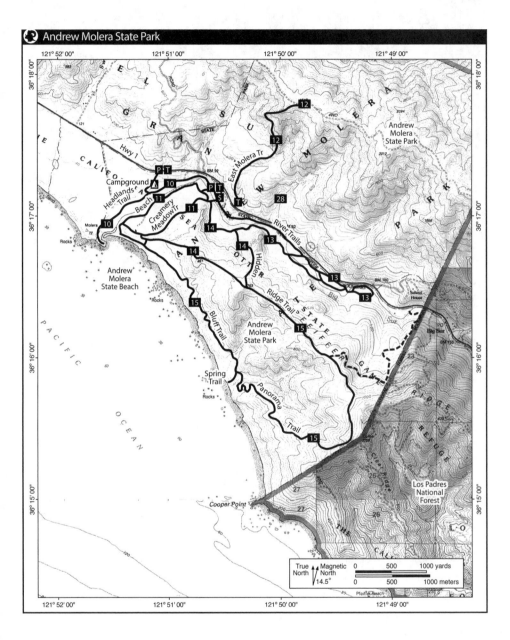

steelhead fishing is permitted from mid-November through February, while surf casting for rockfish and surfperch is permitted year-round. Fishing regulations change from year to year, so contact the Department of Fish & Game at (831) 649-2870 for current information.

The day-use fee is $8/vehicle, or you can park on the highway and hike in for free. The free turnout is on the west side of the highway, 0.1 mile north of the park entrance. A trail

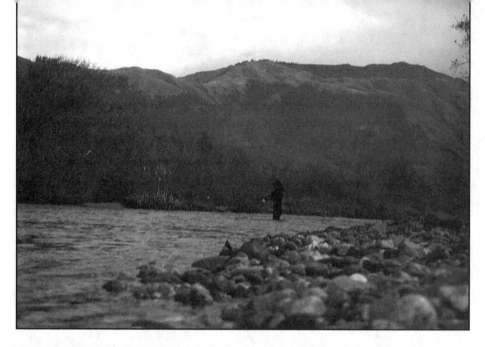

The mouth of the Big Sur River is a dynamic place that is subject to dramatic seasonal changes—be prepared to get your feet or more wet if planning to cross.

leads from the turnout to Cooper's Cabin, just west of Trail Camp. If that turnout is full, there's another 0.3 mile south of the park's entrance. Water and toilet facilities are available at the official park lot.

DIRECTIONS: The park lies at the junction of Highway 1 and Old Coast Road, 22 miles south of Carmel and 4.2 miles north of Pfeiffer Big Sur State Park. The entrance is on the west side of the highway.

VISITOR CENTER: Big Sur Station: (831) 667-2315. The station is on Highway 1, 4.2 miles south of Andrew Molera State Park and just south of Pfeiffer Big Sur State Park. Open daily 8 a.m.–6 p.m. Memorial Day through Labor Day, 8 a.m.–4:30 p.m. the rest of the year.

NEAREST CAMPGROUNDS: The park's Trail Camp walk-in campground (24 sites, $25/night; register at the entrance kiosk) is in a large meadow near the Big Sur River, an easy 0.3-mile walk from the parking lot. Sites are granted on a first-come, first-serve basis and fill up quickly in summer and on holidays. Another option is Pfeiffer Big Sur State Park (218 sites, $25/standard site; $35/river site; reservations recommended in summer and on holidays).

INFORMATION: The park is day use only unless you're camping. Dogs are not allowed on trails or at Trail Camp. Bikes are permitted only on Ridge, Beach, Trail Camp, and Creamery Meadow Trails. Horses are not allowed on the Hidden, Headlands, or Spring Trails, or in Trail Camp. To reserve a guided horseback tour, call Molera Horseback Tours at (831) 625-5486 or visit molerahorsebacktours.com.

WEBSITE: parks.ca.gov | **PHONE:** (831) 667-2315

Trip 10

TRAIL CAMP & HEADLANDS TRAILS

LENGTH AND TYPE: 2-mile out-and-back

RATING: Easy

TRAIL CONDITION: Well maintained, poison oak, good for kids

HIGHLIGHTS: An array of migratory and resident birds, seals, whales, and otters make their home amid the marsh, estuary, and ocean along Molera Beach.

TO REACH THE TRAILHEAD: At the park's entrance kiosk, turn right. The trailhead is at the north end of the parking lot.

TRIP SUMMARY: Among the region's easiest coastal bluff hikes, this hike offers gorgeous overlooks of the Big Sur River, distant peaks, sheer cliffs, and a driftwood-blanketed beach.

Tracing the final mile of the river's 15-mile journey to the Pacific, the trails lead through a walk-in campground nestled in an expansive meadow, past views of the Santa Lucia Range to the east, to emerge at the river mouth. Watch for migrating gray and humpback whales, foraging seals and sea otters amid the kelp, and hundreds of soaring, diving, and foraging seabirds aloft on coastal air currents.

Trip Description

Trail Camp Trail starts on the north end of the parking lot, then turns west along the north bank of the **Big Sur River,** skirting a lush riparian habitat. After 0.2 mile the trail broadens into a road and enters the spacious **walk-in campground.** You'll find 12 primitive sites scattered throughout the meadow. Campers are rewarded with a night's sleep under giant sycamores and a short walk to one of Big Sur's most scenic beaches. Bring a tent, especially in summer, when fog blankets the meadow with condensation.

Facilities include toilets, potable water, tables, and a fire ring. Purchase firewood at the entrance kiosk or at the Big Sur Village store, less than 5 miles south on Highway 1. California State Parks reduced the number of sites from 50 to 12, conforming to state health codes and protecting park resources.

A hundred feet beyond the campground, the trail forks. A short spur on the right leads to historic **Cooper Cabin,** then continues east 0.2 mile to a Highway 1 turnout (a free place to park and still access the park). Continue along the riverbank 0.2 mile through a dense forest of twisted alders and willows. Less than 0.1 mile farther the path narrows and reaches the **Headlands Trail junction** (0.9 mile, 20').

COOPER & THE BUTTERFLIES ■ ■ ■ ■ ■ ■ ■ ■ ■ ■ ■ ■ ■ ■ ■ ■

In 1834 this area was part of a Mexican land grant known as Rancho El Sur, owned by Juan Bautista Alvarado. Six years later Alvarado sold the land to Juan Bautista Rogers Cooper, a Monterey sea captain and merchant. Built in 1861, Cooper Cabin remains the oldest standing structure in Big Sur. Cooper used the land to graze livestock and also launched the first large-scale production of Monterey Jack cheese.

In the late 1800s the narrow wagon road from Monterey went only part way down the coast, so settlers gathered annually near Cooper's riverside cabin to picnic, fish, and dance while awaiting the arrival of supply schooners. Andrew Molera was Cooper's grandson, and in 1965 his sister donated the land in his name.

Visitors still wonder at enormous bluegum eucalyptus trees, planted when the cabin was built. In 1986 state park officials, concerned that this introduced Australian species was crowding out native willows and alders and negatively affecting wildlife, began to remove eucalyptus saplings. Biologists opposed the cutting, as monarch butterflies roost here during their long migration. The biologists and butterflies ultimately prevailed, preserving the giant trees.

From October through January, monarchs return to Big Sur to roost amid the stands of eucalyptus. By day watch them glide from branch to branch in the spacious canopy of this exotic tree.

■ ■

Turn right and head north up the old wooden stairs. You'll find yourself 30 feet above the shoreline as you pass thick patches of poison oak, golden yarrow, and sagebrush. Continue the gentle climb for ever-expanding panoramic views of **Molera Point** and the rugged coastline to the north and south.

Look south to spot sculpted driftwood strewn across the white sand. Look below and see if you can discern where the sand is tinged purple. This purple sediment is eroded almandite, a rare mineral. Also notice the jagged rocks in the surf. These contorted rocks were heavily metamorphosed within the numerous faults that divide, break, and reshape the Big Sur coastline, most all of them associated with the San Andreas Fault.

Skirt the secluded coves and beaches till you reach a bench atop the bluff overlooking 2-mile **Molera Beach,** a great spot to watch for sea lions, seals, and sea otters as they feed and play among the giant kelp beds. California gray whales migrate south to Baja from December through January and return north to Alaska in March and April. Take a moment to enjoy the sweeping view before returning the way you came.

Back at the Trail Camp Trail junction, turn right and continue your route west. In less than a hundred feet, the path emerges on the beach at the mouth of the Big Sur River.

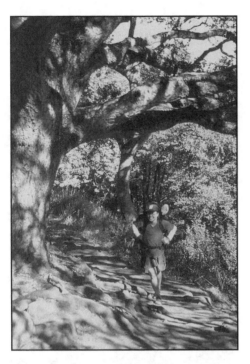

Trail Camp is a short jaunt through massive oaks and sycamores along the Big Sur River.

During the dry season (May through October), when less water flows into the ocean, sand builds up and blocks the river mouth, flooding the lagoon and inland marsh. This diverse ecosystem creates a unique habitat for shorebirds and waterfowl, including great blue herons, egrets, gulls, and pelicans.

Big Sur is also home to steelhead trout (a rainbow trout that spends part of its life in the sea), which migrate upstream to spawn and lay eggs. Each spring thousands of 6-inch steelhead smolt venture downstream into the ocean. For every 100 smolt that reach the sea, fewer than 5% will return as a spawning adult. At dawn and dusk in summer and fall, watch as dozens of young steelhead leap through the air to enjoy a banquet of aquatic insects.

When you're ready, return the way you came. In drier months you could cross the river and head back following the **Beach** or **Creamery Meadow Trails** (see following trip description).

Trip 11

BEACH & CREAMERY MEADOW TRAILS LOOP

LENGTH AND TYPE: 1.8-mile loop

RATING: Easy

TRAIL CONDITION: Well maintained, poison oak, good for kids

HIGHLIGHTS: A barefoot stroll across windswept, driftwood-strewn Molera Beach

TO REACH THE TRAILHEAD: From the park's entrance kiosk, continue straight to the picnic area. The route begins at the bridge across the Big Sur.

TRIP SUMMARY: Adjacent to the Big Sur River, Creamery Meadow is lined with dense riparian woodland. You'll stroll past twisted sycamores, head-high yellow bush lupines, and gnarled redwoods. Once a cattle pasture, today it boasts some of the best bird-watching in California.

Trip Description

From the picnic area, cross the **Big Sur River** on the narrow footbridge. In winter the bridge is removed so steelhead trout can migrate upstream—expect a knee- to waist-high wade. After heavy winter storms, the river may be too swift to cross. If you prefer to stay dry or cannot cross, take the **Trail Camp Trail** to the beach (see page 83).

Once across the Big Sur, turn right and head west on the **Beach Trail** alongside **Creamery Meadow,** a turn-of-the-century pasture for cows that produced Monterey Jack cheese. Park officials are replanting and slowly restoring the area to a beautiful open meadow dotted with willows, cottonwoods, red alders, sycamores, and a few scraggly, salt-stunted redwoods. Abundant wildlife includes coyotes, bobcats, and deer along the trails; lizards, mice, and rabbits in

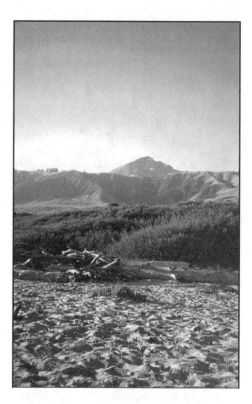

Views from Molera Beach lead toward the triangular marble-topped Pico Blanco.

the high grass; and white-tailed kites, kestrels, and red-shouldered hawks soaring overhead.

Closer to the beach, the wind and salt spray have taken a toll on vegetation. As you turn north toward the river, notice the contorted redwood to your left across the meadow. Farther down the trail you'll pass the rocky end of a bluff midway to the surf. During large swells, waves surge halfway up this stretch, stranding massive logs and driftwood. On your left, just before you reach the beach, you'll pass the **Bluffs Trail** (1.1 miles, 10'), which heads southeast along the edge of a marine terrace.

Before heading back toward the **Creamery Trail,** stroll windswept **Molera Beach**. You'll likely spot sea otters, sea lions, and harbor seals feeding in the nearshore kelp forests. Notice the low bluffs of deformed rocks, part of the Franciscan complex, a mix of sedimentary rocks and basalt slices from the seafloor. The San Andreas Fault and associated faults continually wrench this region and metamorphose the gray, tan, and brown sandstone, and shale. Look closely to spot almandite, a rare mineral that tints the sand purple and pink.

Stroll farther to escape the crowds and find an isolated cove all to yourself. Keep in mind, though, that your hike is tide-dependent—the beach can be impassable or even dangerous in places during high tides. Tide tables are posted on the information sign in the parking lot, or you can check at Big Sur Station, 4.2 miles south of the park entrance road on Highway 1.

PERFECT PEELING WAVES ■ ■ ■ ■ ■ ■ ■ ■ ■ ■ ■ ■ ■ ■ ■

As you stroll Molera Beach, you may notice surfers paddling past marine mammals to greet perfect peeling waves on the north end of the beach. In fact, this stretch is one of Big Sur's most reliable surf spots. The beach is ringed in from all directions except west, in a semi-point setup. The water sculpts and sustains a gravelly sandbar, and prevailing northwest winds create fast right-hand lanes on days that are blown out elsewhere. Access the break by walking nearly a mile from the park entrance. Though the walk deters some surfers, expect a crowded lineup during big west or south swells.

■ ■

Heading back up the Beach Trail, you'll pass thick patches of toxic poison oak amid colorful flowering plants. Many of the latter display vibrant yellow blossoms, including bush lupine, seaside wooly sunflower, sedum, *Dudleya*, and yellow sand verbena. A tenth of a mile from Molera Beach, you'll reach the **Creamery Trail junction.** Turn right on this wide trail to take in the opposite side of Creamery Meadow. In the meadow you'll spot coyote brush, poison hemlock, California poppies, and more lupines, while large coast live oaks, sycamores, and bay trees line the ridge to your right. The trail gradually bends northeast to rejoin the Beach Trail at the footbridge over the Big Sur (1.8 miles, 40').

Trip 12

EAST MOLERA TRAIL

LENGTH AND TYPE: 3.2-mile out-and-back

RATING: Strenuous

TRAIL CONDITION: Clear, poison oak

HIGHLIGHTS: Coastal vistas, sweeping panoramas of the Santa Lucia Range, and a secluded ridge capped with redwoods

TO REACH THE TRAILHEAD: Access the trailhead via either Highway 1 or from the park's official lot.

On Highway 1, the trailhead lies 0.3 mile south of the park entrance road and is marked by a small, worn wooden cattle chute on the east side of the road. Park at either of two turnouts, about 0.1 mile north and south of this chute.

If you're starting from the parking lot, plan to hike another 0.6 mile overall. From the lot, walk up the entrance road 75 feet past the kiosk and take the service road on your right, which heads southeast toward Molera Trail Rides. Follow this road past the barn, where you'll find a signed trailhead. The trail parallels the highway, then passes beneath it through a large culvert. You'll emerge on a dirt road on the east side of the highway. Follow this road a few yards until you reach the East Molera Trail, which rises from the highway turnout, crosses the dirt road, and continues uphill.

TRIP SUMMARY: This trail switchbacks up a sheer hillside to a secluded ridge capped with redwoods. The 1.6-mile trail reaches 1550 feet, offering sweeping views of the coast and Santa Lucia Range. Bring plenty of water and a wide-brimmed hat for the exposed stretch to the ridge, and pack a sweater or windbreaker for the return hike.

Trip Description

The **East Molera Trail** climbs gradually, first beneath the large twisted branches of coast live oaks and then across open grassland. From its junction with the dirt road (0.1 mile, 180'), the trail up to the redwood saddle is 1.5 miles long with nearly 1500 feet of elevation gain. Heading left uphill, the trail climbs less than 0.1 mile past a water-storage tank to rejoin the road. You could stay on the road for a gentler though longer ascent. Over the next 0.2 mile the trail parallels a narrow band of lush redwoods, bays, and oaks that shelter in a narrow gully. This gully hosts a small creek in wet months and channels a ribbon of thick fog in drier months.

Just before the main trail turns left up a steep rise, a narrow **spur** (0.4 mile, 360') branches right to enter the redwood-shaded gully. The spur traverses the gully past redwoods and fragrant bay trees to open oak woodlands. At trail's end, a majestic oak tops a grassy knoll, a peaceful spot to picnic, offering views south along the **Big Sur River,** north to **Point Sur Lighthouse,** and west to **Molera Beach.**

From the spur junction, continue up the road to your left, where the ascent quickly turns strenuous, climbing nearly 1000 feet in about a mile. The trail switchbacks and climbs directly up a ridge. After a steep climb east, the trail ascends another ridge. From here you can see the redwood saddle, less than 0.1 mile away. The views only improve, and hints of even better ones urge you on.

The final 0.1 mile gradually ascends grassy slopes that in spring are blanketed in the deep purple and orange hues of abundant lupines and poppies. The trail ends on a **ridge crest** (1.6 miles, 1550') amid towering redwoods, which seem blatantly out of place. The cool shade is a blessing, especially after strenuous hikes on hot summer days. In summer, fog may obscure the view, but in spring and fall you'll likely be rewarded with stunning views. Northeast is the narrow **South Fork Little Sur River** canyon and the massive marble **Pico Blanco,** southeast lies the **Big Sur River** watershed, and the park stretches south and southwest to the Pacific. When you're rested, head back down the trail.

NORTH MEETS SOUTH ▪ ▪ ▪ ▪ ▪ ▪ ▪ ▪ ▪ ▪ ▪ ▪ ▪ ▪ ▪ ▪ ▪ ▪

Northern and southern biogeographical regions converge in Andrew Molera State Park, forming a kind of suture zone with sharp differences in vegetation. Canyons filled with redwoods, lush ferns and mosses, slithering salamanders, and chatty winter wrens lie adjacent to semiarid grasslands dotted with yuccas, scurrying alligator lizards, and rufous-crowned sparrows. This blend of distinct zones, along with the park's mild climate, topographic diversity, and proximity to the ocean, supports a remarkable 17 distinct plant communities.

If you'd like to hike farther, the trail continues up an overgrown **fire road.** Heading southeast, this road stretches 2 miles to the park boundary, marked by an old fence line, then climbs through Forest Service land another 1.25 miles to **Post Summit.** Be aware that the summit trail is steep, overgrown, and hard to follow. Diehards will be rewarded with spectacular views of the coast, the **Little Sur River** drainage basin, and the crags of **Ventana Double Cone.** The rocky gorge below shelters a pristine stand of Santa Lucia firs, endemic only to the Santa Lucia Range.

Trip 13

RIVER TRAIL LOOP

LENGTH AND TYPE: 4-mile loop

RATING: Easy

TRAIL CONDITION: Well maintained, poison oak

HIGHLIGHTS: This oasis within the Big Sur River canyon offers a chance for a refreshing dip in a natural swimming hole.

TO REACH THE TRAILHEAD: From the park's official parking lot, walk up the entrance road 75 feet past the kiosk and turn right on the road toward Molera Trail Rides and the Ventana Wilderness Society. Considered the start of the Bobcat Trail, this road leads 0.3 mile to a horse corral. From there the trail narrows and follows the river.

TRIP SUMMARY: Skirting crystal clear water amid a verdant canyon, these riverside trails promise a wonderful year-round stroll. In fall a radiant display of sycamore, maple, alder, and cottonwood leaves brightens the river's course. Following winter storms, the 15-mile Big Sur River provides critical habitat for steelhead trout and a variety of other wildlife. In spring new life abounds, as bare golden hills sprout carpets of blooming wildflowers. Summer welcomes perfect weather for a picnic and swim.

Trip Description

From the trailhead at the horse corral, the **Bobcat Trail** narrows and begins a gentle climb alongside the **Big Sur River,** passing dense thickets of blackberry and poison oak. These are often mistaken for one another due to their similar three-leaf arrangement (blackberries have thorny stems). At the first **junction** (0.1 mile, 150'), a spur leads right (south) to the river. If you prefer an easy 1-mile loop, this spur leads to the **River Trail,** then back to the parking lot. The spur heads upstream a few feet, crosses the river, climbs the south bank, and eventually joins the River Trail. From there walk downstream to the parking lot.

Back at the junction, another short spur climbs east to a Highway 1 parking turnout, 0.75 mile south of the park entrance road. For the next 0.1 mile the Bobcat Trail parallels Highway 1, which drowns out the river and birdsong. The trail soon leaves the highway and emerges at an open meadow (1 mile, 150'). Large yellow and purple lupine bushes dot the meadow amid a colorful tapestry of California poppies, shooting stars, Indian paintbrush, blue dicks, and wild oats. Deer often graze here at dawn and dusk.

The trail crosses the meadow and rejoins the river at a **junction** with two spurs (1.2 miles, 170'). Both spurs offer optional 2.5-mile loops back to the parking lot. The first spur crosses the river diagonally, meets the opposite bank beneath a small cliff, then leads 200 feet downstream to the River Trail. A few feet upstream, the second spur heads across a bend in the Big Sur and also joins the River Trail.

Past this junction, the Bobcat Trail briefly follows the east bank, heads north up a shallow seasonal creek, then branches at **Coyote Flat,** an expansive meadow. The left branch skirts the meadow and leads to turnouts along Highway 1 (2 miles south of the park entrance road) before rejoining the main trail. The more scenic main trail branches right along the meadow's southeast edge to another fork. At this **junction** (1.5 miles, 180'), a spur leads southwest, crossing a narrow stretch of the Big Sur. Here a large outcrop channels water into a deep emerald **swimming hole,** an ideal spot for a summer picnic and swim.

Back at the junction, continue along the Bobcat Trail across the river to the Cooper Loop (1.8 miles, 180'), a 0.3-mile circuit through a redwood grove carpeted in dense ferns, mosses, and redwood sorrel. Pfeiffer Ridge and Franciscan cliffs just west of the river flats shelter these trees from harsh ocean winds and salt spray.

Complete the loop, recross the river, and head to the swimming hole mentioned above (2.3 miles, 180'). You'll have to wade across here to hook up with the **River Trail**. After heavy winter storms, the water may rise dangerously high, in which case you'll have to retrace your steps to the parking lot via the Bobcat Trail.

Across this ford, the River Trail winds downstream beside cottonwoods, bigleaf maples, and western sycamores, heading northwest to a junction with the **Hidden Trail** (3.1 miles, 170'). Continue on the River Trail past live oaks and coyote brush for a gentle descent alongside **Creamery Meadow**. North of the meadow, a spur on your right leads across the river to the Bobcat Trailhead, sparing you 150 yards of extra walking. For more exercise, continue northwest 0.1 mile to a junction on the left with the **Creamery Meadow Trail**. A few yards past this junction, the route darts east across the Big Sur back to the parking lot.

Trip 14

CREAMERY MEADOW, RIVER, HIDDEN, & RIDGE TRAILS LOOP

LENGTH AND TYPE: 3.6-mile loop

RATING: Moderate to strenuous

TRAIL CONDITION: Well maintained, poison oak

HIGHLIGHTS: Panoramic views from Pfeiffer Ridge of marble-rimmed ridges carved by the meandering Big Sur River and broad marine terraces that slope down to Point Sur

TO REACH THE TRAILHEAD: From the park's entrance kiosk, continue straight to the picnic area. The route begins at the bridge across the Big Sur.

TRIP SUMMARY: The route crosses the Big Sur and follows the river past mature sycamores, cottonwoods, maples, and alders before climbing high above the coastal bluffs. The Hidden Trail ascends Pfeiffer Ridge for 360-degree views of the region's diverse topography and vegetation. The Ridge Trail gently descends to Molera Beach, offering sweeping ocean views. Bring your binoculars, as you may glimpse migrating gray whales in spring. Hundreds of bird species make this one of the state's best bird-watching spots.

Trip Description

From the picnic area, cross the **Big Sur River** on the narrow footbridge. In winter the bridge is removed so steelhead trout can migrate upstream—expect a knee- to waist-high wade. After heavy winter storms, the river may be too swift to cross. If you prefer to stay dry or cannot cross, take the **Trail Camp Trail** to the beach (see page 83).

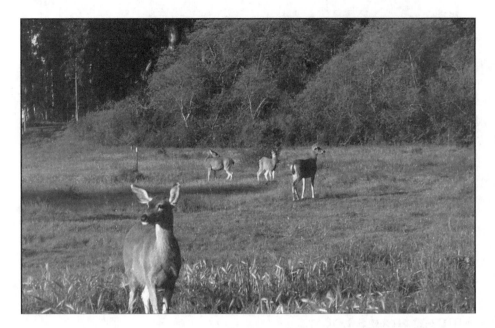

A healthy and stable population of native mule deer can now be seen along Creamery Meadow, once grazed by cattle that supported the Monterey Jack cheese creameries.

Once across the river, head left on **Creamery Meadow Trail** about 100 yards southwest to a junction. The right fork follows the **Beach Trail**. Instead, veer left along the Creamery Meadow Trail, passing both the meadow and a junction with a dirt road (the continuation of the Creamery Meadow Trail).

Continue southeast on the **River Trail** along the south bank of the Big Sur. For its first 0.1 mile the trail follows a level dirt road south to the broad meadow at **Coyote Flat**. At dawn and dusk, coyotes stalk the shoulder-high bush lupine in search of scurrying rabbits, voles, and mice, while black-tailed deer (also known as mule deer for their large ears, which twitch and turn at any sound) feed on herbs and grasses. Past the meadow, the vegetation quickly changes to sprawling live oaks amid thickets of coyote brush. Pause to gaze across the river toward 3709-foot marble-topped Pico Blanco.

After 0.8 mile you'll reach the **Hidden Trail junction**. This 0.7-mile trail is steep and strenuous, with an average 15% grade. The first 0.1 mile is a moderate ascent beneath live oaks, followed by a steep stretch that climbs beyond the oaks to slopes covered in coyote brush. Stop to catch your breath and admire the rugged foothills and folds of the Santa Lucia Range.

Hidden Trail climbs the spine of **Pfeiffer Ridge** to the **Ridge Trail junction** (1.5 miles, 720'). On a clear day you'll see **Point Sur,** which rises from broad marine terraces 10 miles north. Turn right onto the Ridge Trail and head west toward **Molera Point**. The trail slopes gently 1.1 miles down Pfeiffer Ridge (aka **Molera Ridge**) toward **Molera Beach** and the Creamery Meadow Trail. Hit the beach to stroll barefoot in the sand and wonder at the sculpted driftwood before turning right (northeast) on the Creamery Meadow Trail.

The trail skirts a mile of **Creamery Meadow,** a former pasture that once supported cattle raised to produced Monterey Jack cheese. Recent restoration efforts have attracted abundant wildlife. Watch for grazing black-tailed deer, elusive coyotes and bobcats, hundreds of small songbirds, and soaring raptors overhead. Just past the meadow is the familiar River Trail junction. Head left to recross the Big Sur on the footbridge (or ford in the wet season).

Trip 15

BLUFFS, SPRING, PANORAMA, & RIDGE TRAILS

LENGTH AND TYPE: 8.4-mile loop

RATING: Moderate

TRAIL CONDITION: Well maintained, poison oak

HIGHLIGHTS: Spectacular views of marble mountains and secluded coves awash in foamy surf

TO REACH THE TRAILHEAD: From the park's entrance kiosk, continue straight to the picnic area. The route begins at the bridge across the Big Sur. You'll need to follow the first mile of the Beach Trail to reach the Bluffs Trail junction.

TRIP SUMMARY: This hike leads to an idyllic cove at the west end of the Spring Trail, where the sand is tinged with pink and purple hues. The return along the Panorama and Ridge Trails promises spectacular views as you cross golden grasslands and pass beneath robust redwoods, oaks, and bays. Seals and sea otters feed in the nearshore kelp forests, raptors soar overhead, rabbits and lizards scurry into the brush, and elusive bobcats slink past the trails.

Trip Description

From the picnic area, cross the **Big Sur River** on the narrow footbridge. In winter the bridge is removed so steelhead trout can migrate upstream—expect a knee- to waist-high wade. After heavy winter storms, the river may be too swift to cross. If you prefer to stay dry or cannot cross, take the **Trail Camp Trail** to the beach (see page 83).

Once across the Big Sur, turn right and head west on the **Beach Trail** alongside **Creamery Meadow.** About a mile down the trail on your left, just before you reach **Molera Beach,** you'll meet the **Bluffs Trail junction,** which heads southeast along the edge of a marine terrace.

The trail begins with a half dozen stairs and a steep 100-yard climb atop bluffs formed by uplifted marine terraces. Pause to watch stout waves slam into the boulder-strewn beach.

A spur on the right skirts the cliffs for daunting views, then loops back to the main trail. At this point (1.2 miles, 50') the trail widens into a road, leaving plenty of room for passing hikers, bicyclists, and equestrians.

The Bluffs Trail is a kaleidoscopic experience, a blend of glistening blue ocean, golden grasses, rich rust-colored earth, and coastal brush in varying hues of green, yellow, orange, and purple. The trail crosses two small gullies, dry in all but the wettest months of the year. Bicyclists are not allowed past the second gully, as posted on a sign. The trail narrows and then widens as it crosses a barren sandstone landscape, perhaps a beach during the Ice Age, when ocean levels were several feet higher. California poppies thrive here, among few plants capable of surviving such harsh conditions. The trail ends at the **Spring Trail junction** (2.8 miles, 50').

The Spring Trail leads 0.1 mile down a narrow, slightly overgrown trail, following a small gully to a dramatic beach, one of my favorites along the Big Sur coast. After heavy winter storms, a tangle of driftwood blankets the beach entrance, creating a beautiful obstacle course of water-sculpted roots, limbs, and trunks. Under high tide and large winter surf, much of the beach disappears, but most other times you can enjoy a barefoot stroll nearly half a mile in either direction (north toward **Molera Point** or south toward **Cooper Point**). Beyond that, the beach is too narrow and dangerous to traverse in all but the lowest tides. Check tide tables at the entrance kiosk before setting your sites on a long stroll. To reach the Bluffs and Panorama Trails, return to the Spring Trail junction.

At this junction, the 1.9-mile **Panorama Trail** begins. The trail crosses the previously mentioned gully, then gradually switchbacks inland, ascending to a ridge capped by a cluster of stunted redwoods that hardly resemble the species renowned as the world's tallest tree. This close to the ocean, the redwoods are exposed to salt spray and gale-force winds that warp the trees into their gnarled state.

The trail follows a minor depression, then ascends to one of the park's best viewpoints, allowing plenty of time to catch one's breath and enjoy the hike (4.3 miles, 930'). Following a 200-foot climb, you'll be rewarded with panoramic views of Point Sur to the northwest, Pico Blanco to the north, and Cone Peak lording over the southeastern horizon some 40 miles away.

Pressing on, you'll reach a junction with a 200-foot spur (4.4 miles, 950'), which leads south toward a cluster of homes nestled along a hillside beside the fence and road. The steep ascent continues 0.3 mile to the **Ridge Trail junction** (4.7 miles, 1050') and the park's highest viewpoint west of Highway 1. Find the well-placed bench in the shade of a Monterey cypress to rest and take it all in.

The 2.75-mile Ridge Trail gently descends a closed fire road through incredibly diverse plant communities of coyote brush, sagebrush, coffeeberry, and the ubiquitous poison oak,

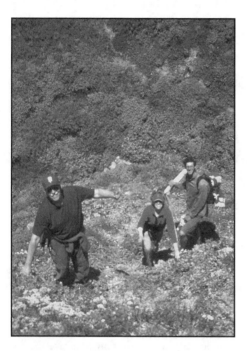

From Bluffs Trail, follow the spurs for dramatic vistas atop coastal bluffs.

then past clustered tanoaks and sprawling coast live oaks draped with lacy sage-colored lichen. Next come stately redwoods accompanied by redwood sorrel (a large four-leaf clover) and sword fern, easily identified by its large serrated fronds.

In half a mile the trail reaches the **South Boundary Trail junction** (5.2 miles, 900'). For a change of scenery and a chance to commune with nature, you could descend this lightly used 1.9-mile spur to the **Big Sur River** and Highway 1. Refrain from hiking the 2 miles along Highway 1 back to the parking lot, however, as narrow lanes leave little room between speeding cars and you.

Continuing along the Ridge Trail, you'll reach the **Hidden Trail junction** (6.3 miles, 730'). Pause to admire an awesome view that encompasses the lower Big Sur watershed, bordered by sprawling willows, alders, cottonwoods, and bigleaf maples against a backdrop of prominent peaks along the **Santa Lucia Range.** To the southeast, **Manuel Peak** (3379') rises amid a dark green patchwork of redwoods that border the Big Sur on its way through a narrow gorge. On a clear day you'll also see **Cone Peak** (5155'), which rises from the shoreline some 40 miles southeast. Less steep but perhaps more impressive, conical, marble-capped **Pico Blanco** (3709') towers over the nearby Santa Lucia foothills.

The return to your vehicle via the Hidden and River Trails, then across the Big Sur along the final stretch of the Creamery Meadow Trail (see TRIP 14 Creamery Meadow, River, Hidden, & Ridge Trails Loop, page 91, for details), is a half mile less than if you continue on the Ridge Trail to the Creamery Meadow Trail.

If you do continue on the Ridge Trail (6.3 miles, 730'), your route will follow a nearly level traverse until it descends south to the Creamery Meadow Trail junction. Turn right and hike the final mile to the parking lot.

Pfeiffer Big Sur State Park

■ ■

AT THE NAME BIG SUR, many picture a landscape of ancient redwoods along clear creeks that cascade down to the Pacific. Others immediately think of Pfeiffer Big Sur State Park, the region's most popular park, a top spot to camp, picnic, hike, and swim. Hikers come for redwood-lined gorges, oak woodlands, lush forests of sycamores, maples, alders and willows, open meadows blanketed in spring wildflowers, and a deep, narrow canyon along the Big Sur River that offers opportunities to swim and sunbathe. Although the park lies along Highway 1, it's more than a mile inland—a blessing for those hoping to escape the fog that blankets the coast most summer days.

Sweeping panoramas of jagged ridgetops slice the headwaters between the Carmel and Big Sur Rivers east of Manuel Peak.

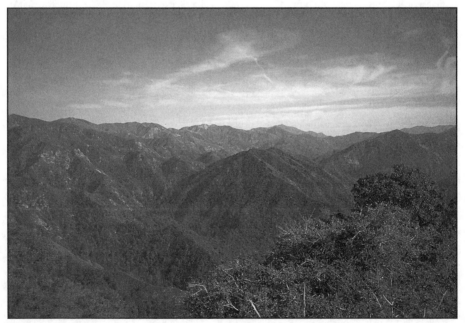

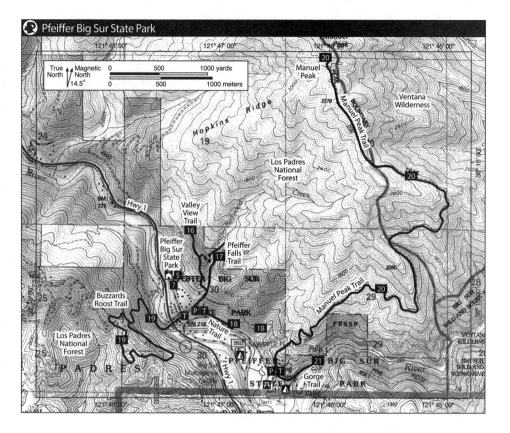

This parcel belonged to John Pfeiffer, son of Michael and Barbara Pfeiffer, who in 1869 became the first European immigrants to permanently settle in the region. John's wife, Florence, launched the first resort in Big Sur after deciding to charge freeloading guests for room and board. The Big Sur Lodge stands on this site, while the couple's 1884 homestead cabin lies along the Oak Grove Trail. In 1930 a Los Angeles developer offered John Pfeiffer $210,000 for his 1200-acre property, with the intent to parcel it off as a subdivision. Fortunately, the offer was rejected, and in 1933 the State of California purchased 700 acres and named the new park in Pfeiffer's honor.

DIRECTIONS: The park is on the east side of Highway 1, 26 miles south of the Carmel Valley Road (County Road G16) junction in Carmel and 28 miles north of the Nacimiento-Fergusson Road junction near Kirk Creek Campground.

VISITOR CENTER: Big Sur Station: (831) 667-2315. The station is on Highway 1, a half mile south of the park entrance. Open daily 8 a.m.–6 p.m. Memorial Day through Labor Day, 8 a.m.–4:30 p.m. the rest of the year.

NEAREST CAMPGROUND: Pfeiffer Big Sur State Park (218 sites, $35/standard site, $45/river site; reservations recommended in summer and on holidays). For more information call Reserve America at (800) 444-7275 or visit ReserveAmerica.com.

INFORMATION: Open daily 9 a.m.–8 p.m. There's a $10/vehicle entrance fee. No dogs or bikes allowed on park trails. No overnight camping.

WEBSITE: parks.ca.gov

PHONE: (831) 667-2315

Trip 16

VALLEY VIEW TRAIL

LENGTH AND TYPE: 1.6-mile loop

RATING: Easy

TRAIL CONDITION: Well maintained, poison oak, good for kids

HIGHLIGHTS: Sweeping views of the Big Sur River gorge, Point Sur, and Andrew Molera State Park

TO REACH THE TRAILHEAD: Pass the park's entrance kiosk and turn left at the stop sign, following signs to Pfeiffer Falls. After 100 feet the road will fork. Veer right past Ewoldsen Memorial Nature Center to the parking lot at road's end. The Valley View Trail begins either 0.1 mile from the start of the Pfeiffer Falls Trail or from the base of the falls, 0.4 mile down the same trail.

TRIP SUMMARY: Beginning alongside Pfeiffer Redwood Creek, this semi-loop route meanders past some of the park's largest coast redwoods. Climbing above the canyon floor, the trail offers views down the Big Sur River gorge.

Trip Description

The Pfeiffer Falls Trail begins beneath old-growth redwoods alongside Pfeiffer Redwood Creek. The narrow, well-used path gently ascends the canyon, soon reaching the Valley View Trail junction (0.1 mile, 400'). From the junction, the Valley View Trail branches west, crosses a wooden footbridge, and ascends Pfeiffer Redwood Canyon.

Rising above the canyon floor, you'll pass beneath some of the park's grandest redwoods. Over thousands of years, creek sediments have formed the rich alluvial soils necessary to support these trees. Over the next 0.1 mile a trio of switchbacks leads out of the canyon. Farther from the creek, these drier slopes support an entirely different group of plants. Twisted live oaks, scraggly brush, and spring displays of deep purple wild iris blanket the hillside (0.2 mile, 570').

As the trail climbs to the ridge, you'll glimpse the **Big Sur River** gorge off to the west. Three more switchbacks lead to a trail junction—the route to the right leads 0.2 mile to **Pfeiffer Falls,** while the route left leads 0.3 mile to the **Valley View Vista** (0.5 mile, 630'). Veer left toward the vista, climbing to a ridge that offers oak-filtered views to the north, east, and west.

The **viewpoint** (0.8 mile, 700') rewards you with panoramic views of the **Santa Lucia Range** and down the Big Sur River gorge to the Pacific. **Point Sur** rises over the rolling hills of Andrew Molera State Park, 7 miles northwest. In the canyon and on the river flats, dark redwoods stand beside alders, sycamores, bigleaf maples, black cottonwoods, and willows, which boast vibrant greens in spring and deep hues of orange, red, and yellow in fall. Sprawling oaks dot hillsides and ridges of golden grass, while tanoaks, live oaks, madrones, and bays fill the cool, moist, north-facing slopes and ravines. Offering contrast on the hot, dry south-facing slopes are the velvety greens and browns of the chaparral, dominated by chamise, ceanothus, manzanita, and coffeeberry. Take in the view and return the way you came.

WORLD'S TALLEST TREE ■ ■ ■ ■ ■ ■ ■ ■ ■ ■ ■ ■ ■ ■ ■ ■ ■ ■

Exceeding 300 feet in height, coast redwoods (*Sequoia sempervirens*) are the world's tallest trees. Big Sur marks the species' southernmost range. These moisture-loving giants thrive in the region's narrow river gorges. Farther south, temperatures are too hot and precipitation too low to sustain them. The remaining trees represent a fraction of the original groves.

Coastal Indians were the first to make use of the trees, stripping the roots of their strong fibers for use as thread in basketry. In subsequent settler days the land was ill managed. Many old-growth groves were lost when the Ventana Power Company operated a sawmill here in the late 19th century. About the same time, John and Florence Pfeiffer opened Pfeiffer Ranch Resort. To supply guests with lodging and warmth, the Pfeiffers turned to the mill for their lumber needs. Decades later, when Highway 1 was being built, the mill supplied lumber for worker housing.

■ ■

Trip 17

PFEIFFER FALLS TRAIL

LENGTH AND TYPE: 1.4-mile round-trip

RATING: Easy

TRAIL CONDITION: Well maintained, good for kids

HIGHLIGHTS: Ancient redwoods flank this spectacular 60-foot waterfall.

TO REACH THE TRAILHEAD: Pass the park's entrance kiosk and turn left at the stop sign, following signs to Pfeiffer Falls. After 100 feet the road will fork. Veer right past Ewoldsen Memorial Nature Center to the parking lot at road's end.

TRIP SUMMARY: Unquestionably one of the most popular hikes in Big Sur, this short, easy 0.7-mile trail leads past ancient redwoods to the base of the 60-foot cascade. Expect crowds in summer, when the park campground often fills. The falls are most impressive during the winter wet season, when lush ferns, fungi, and mosses line the canyon.

Trip Description

Pfeiffer Falls Trail begins beside **Pfeiffer Redwood Creek,** shaded by the park's most magnificent redwoods. Once comprising some 2,000,000 acres of fogbound coast between Big Sur and southern Oregon, most of the old-growth redwood forests were heavily logged, and now only small stands of these ancient trees remain in an area of less than 300,000 acres. A 6-foot diameter cross-section of a 1000-year-old felled redwood rests beside the upper trailhead. Although enormous, it's an average size and age for this region. Throughout their range in central California, redwoods rarely exceed 1500 years old, 10 feet in diameter, or 250 feet in height. It's the celebrated redwoods in Northern California's Coast Ranges that commonly exceed 2000 years old, 15–20 feet in diameter, and 300 feet in height.

A gentle ascent up the narrow, well-used path beside **Pfeiffer Redwood Creek Canyon** leads to the **Valley View Trail junction** (0.1 mile, 400'), on your left. Both trails lead to the falls, but the Pfeiffer Falls Trail is less steep and a quarter mile shorter than the Valley View Trail. Pass this junction and you'll soon reach steps that ascend to the **Oak Grove Trail junction** (0.2 mile, 470'), which veers sharply south. Stay on course to reach the first of four scenic wooden footbridges that cross the creek.

A PFEIFFER ON EVERY HILL ■ ■ ■ ■ ■ ■ ■ ■ ■ ■ ■ ■ ■ ■ ■ ■ ■

Still standing along the Oak Grove Trail, the Homestead Cabin was built in 1884 by homesteader John Pfeiffer. John was 7 years old when his family arrived in Big Sur in 1869, becoming the first European immigrants to settle here permanently. By the turn of the century, the Pfeiffers were operating a sawmill and boarding house on the property. In 1933, John and wife Florence Pfeiffer sold most of the surrounding land to the state, stipulating that it be preserved as a park. Florence and seven of her children are buried in a cemetery near the Homestead Cabin.

■ ■

Pfeiffer Redwood Creek cascades 60 feet along its path toward the confluence of the Big Sur River farther downstream.

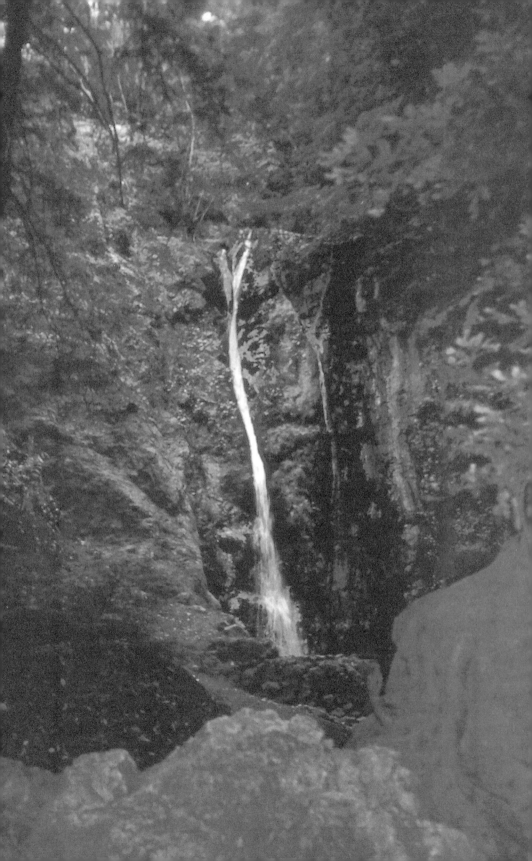

Soon after crossing the fourth footbridge, you'll reach the northern **Valley View Trail junction** (0.4 mile, 590'), which leads northwest across a fifth bridge. Once again, continue straight and follow the burbling creek through its narrow, steep-walled canyon. You'll ascend more than 40 steps to the base of the 60-foot falls, where visitors pause on a wooden platform to watch water plunging over the mossy granite cliff into the crystal clear pool below. Benches on the platform offer a great picnic spot, though you shouldn't expect solitude.

Trip 18

NATURE TRAIL

LENGTH AND TYPE: 0.6-mile out-and-back

RATING: Easy

TRAIL CONDITION: Well maintained, good for kids

HIGHLIGHTS: Stroll through oak woodlands and ancient redwood groves on this 30-minute self-guided nature tour.

TO REACH THE TRAILHEAD: From the park entrance, head to the stop sign, then continue straight past Big Sur Lodge. Immediately past the lodge, the road forks. Continue straight for 0.1 mile to the next fork, then veer left. Drive a quarter mile farther, bypassing the campfire center parking lot for the smaller lot beside a picnic area. The trailhead is opposite this lot.

TRIP SUMMARY: This self-guided, 30-minute stroll through oak woodlands and a magnificent redwood forest is the perfect way to experience the park's diverse plant life. Informative pamphlets at either end of the trail describe two of the five major resident plant communities. Your $0.25 donation supports the Big Sur Natural History Association.

Trip Description

You'll start on a level trail that meanders beneath sprawling **live oaks,** fragrant bay trees, and twisting sycamores, whose bark may remind you of a jigsaw puzzle. A dozen numbered posts correlate to brochure entries, helping you identify plants and animals common to these unique forest communities.

By the tenth post (0.2 mile, 300'), you'll have entered a **redwood grove,** marked by dramatic changes in vegetation. Little sunshine penetrates the dense redwood canopy, creating a dark, cool microclimate. These ancient giants lie at the southern limit of their range, in a much warmer, drier climate than that associated with Pacific Northwest redwood groves. Only along the small creeks and rivers that slice the Big Sur coast are they able to find adequate moisture to survive. The adverse conditions prevent these redwoods from obtaining the impressive size and lifespan of their northern counterparts. Nonetheless, redwoods have thrived along the **Big Sur River** for thousands of years, their broad shallow roots taking hold in rich deposits of alluvial soil along the riverbank.

The trail crosses the roadway just past the eleventh post (0.25 mile, 300') and leads to one of the park's largest trees, which towers nearly 300 feet. Most trees at the trail's end are 500–800 years old, hardly record-breaking for a species that can live more than 2000 years and exceed 300 feet in height. The trail emerges at the visitor lot beside park headquarters. Retrace your steps to the trailhead.

Trip 19

BUZZARDS ROOST TRAIL

LENGTH AND TYPE: 3.1-mile loop

RATING: Moderate

TRAIL CONDITION: Clear, poison oak

HIGHLIGHTS: Summit views overlook prominent ridgelines east to the Big Sur River gorge and west to Sycamore Canyon and the vast blue ocean.

TO REACH THE TRAILHEAD: From the park entrance, head to the stop sign, then continue straight past Big Sur Lodge. Immediately past the lodge, the road forks. Bear right on the two-lane bridge over the Big Sur River. The parking lot is on the left just past the bridge. The trail begins on the west bank beneath the bridge.

TRIP SUMMARY: This trail follows the south bank of the Big Sur beneath a canopy of redwoods and tanoaks before climbing Pfeiffer Ridge. Despite the promise of gorgeous overlooks of the Santa Lucia Range and Pacific, the trail is little used. You may find yourself alone at the top with large turkey vultures that roost in the redwoods below. In summer, fog envelops the coast, obscuring views. Fog is less likely in the spring and fall, while winter views between storms are often spectacular. Strong winds are always a factor atop the open ridge—bring a windbreaker or sweater year-round.

Trip Description

From the trailhead, the **Buzzards Roost Trail** crosses beneath the bridge to follow the banks of the **Big Sur River**. Autumn visits are highlighted by deep yellow and orange hues from the large sycamores, alders, bigleaf maples, and willows that flank the river. A short, gentle descent downstream brings you to a spur that leads straight 0.1 mile to a riverside group camp.

From this **spur junction** (0.2 mile, 310'), the main trail forks uphill toward **Pfeiffer Ridge**. A riparian woodland dominated by broadleaf deciduous trees quickly gives way to a dense, shady redwood-tanoak forest. The redwoods persist despite a drier environment than that found in their northern range. As a result, much of the expected dense understory of ferns and mosses is not present here.

At a sign marked BUZZARDS ROOST TRAIL (1.4 miles, 550'), the route forks to become a 1.7-mile loop. Bear right on the more direct, well-graded ascent to **Buzzards Ridge**. The shaded path passes beneath young redwoods and thin, dense stands of bay trees. Closer to the ridgeline, the redwoods are stunted, perhaps from nutrient-poor soil or lack of water. You'll encounter a dramatic vegetation shift atop the ridge (1.9 miles, 1000'), as you enter dry thickets of manzanita and chamise.

The path crosses the ridge to a narrow **spur junction** (2 miles, 1010'), which bears right and climbs 50 feet to the **summit,** topped by a large antenna. Turn your back to the obtrusive antenna for beautiful views down **Sycamore Canyon** to the Pacific. Gaze east to take in the steep narrow Big Sur River gorge and the **Manuel Peak Trail,** which switchbacks and ascends the gorge's sheer north walls.

Back on the main trail, you'll skirt the ridgeline south for 200 feet, then descend a few large steps to reenter dense stands of redwoods, bays, and tanoaks. The next 0.7 mile is a gradual descent with limited views across the river gorge. From the loop junction, retrace your steps 1.4 miles to the trailhead.

Atop Buzzard's Roost, keep an eye out for the 9-foot wingspan of the California condor.

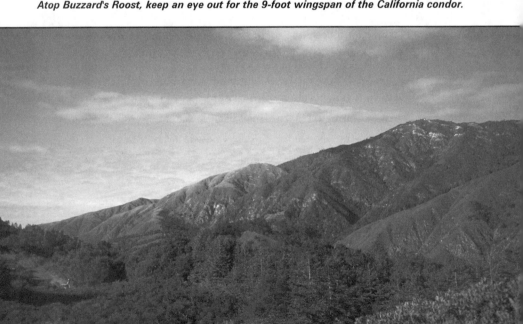

Trip 20

MANUEL PEAK TRAIL

LENGTH AND TYPE: 10.8-mile out-and-back

RATING: Challenging

TRAIL CONDITION: Passable to difficult, poison oak

HIGHLIGHTS: Panoramic views from a secluded peak deep within the Big Sur watershed.

TO REACH THE TRAILHEAD: From the park entrance, head to the stop sign, then continue straight past Big Sur Lodge. Immediately past the lodge, the road forks. Bear left and drive 0.7 mile past the picnic areas. Bear left at the next fork and park across from the trailhead at the base of a closed road, labeled on the park map as the Gorge Trail.

TRIP SUMMARY: Offering an overview of the Ventana Wilderness, this steep trail averages an 11% grade, reaching 3379' in 5.4 miles at the peak's scenic viewpoint. You'll ascend past sun-scorched chaparral, cool redwood groves, and oak woodlands. From May through October, this is often a sunny, dry trek, so bring a wide-brimmed hat and plenty of extra water. Despite the hot climb, wear long pants for protection from ticks, brush, and poison oak. In summer, the coast is often fogbound, though views inland remain unobscured.

Trip Description

The trailhead for the **Gorge Trail, Manuel Peak Trail,** and south end of the **Oak Grove Trail** begins at the base of the closed paved road across from the parking lot. Climb the service road 0.1 mile till it curves north at a junction with a dirt road. The main road continues straight as the Gorge Trail. Turn left (west) on the dirt road past John Pfeiffer's **Homestead Cabin.** Follow the Oak Grove Trail 50 feet north of the cabin, where it narrows to a single lane and leads 0.4 mile farther to the Manuel Peak Trail junction.

The trail makes an initial switchback east to meet a **spur** (0.2 mile, 220') that leads down to one of the picnic area parking lots. Continue your moderate ascent beneath a dense canopy of gnarled live oaks, tanoaks, and bays. In summer this short stretch of shade provides welcome relief from the mostly exposed Manuel Peak Trail.

Past an enormous downed oak, you'll clamber up a minor ridge to a **fork** (0.6 mile, 560'). A sign warns that from here the Manuel Peak Trail is a strenuous climb that ascends nearly 3000 feet in 4 miles. While largely well graded to the summit, the last mile is overgrown and requires brushing past, at times, shoulder-high shrubs. In winter and spring keep watch for hitchhiking ticks.

Take the right fork upslope along the Manuel Peak Trail, which soon leaves the shade on a steady climb through fragrant coastal scrub past chamise, sage, poison oak, coyote brush, and toyon. You'll switchback five times and climb 400 feet before catching your first glimpse of the jagged Big Sur coast and glistening Pacific, spurring you to continue your ascent. Trail switchbacks stand out clearly against the south-facing slopes, while the narrow river gorge below drops precipitously, seemingly the result of landslides in places. The **Pine Ridge Trail** traces the cool, forested north-facing slopes across the gorge. In summer and early fall, fog envelops the valley, obscuring views.

After 2.5 miles the trail turns north and enters a canopy of live oaks, madrones, and stately redwoods. Traversing the redwood-lined gully, the route descends into a smaller but more significant **gully** (3.4 miles, 1720'), home to a small seasonal creek—though in dry months (April through October), this is little more than a muddy seep.

From this minor gully, you'll climb east and enter the **Ventana Wilderness**. After 0.3 mile (3.7 miles, 2200'), turn north for your first views toward the scraggly bald peaks of **Ventana Double Cone** (4853') and neighboring summits. The trail is not regularly maintained from here to the summit, though it's still easy to identify through the overgrown brush. You'll have to scramble across a few downed trees and dry washes.

Continue your ascent through dense, sometimes shoulder-high thickets of coastal chaparral (4 miles, 2200'). Dominating the trailside is wartleaf, which bears pungent sawtooth leaves. After 0.4 mile passage through this moderate overgrowth, the trail opens and climbs west across a north-facing ridge studded with oaks and madrones. You'll soon crest the ridge with views of the Pacific (or perhaps fogbanks in summer) to the west and the rugged **Santa Lucia Range** to the east.

MANUEL INNOCENTI ■ ■ ■ ■ ■ ■ ■ ■ ■ ■ ■ ■ ■ ■ ■ ■ ■ ■ ■

Manuel Peak is named for Manuel Innocenti, an Esselen Indian from Big Sur who was raised and educated at the Santa Barbara Mission in Southern California. In 1868 he returned to this area, purchasing land and a cabin near Manuel Peak for $50.

Tragically, though the land and the sea had provided Manuel's tribe with an abundance of all they needed to survive—deer, rabbits, fish, shellfish, wild flax, tule reeds, berries, acorns, bulbs, quail—his people had vanished. From 1770, when Father Junipero Serra and Captain Gaspar de Portola founded a mission and presidio at Monterey, the "pagan souls" of the coast had been brought into the mission system. Most either assimilated, succumbed to disease, or were killed in warfare.

Manuel became head vaquero at Juan B.R. Cooper's Rancho El Sur, at present-day Andrew Molera State Park. Manuel and wife Francisca had seven children, none of whom reached adulthood.

The trail switchbacks up a steeper crest, then makes a short ascent on an easier grade to a spur for the **Manuel Peak viewpoint** (5.3 miles, 3379'), capped with white marble rubble and a small scraggly live oak. The open summit offers a nearly 360-degree view of the Ventana Wilderness and neighboring **Big Sur State Park**. For relief in the shade, retreat to a dense stand of Coulter pines past a conspicuous, yet camouflaged reflector a few paces north of the viewpoint. Once rested, head back down the trail.

For those headed to Bottchers Gap, 12.7 miles farther north, reverse the trail description in TRIP 42 Manuel Peak & Pfeiffer Big Sur State Park (page 169). Be forewarned: The trail from Manuel Peak to Launtz Creek Camp is heavily overgrown and not recommended.

Trip 21

GORGE TRAIL

LENGTH AND TYPE: 1-mile out-and-back

RATING: Easy to challenging

TRAIL CONDITION: Well maintained, poison oak

HIGHLIGHTS: This steep, narrow canyon features large granite boulders amid brisk, refreshing swimming holes.

TO REACH THE TRAILHEAD: From the park entrance, head to the stop sign, then continue straight past Big Sur Lodge. Immediately past the lodge, the road forks. Bear left and drive 0.7 mile past the picnic areas. Bear left at the next fork and park across from the trailhead at the base of a closed road.

TRIP SUMMARY: This short trail skirts the Big Sur River to some of the region's best swimming holes. The gorge is easy to traverse in summer, when campers and hikers descend en masse to lounge poolside and bask on sunny boulders. During heavy winter storms, however, the river can rise several feet in just a few hours, flooding the trail.

Trip Description

Head southeast up the paved fire road through the gate and gradually ascend to the **Homestead Cabin** (0.2 mile, 340'), built in 1884 by John Pfeiffer. Continue along the paved road and cross the large bridge over the **Big Sur River** into the northern section of the park campground (0.3 mile, 300').

Officially, the **Gorge Trail** ends here, though you have yet to enter the gorge. Starting beside the bridge, two trails lead upstream along either the east or west banks to the gorge. Passage is easiest in summer and fall, when water levels are low.

To avoid hiking through people's campsites, take the west bank, which leads upstream 0.1 mile to a refreshing pool, followed by a steep granite wall. On summer afternoons, the surrounding granite rocks make warm, smooth sunbathing platforms. Water temperatures on even the hottest summer day remain in the low to mid 60s Fahrenheit, while on warm fall and spring days, temps linger in the mid to high 50s. Despite the brisk water, dozens of swimmers frequent these pools in summer.

If you prefer more solitude, head farther upstream, though steeper walls allow only slivers of sunshine to reach the canyon floor. The park discourages climbing here due to loose rock and unstable soil. Clambering atop the slick granite boulders that line the canyon floor is equally dangerous. During winter storms, the river can swiftly rise several feet above its normal level. Be aware of the weather and never enter the gorge when storm clouds are approaching.

Trip 22

PFEIFFER BEACH

LENGTH AND TYPE: 1-mile out-and-back

RATING: Easy

TRAIL CONDITION: Well maintained, good for kids

HIGHLIGHTS: Stroll barefoot along one of Big Sur's finest windswept beaches to commune with the sea.

TO REACH THE TRAILHEAD: The road to Pfeiffer Beach lies at a saddle with two roads on the west side of Highway 1, a quarter mile south of Big Sur Station and 1.1 miles north of the Ventana Inn entrance. Turn west on Sycamore Canyon Road, a narrow, winding stretch that leads 2.2 miles to the beach parking loop. There's a $5 day-use fee. You'll find water and bathrooms at the trailhead.

TRIP SUMMARY: This hike leads to one of the region's most striking beaches. In spring the coastal bluffs boast a colorful tapestry of wildflowers, including California poppies, sticky monkeyflowers, yellow sand verbena, Indian paintbrush, and lupines. Foaming surf crashes through dramatic nearshore arches, highlighting the gorgeous sunsets.

Trip Description

From the west end of the parking lot, follow Sycamore Creek 0.1 mile down to the ocean. Redwoods, bays, and buckeyes line the stream, soon giving way to a wind-sculpted stand of Monterey cypress, whose roots anchor in the steep dunes.

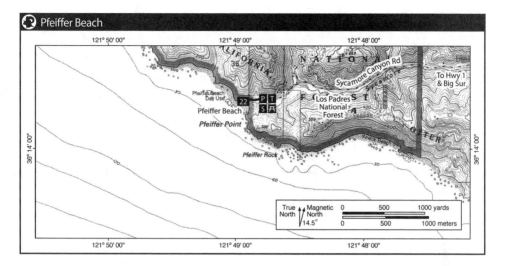

At the creek mouth, the trail emerges on the wide beach. Leave your own footprints in the soft sand. Just offshore, waves crash against rugged rocky outcrops, some carved over time into natural arches. These dramatic formations offer a natural barrier from the crashing surf, sheltering shallow tide pools for waders of all ages. Water temps remain a nippy 50s Fahrenheit year-round.

Enjoy a barefoot beach stroll along Pfeiffer Beach, one of the most incredible wave-washed beaches of Big Sur.

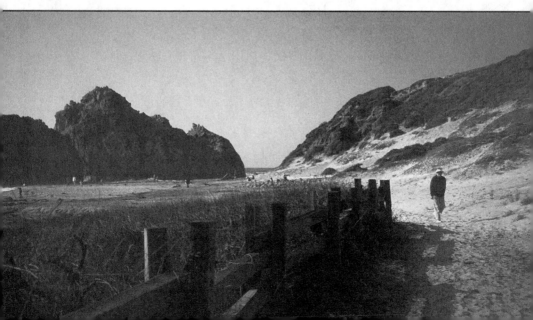

PFEIFFER BEACH GEOLOGY ▪ ▪ ▪ ▪ ▪ ▪ ▪ ▪ ▪ ▪ ▪ ▪ ▪ ▪ ▪ ▪

Referred to as the Pfeiffer Beach Slab, these low bluffs and loosely consolidated cliffs expose the variegated hues of ancient deformed rocks. The predominant rock at Pfeiffer Beach is sandstone, ranging in color from tan or gold to gray. Carved with numerous arches, the nearshore rocks are remnants of massive sandstone blocks that continue to erode with each pounding wave.

While part of the Franciscan complex, they have been less heavily metamorphosed than similar formations farther north. Geologists believe these differences are due to the numerous northwest-trending faults associated with the San Andreas Fault, which rends the Big Sur region.

▪ ▪

Sea arches and sunsets are not to be missed along Pfeiffer Beach.

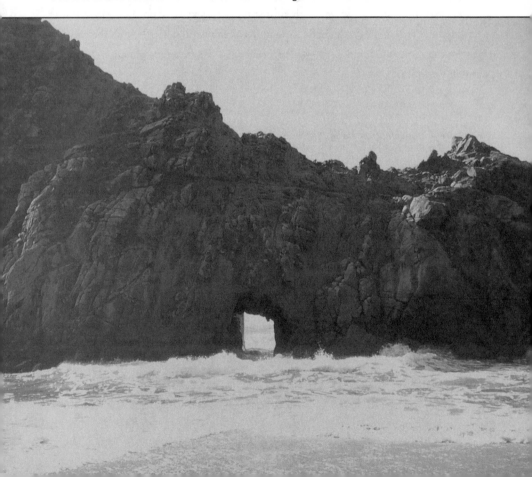

Julia Pfeiffer Burns State Park

■ ■ ■ ■ ■ ■ ■ ■ ■ ■ ■ ■ ■ ■ ■ ■ ■ ■ ■

JULIA PFEIFFER BURNS STATE PARK epitomizes Big Sur's natural scenic grandeur. This exquisite 3.75-square-mile parcel preserves a dramatic convergence of coastal and mountain features. Rocky points rise thousands of feet above rich underwater canyons, streams flow down steep gorges shaded by ancient redwoods, and a ribbony waterfall plunges over a granite lip to the sand of a pristine cove.

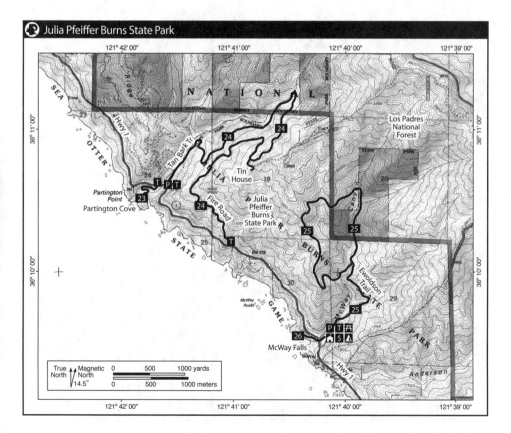

Julia Pfeiffer Burns State Park

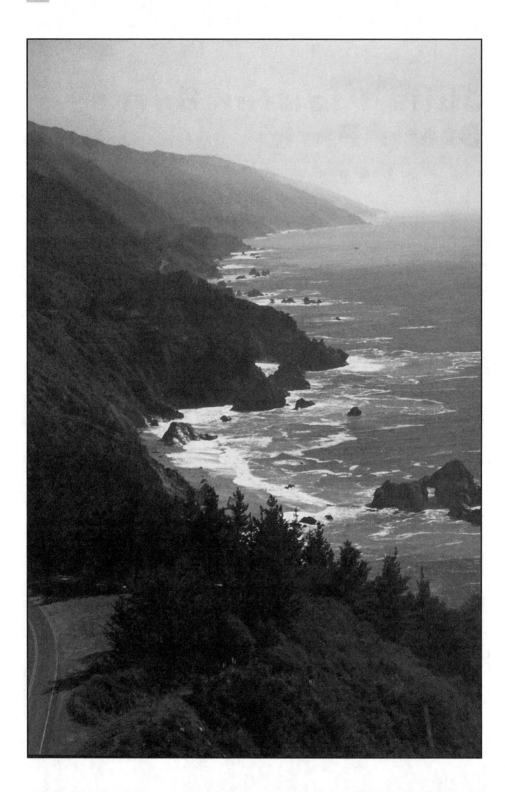

In addition to its 10 miles of coastline and 1860 acres of mountains, meadows, and valleys, the park also contains a 1680-acre underwater reserve that hosts diverse marine life. Scan the thick nearshore kelp beds to spot foraging seals, sea lions, and sea otters. You may also witness the annual winter migration of California gray whales, which journey south to breeding and calving grounds in Baja between November and January, then migrate north to Alaskan feeding grounds between February and April. In spring, females steer their calves close to shore for protection from predators. McWay Cove is an excellent vantage point.

The park is named for Julia Pfeiffer Burns, a respected Big Sur pioneer. She was less than a year old in 1869 when her parents, Michael and Barbara Pfeiffer, journeyed to this wild coast to become Big Sur's first permanent white settlers. The Pfeiffer family grew, prospered, and homesteaded so much of the surrounding land that it was often said, "There was a Pfeiffer on every hill."

In the late 1870s, Christopher McWay arrived to settle the adjacent canyon. Fifty years later, Lathrop Brown, a former New York congressman, and wife Helen Hooper Brown purchased McWay's Saddle Rock Ranch and built a home atop what today is the waterfall overlook. Helen Brown donated the ranch to the state of California in 1961, choosing to name the park in honor of Julia, the strong, self-sufficient pioneer.

DIRECTIONS: The park entrance is on the east side of Highway 1, 37 miles south of the Carmel Valley Road (County Road G16) junction in Carmel and 11 miles south of Big Sur State Park.

VISITOR CENTER: Big Sur Station: (831) 667-2315. The station is on Highway 1, 10 miles north of the park entrance. Open daily 8 a.m.–4:30 p.m. Memorial Day through Labor Day, 8 a.m.–6 p.m. the rest of the year.

NEAREST CAMPGROUND: The park's walk-in campground lies on the south side of the McWay Falls promontory, 0.3 mile from the parking lot. Two primitive sites ($30/night; reservations required) hold a maximum of eight people each. For more information call Reserve America at (800) 444-7275 or visit ReserveAmerica.com.

INFORMATION: Open 7 a.m.–10 p.m. There is a $10 day-use fee. Restrooms and water are available at the parking lot. No pets allowed except seeing-eye dogs.

WEBSITE: parks.ca.gov

PHONE: (831) 667-2315

Feel the raw elements of fog, wind, and sunshine along the jutting coastal cliffs within Julia Pfeiffer Burns State Park.

Trip 23

PARTINGTON COVE TRAIL

LENGTH AND TYPE: 0.6-mile out-and-back

RATING: Easy

TRAIL CONDITION: Well maintained, poison oak, good for kids

HIGHLIGHTS: Coastal access to a dramatic stretch of pounding surf, jagged granite rocks, and sheer cliffs

TO REACH THE TRAILHEAD: The trailhead is 2 miles north of the park entrance on Highway 1, at the west end of Partington Creek Bridge. There are small turnouts on either side of the bridge. A cattle gate on the ocean side of the road marks the trailhead. You won't find water or restrooms, save for two outhouses at Partington Cove.

TRIP SUMMARY: This short, steady descent traces Partington Creek's final yards to sea, emerging in a cove with stunning natural features and rich cultural history. In the 1870s the site served as a port from which tanoak bark was shipped to the tanning industry in San Francisco. Local legend has it the cove was also used as a booze smuggling port during Prohibition in the 1920s. Expect crowds in summer and on weekends.

Trip Description

From the cattle gate near the northwest end of **Partington Creek Bridge** (240'), you'll descend a steep grade 0.2 mile along a fire road to a small flat beside the creek. The trail narrows as you reach a **spur** (0.25 mile, 60') that leads upstream 100 feet toward an outhouse beside a dense stand of redwoods.

Continue downstream 100 feet to another **spur** (0.3 mile, 50'), which leads 200 feet to the narrow west cove at **Partington Point**. Taking this spur, you'll pass a cluster of grizzled redwoods that struggle against the salt spray and pounding surf.

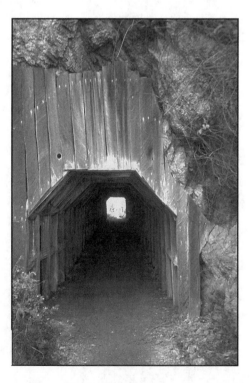

Local legend has it that the Partington Cove tunnel was used to smuggle booze during Prohibition.

The spur emerges on the beach, where you'll have to clamber over a few granite boulders onto coarse sand washed by exceptionally clear emerald water. Dominating the cove is Salinian block granite, formed 80 million years ago in Mexico and carried here along the San Andreas Fault. This granite is extremely erosion resistant, leaving the water largely free of sediments that cloud water elsewhere along the coast.

From the prior junction, the main trail bears left and threads through a 100-foot tunnel to the east cove. Built in the 1870s by John Partington, the hand-split redwood tunnel leads to **Partington Landing**. Here the canyon's redwoods and oaks were loaded onto waiting ships. Redwood was used to build homes, roofs, and fences in rapidly growing San Francisco, while tanoak bark was used to tan leather. Today, this is an ideal spot to have a picnic, watch for whales and sea otters, and soak up magnificent sunsets. Return the way you came.

Trip 24

TAN BARK TRAIL & FIRE ROAD LOOP

LENGTH AND TYPE: 6.6-mile out-and-back or 5.6-mile loop

RATING: Moderate to strenuous

TRAIL CONDITION: Clear, poison oak

HIGHLIGHTS: Old-growth redwoods and sweeping Pacific vistas.

TO REACH THE TRAILHEAD: The Tan Bark Trail starts at the east end of Partington Creek Bridge, 2 miles north of the park entrance on Highway 1. There are small turnouts on either side of the bridge. The Fire Road emerges near Vista Point at Mile 37 on Highway 1. The road lies 70 yards east of the parking area. Neither trailhead offers restrooms or water.

TRIP SUMMARY: Choose between a 6.6-mile out-and-back hike via the Tan Bark Trail or a 5.6-mile loop that traverses the Tan Bark Trail and Fire Road back to Highway 1. The 3.3-mile Tan Bark Trail is a longer, more scenic route to the Tin House and is better graded than the wide, steep Fire Road. That said, it starts lower and thus climbs more than 2000 feet versus the Fire Road's 1580-foot climb. The 2.2-mile Fire Road is a steep climb past sunny hilltops with coastal views. The following description starts on the Tan Bark Trail, ascends to the Tin House, then descends the Fire Road to Highway 1.

Trip Description

From the southeast end of **Partington Creek Bridge** (210'), the **Tan Bark Trail** follows **Partington Creek** as it tumbles over granite boulders beneath towering redwoods. In 0.1 mile a spur bears left across the creek on a **wooden bridge** (0.1 mile, 170'). This spur leads back downstream to the west end of the bridge. Continue straight along the south fork of Partington Creek, taking in the persistent cries of tiny brown winter wrens.

The trail follows the south bank in the cool shade of redwoods, tanoaks, and bays. After 0.3 mile the trail reaches another spur that darts upstream 100 feet to the creek. At this junction, the main trail turns east through the **Donald McLaughlin Memorial Grove** (0.3 mile, 350'). The trail then begins its major ascent, climbing a series of steep switchbacks past a minor gully that hosts a creek only during the wettest months. Glance across canyon at the sun-baked south-facing slopes, dotted with homes in the **Partington Ridge** subdivision.

The trail continues northeast, switching from redwoods amid lush sorrel and sword ferns to drier stands of oaks and bays. Sadly, most of these oaks are dead or dying from sudden oak death. The main trail is clearly marked and well trodden in contrast to the numerous spurs, remnants of trails once used to haul out batches of tanoak bark.

BIG SUR LUMBER ▦

The redwoods along Partington Creek are among Big Sur's largest, survivors of a lumber industry that clear-cut whole stands along the Coast Ranges. Redwood is highly valued as a building material, but these gnarled old-growth trees were unsuitable for lumber and spared from the axe.

Tanoaks, however, were extensively harvested for the leather-tanning industry. The trees were clear-cut in this canyon, then shipped from Partington Cove to tanneries in Santa Cruz and San Francisco. The harvest was hard on the forest. Tanoaks didn't grow in pure stands, so loggers forged rough trails to reach the trees. Although tanoak wood is usable as a building material or firewood, loggers were only after the bark and left the trees to rot.

Yet today, extensive stands dominate Partington Canyon along the Tan Bark Trail. This recovery is due to tanoak's reproductive capacity to "stump sprout" from the roots of a felled tree. These sprouts grow at the same time, establishing multiple trunks from a common root system.

▪ ▪

Just past a minor confluence of the **south fork** (2 miles, 1550'), note the enormous old-growth redwoods, some nearly 10 feet in diameter. Continue your gentle ascent through the glade to a creek that flows in all but the driest months. Ignore the overgrown trail to the northeast and follow the main trail southeast to a bench beside the creek. Check the path for obvious stonework (2.3 miles, 1680'), remnants of **Swiss Camp,** built by settler Gunder Bergstrom in the 1920s. The most strenuous climbing is now behind you.

For the next 0.7 mile you'll climb a gentle grade, soon reaching a junction with a **spur** (3 miles, 2110') that climbs a prominent ridge on private property. Stay on the main trail and follow it downhill 200 yards till you merge with the wide Fire Road. From here you'll bear left and descend another 200 feet to the **Tin House** (3.3 miles, 1960'), perched on a ridge crest.

Built during World War II from tin scavenged from a defunct gas station, the Tin House is a peculiar structure with an obscure history. In wartime, tin was a tightly controlled material, so it's unusual to find so much tin in a house from that era. The previous landowner was Lathrop Brown, a politician who served in Congress and the Department of the Interior. Locals insist Brown built the house as a retreat for friend and college classmate Franklin D. Roosevelt. Others believe it served as the Browns' second home. Regardless, this is a beautiful spot for a picnic, atop a golden hilltop that offers sweeping views of the coast.

When rested, you can return the way you came or finish the loop via the **Fire Road,** a 2.2-mile descent to **Vista Point** on Highway 1, a mile north of Partington Creek Bridge. From the Tin House, head back uphill 0.2 mile to the Tan Bark Trail **junction** (3.5 miles, 1980'), then turn north to descend the canyon's east side. Over the next 0.6 mile the steep road switchbacks in the shade of tanoaks and redwoods. After 1.4 miles the road reaches a prominent **ridge** (4.7 miles, 1030'), with excellent views across steep, narrow **Partington Canyon.** Leaving the shade, the road emerges amid fragrant coastal scrub that flaunts colorful wildflowers in the spring, when abundant lupines, golden yarrow, and poppies paint the hillsides in yellow, purple, and orange hues.

The coastal views continue to impress as you descend the Fire Road, weaving past gullies to a minor spring flanked by redwoods and lush ferns. It's a 200-foot jaunt from here to the Fire Road gate and Highway 1.

If you parked at Vista Point, cross the highway and walk 200 feet north to the lot. If you parked at Partington Creek Bridge, continue walking a mile north on Highway 1. Use caution, especially when walking with children, as the shoulder narrows in places.

Trip 25

EWOLDSEN TRAIL

LENGTH AND TYPE: 5.7-mile loop

RATING: Moderate

TRAIL CONDITION: Restored in 2013 after the 2008 Basin Complex Fire, poison oak

HIGHLIGHTS: Wind past some of Big Sur's oldest, largest redwoods and admire coastal views from hillsides covered in wildflowers and oaks.

TO REACH THE TRAILHEAD: The trailhead is at the far end of the upper parking lot on the north side of McWay Creek. Restrooms and water are available at the trailhead.

TRIP SUMMARY: This hike is a semi-loop with gorgeous coastal views. You'll follow boulder-laden McWay Creek in the shade of redwoods before ascending a ridgetop more than 1600 feet above the sea. In winter and spring, gray whales skirt the shore on their migration route between Baja and Alaska. Watch for their blowholes and arching backs from the open bluffs.

Trip Description

The **Ewoldsen Trail** begins at the far end of the upper parking lot (260'), following **McWay Creek** through a lush canyon of redwoods to a creekside **picnic area** (0.1 mile, 280'). A few feet farther the trail skirts past a dilapidated barn and crosses the creek on a rustic wooden bridge, one of many along the creek.

You'll soon pass redwoods bearing fire scars at the base of their trunks. In 1985 the Rat Creek Fire raged through much of the canyon. Thanks to their thick, fire-resistant bark, these redwoods endured the heat and flames with only minor burns. This unique adaptation has enabled the trees to survive for thousands of years in fire-prone areas. Ecologists believe that prior to permanent European settlement, fires hit the Big Sur every 12–20 years, and as a result, the dominant vegetation evolved to adapt to fire.

CONDOR COMEBACK ■ ■ ■ ■ ■ ■ ■ ■ ■ ■ ■ ■ ■ ■ ■ ■ ■

By the early 1900s, after decades of habitat loss, hunting, and poisoning, California condors were severely threatened. In 1987 researchers rounded up the last of the state's 27 remaining wild condors and laid the groundwork for a captive breeding and reintroduction effort. Under the auspices of the U.S. Fish & Wildlife Service, the California Condor Recovery Program is a multi-entity effort to recover the wild condor population. There are three release sites in California, including one in Big Sur, managed by the Ventana Wilderness Society, a nonprofit research, education, and restoration organization.

In 2012 the total California condor population reached 186 birds, 126 of those in the wild. Visitors and researchers regularly spot condors along the ridgeline atop the Ewoldsen Trail.

For more information about restoration efforts and how you can help, contact the Ventana Wilderness Society in Salinas: (831) 455-9514, info@ventanaws.org.

■ ■

A quarter mile up the trail, you'll reach the **Canyon Trail junction** (0.25 mile, 390'). This worthwhile spur leads 0.1 mile farther upstream along the south fork of McWay Creek. A few feet past a confluence with the main creek, you'll reach a bench that overlooks a waterfall.

From the Canyon Trail junction, the Ewoldsen Trail branches right and ascends the canyon. Switchbacks thread deep into the redwoods high above McWay Creek, often at eye level with the forest canopy. Watch for birds that rarely visit the canyon floor, such as the golden-crowned kinglet, which hovers to glean insects from the tips of branches. This tiny insectivore has a boldly striped face and bright yellow crown. Woodpeckers' raucous chatter permeates the silence, as they busily carve insects out of trees. Acorn woodpeckers store acorns in their bore holes, providing food for insects, which in turn provide the woodpecker a scrumptious meal of fattened grubs.

You'll exit the south fork canyon along four switchbacks, cross the creek on a stable bridge, and emerge from the shady groves amid dry, exposed chaparral. The vegetation switches back just as quickly once you hike 0.1 mile into the main fork watershed. As you approach the gurgling creek in the shade of redwoods, you'll reach the **loop junction** (1.5 miles, 800').

The loop is 2.1 miles. The left fork climbs a mile along an exposed trail to the viewpoint spur, while the right fork climbs 1.1 miles in the shade of oaks, bays, redwoods, and madrones to the same junction. Ascend the right fork along redwood-lined **McWay Canyon**. You'll soon turn west on a steep grade through dense oak woodland, then curl south to a minor ridge that offers stunning coastal views.

Continue across an oak-clad ridge to the spur in a shallow **saddle** (2.6 miles, 1700'). Follow the VIEWPOINT sign northwest up this 0.3-mile spur, which ends atop a marble-crested ridge with dramatic views north and south along the coast. Keep watch for red-tailed hawks, American kestrels, and, if luck is on your side, endangered California condors in search of tasty rotting flesh. When ready, head back to the spur junction.

The loop continues southwest on a gentle grade along a ridge crest of exposed marble, easily identified by its white to gray coloring and sugary texture. You'll soon emerge on bare golden hillsides that in spring display decadent carpets of wildflowers. The path plunges south and passes a huge, temporarily stabilized landslide scar above Highway 1. A mile farther you'll arrive at a bridge near the loop junction. From here retrace your steps to the trailhead.

Trip 26

MCWAY FALLS

LENGTH AND TYPE: 1-mile out-and-back

RATING: Easy

TRAIL CONDITION: Well maintained, poison oak, good for kids

HIGHLIGHTS: Unforgettable overlook of an 80-foot waterfall that drops from a granite precipice into a serene cove

TO REACH THE TRAILHEAD: The trailhead is on the east end of the main parking lot.

TRIP SUMMARY: This is one of Big Sur's shortest, most spectacular, and most popular trails. You'll follow McWay Creek a half mile to the viewpoint atop an open bluff for stunning views of the cove and open coastline. Summer crowds are elbow to elbow along this heavily used trail.

Trip Description

From the east end of the parking lot, the **Waterfall Overlook Trail** crosses a bridge over **McWay Creek** to a **spur junction** (0.1 mile, 250'). Turn left on this spur and walk 50 feet to see the Pelton Wheel, a vintage hydroelectric plant that once harnessed steep, low-volume McWay Creek to generate electricity. It supplied Saddle Rock Ranch (now part of the state park) with all of its power needs until 1952, when Pacific Gas & Electric brought in power.

McWay Falls plunges 80 feet over a granite precipice to pristine McWay Cove.

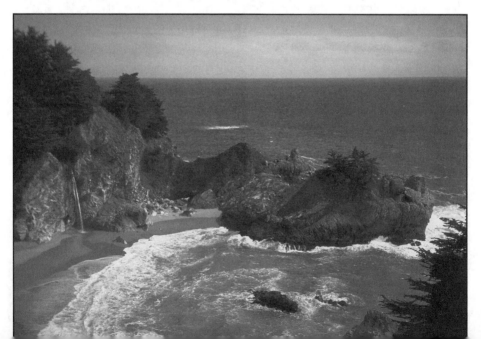

From the spur junction, the main trail heads southwest through a tunnel beneath Highway 1, emerging on the north end of **McWay Cove,** one of Julia Pfeiffer's favorite places to sit, wander, and explore. At one time, a trail descended to the cove, but access is no longer permitted down the rocky, unstable cliffs. Trespassing on the beach can also interrupt the feeding and breeding patterns of sea otters, peregrine falcons, and other protected species.

Bear right for the best vantage point of 80-foot **McWay Falls,** which plunges over a narrow notch in the granite cliff face to the wave-washed crescent of sand below. Fragrant coastal scrub flanks the trail, highlighted in spring by the orange and yellow blossoms of paintbrush, golden yarrow, and sticky monkeyflowers. Palms, bluegum eucalypti, and a number of other exotic species are remnants of a garden planted by the Browns, former owners of Saddle Rock Ranch.

In the 1920s, Lathrop and Helen Hooper Brown purchased the ranch from Christopher McWay, who had settled here in the late 1870s. The Browns built a simple redwood cabin on this overlook, replacing it in 1940 with a larger dwelling called the **Waterfall House.** Helen Brown donated the property for parkland in 1961, and the spectacular house was later demolished. The trail ends at the former homesite, a great spot to watch for the spouts of migrating gray whales.

WHALE-WATCHING ■ ■ ■ ■ ■ ■ ■ ■ ■ ■ ■ ■ ■ ■ ■ ■ ■ ■

Don't miss some of the best opportunities for whale-watching along the Big Sur coast at the bend at the end of Overlook Trail. In December and January, the gray whales migrate southward to their breeding and calving grounds off the Baja California coast. Watch for their high, bushy, heart-shaped blow up to 15 feet and the occasional fluke lifted out of the water prior to a deep dive. These gray whales undertake one of the longest annual migrations of any mammal, traveling some 9,300–12,500 miles (15,000–20,000 km) round-trip. Many whales pass close to shore at this point, and occasionally one will come into the mouth of the cove. In March and April, they can be seen returning north to their summer feeding grounds in the North Pacific.

■ ■

CHAPTER twelve

Limekiln State Park

C RUISING HIGHWAY I, most visitors overlook Limekiln State Park. Yet the sheer, jagged cliffs that make coastal access so difficult along most of the Big Sur coast are not an issue at Limekiln, where you can step a few yards from a shady redwood canyon for a barefoot stroll on the beach.

Once exploited and then forgotten, the park boasts a rich history of homesteaders and entrepreneurs who tramped down the lonely, isolated coast in the late 1800s in search of opportunity. Today, hikers stroll in peaceful solitude amid forests that once supported timber harvesting and limestone extraction and a beach that once flanked a busy shipping port.

Added to the state park system in 1995, Limekiln comprises 716 acres and offers three short hiking trails that follow Limekiln Creek through redwood-lined canyons to a spectacular waterfall and historic limekilns that lend the park its name. The park is open for day use and overnight camping.

DIRECTIONS: The park entrance is on the east side of Highway 1, 56 miles south of Carmel, 2 miles south of Lucia, and 94 miles north of San Luis Obispo.

VISITOR CENTER: Big Sur Station: (831) 667-2315. The station is on Highway 1, 30 miles north of park entrance and just south of Pfeiffer Big Sur State Park. Open daily 8 a.m.–6 p.m. Memorial Day through Labor Day, 8 a.m.–4:30 p.m. the rest of the year.

NEAREST CAMPGROUND: The park campground (33 sites, $35/night; reservations recommended in summer and on holidays) offers developed sites with picnic tables and fire rings. Some sites accommodate RVs and trailers. There are showers, picnic areas, and flush toilets. For more information call Reserve America at (800) 444-7275 or visit ReserveAmerica.com.

INFORMATION: Open daily 9 a.m.–7 p.m. Memorial Day through Labor Day, 10 a.m.–5 p.m. the rest of the year. There is a $10 day-use fee. No dogs or bikes allowed on park trails.

WEBSITE: parks.ca.gov

PHONE: (831) 667-2403

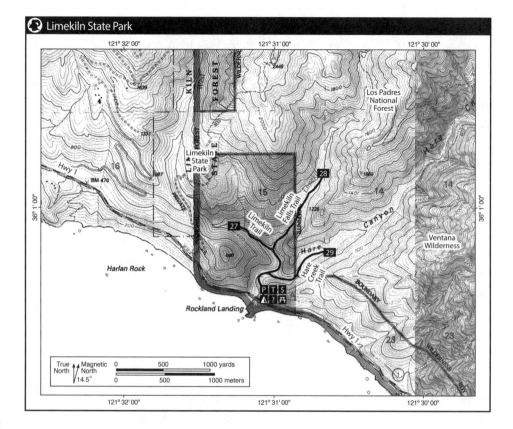

Limekiln State Park

Trip 27

LIMEKILN TRAIL

LENGTH AND TYPE: 0.8-mile out-and-back

RATING: Easy

TRAIL CONDITION: Well maintained, good for kids

HIGHLIGHTS: Historic limekilns nestled in a peaceful redwood grove

TO REACH THE TRAILHEAD: Day-use parking is immediately past the kiosk, adjacent to the restrooms. Park your vehicle and stroll past the north end of the campground (sites 23–34), where all three of the park's trails begin.

TRIP SUMMARY: This hike meanders along Limekiln Creek's West Fork amid dense redwood groves, once home to a vigorous lumber and lime manufacturing industry. Early settlers used harvested trees to fuel kilns that purified, or "slaked," limestone extracted from rich deposits in the canyon. The lime was then loaded in barrels and hauled to Rockland Landing, near Limekiln Beach. Schooners transported the lime to Monterey and San Francisco, where it was used to make cement. Schooners also brought in heavy goods and supplies to sustain the growing population. Today, all that remains are four stone-and-steel furnaces from which the creek and park takes its name. The trail roughly follows an old wagon trail to the kilns.

FIFTY CENTS A DAY ■ ■ ■ ■ ■ ■ ■ ■ ■ ■ ■ ■ ■ ■ ■ ■ ■ ■ ■

Only the hardiest, most self-reliant settlers successfully homesteaded the seemingly impenetrable Santa Lucia Range. These early explorers, adventurers, and entrepreneurs forged a loose network of trails to cultivate flood-prone land and raise livestock, relying on one another for bartered goods and services. When there was a need for money, companies such as Rockland Lime & Lumber offered hard work. Whether they were harvesting redwoods to fuel the limekilns or building wagon trails along Limekiln Creek, men in 1920 made $.50 a day during a typical 10-hour workday.

■ ■

Trip Description

From the trailhead (70'), you'll cross a large wooden footbridge over **Hare Creek**. A few paces beyond the bridge, the trail passes a junction with the eastbound **Hare Creek Trail**. Bear left and climb above the confluence of Hare Creek and **Limekiln Creek,** which flow clear as glass past lush carpets of ferns and mosses. You'll soon pass the remains of an old-growth forest, logged to sustain the appetite of Rockland Lime & Lumber Company. Continue 150 feet past the confluence of the **West Fork** and Limekiln Creek to a junction with the **Limekiln Falls Trail** (0.25 mile, 110') on your right.

Skirting the west bank of the West Fork, the main trail continues straight, turns north, then crosses the creek on a **wooden bridge** (0.3 mile, 170'). A minute farther a split rail fence marks the site of the large stone-and-steel **kilns** (0.4 mile, 240'), built at the base of a natural limestone deposit. Take a moment to explore

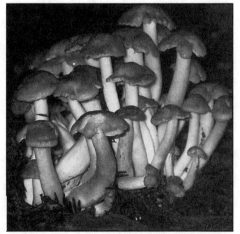

A diverse array of fungi live within the damp, dark, dense redwood forests that shade Limekiln Creek.

the ruins before returning the way you came. Please don't hike off-trail, as canyon walls are steep, poison oak is abundant, and the kilns may be unstable.

Trip 28

LIMEKILN FALLS TRAIL

LENGTH AND TYPE: 1-mile out-and-back

RATING: Easy

TRAIL CONDITION: Well maintained, good for kids

HIGHLIGHTS: A 100-foot waterfall cascading down vertical limestone cliffs

TO REACH THE TRAILHEAD: Day-use parking is immediately past the kiosk, adjacent to the restrooms. Park your vehicle and stroll past the north end of the campground (sites 23–34),

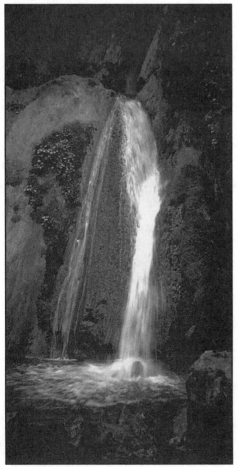

where all three of the park's trails begin.

TRIP SUMMARY: This hike traverses the steepest coastal canyon in the Lower 48, where Limekiln Creek's headwaters pour down from Cone Peak, nearly a mile above sea level and just 3.2 miles from the Pacific. The short, easy trail leads to the base of the falls.

Trip Description

From the trailhead (70'), cross the large wooden footbridge over **Hare Creek**. Bear left past the **Hare Creek Trail junction** and climb past the remains of an old-growth forest. You'll soon reach the **Limekiln Falls Trail junction** (0.25 mile, 110'), 150 feet past the confluence of the **West Fork** and **Limekiln Creek**. Bear right and head northeast.

The trail descends a few steps, then crosses the creek on a narrow wooden

Limekiln Falls plunges 100 feet past limestone cliffs as it descends the steepest coastal canyon in the continental US.

footbridge. Follow the east bank, then turn northwest across another small **footbridge** (0.3 mile, 140'). The trail crosses the creek once more and climbs a small set of stairs past a wooden retaining **wall** (0.4 mile, 170'). Follow the sound of falling water 0.1 mile uphill to the base of these spectacular 100-foot falls. Visitors gaze in silence as water cascades down the moss- and fern-covered limestone cliffs. Rest and feel the mist on your face before heading back.

Trip 29

HARE CREEK TRAIL

LENGTH AND TYPE: 0.6-mile out-and-back

RATING: Easy

TRAIL CONDITION: Well maintained, poison oak, good for kids

HIGHLIGHTS: A fertile coastal river canyon lined with majestic old-growth redwoods

TO REACH THE TRAILHEAD: Day-use parking is immediately past the kiosk, adjacent to the restrooms. Park your vehicle and stroll past the north end of the campground (sites 23–34), where all three of the park's trails begin.

TRIP SUMMARY: This hike begins amid a narrow band of redwoods along Hare Creek. Though you'll find a few mature old-growth trees, most of the redwoods are relative toddlers. These stands are rebounding from heavy logging in the late 1800s, when Rockland Lime & Lumber harvested dozens of ancient trees to fuel nearby kilns used to purify commercial limestone. Today, the trail leads past quiet, undisturbed groves.

Trip Description

From the trailhead, you'll cross the large wooden footbridge over **Hare Creek**. Thirty feet beyond the bridge, the trail reaches the **Hare Creek Trail junction**. Turn right and head east along the north bank. The trail skirts the clear creek, sheltered by sheer canyon walls and a dense redwood canopy. Shrouded in darkness, your surroundings suggest a vast forest, but this narrow band of trees is restricted to the canyon floor.

The trail soon emerges on open slopes that support oaks, shrubs, and grasses, then ascends **rock steps** (0.2 mile, 160') past lush ferns, redwood sorrel, blackberries and thimbleberries. Steep cliff faces across the canyon are draped with a vibrant green tapestry of mosses and ferns. Head back when you reach the END OF TRAIL sign beside a large downed **redwood** (0.3 mile, 200'). Avoid hiking off-trail, as poison oak is abundant and the canyon walls are steep and unstable.

STEELHEAD MIGRATION ▪ ▪ ▪ ▪ ▪ ▪ ▪ ▪ ▪ ▪ ▪ ▪ ▪ ▪ ▪ ▪ ▪

Serving as a vital habitat for southern steelhead trout, the entire Limekiln and Hare watershed is free flowing (i.e., no dams). Slowly approach small trailside pools and you may spot an immature steelhead darting amid shadows along the creek bottom.

Part of the family *Salmonidae*, which includes all salmon and trout, steelhead are the anadromous form of rainbow trout, which means the fish are born in freshwater and migrate to the ocean as adults. They spend their first one to three years here before heading out to sea from Limekiln Beach. After one to four years in the Pacific, they return to their native creeks to spawn.

In California most steelhead spawn from December through April. Limekiln State Park supports a significant run of southern steelhead trout. Contact the California Department of Fish & Game for local fishing regulations: (831) 649-2870, dfg.ca.gov.

CHAPTER thirteen

Pacific Valley to San Simeon State Park

■　■　■　■　■　■　■　■　■　■　■　■　■　■

THIS CHAPTER DESCRIBES state and federal day-use lands from Pacific Valley south to Sand Dollar Beach, Jade Cove, Ragged Point, Piedras Blancas, Hearst Memorial State Beach, and San Simeon. This stretch of coast is a premier hiking destination. Trails meander through wind-sculpted pine forests, across slopes of fragrant coastal scrub and spring wildflowers, and down to driftwood-strewn beaches. You'll also find plenty of the trademark ocean views that draw people up and down Highway 1.

Pacific Valley to Jade Cove

Pacific Valley's rocky bluffs and rolling prairie overlook a prominent marine terrace punctuated by archways and pounding surf. Several intriguing trails cut through golden grasslands and dense coastal shrub to secluded coves and dramatic views. Farther south off Highway 1, Sand Dollar Beach and Jade Cove offer access to beachcombers, anglers, surfers, scuba divers, and rock hounds in search of the coveted green gemstone.

> **DIRECTIONS:** This coastline is accessible via pullouts along Highway 1, some 60 miles south of Rio Road in Carmel and 30 miles north of Hearst San Simeon State Historical Monument (Hearst Castle).
>
> **VISITOR CENTER:** Pacific Valley Station: (805) 927-4211. Open daily 8 a.m.– 5 p.m. The station is on the east side of Highway 1, 3 miles north of the Sand Dollar Beach Day-Use Area, 60 miles south of Carmel, and 30 miles north of Hearst Castle.
>
> **NEAREST CAMPGROUND:** Plaskett Creek Campground (41 sites, $22/night; 3 group sites, $80/night; reservations recommended in summer and holidays) is on the east side of Highway 1, 0.1 mile south of the entrance to the Sand Dollar Beach Day-Use Area. There's a maximum of eight people per site. Each site includes a picnic

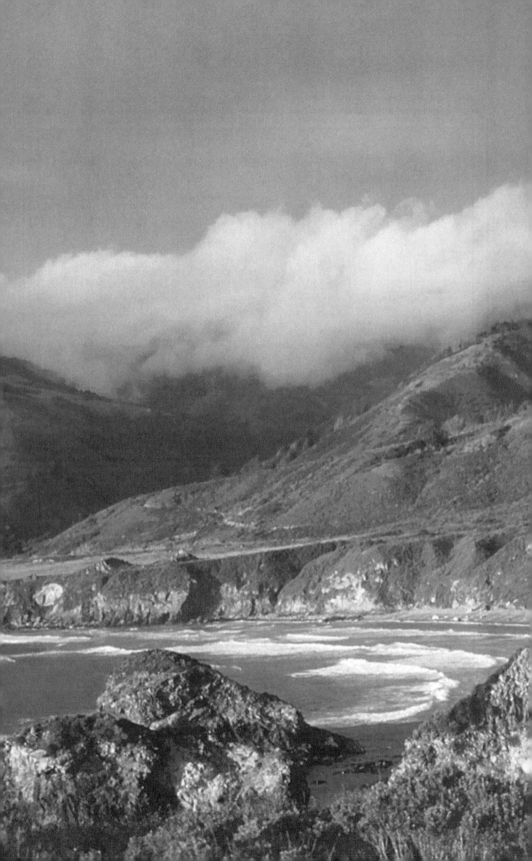

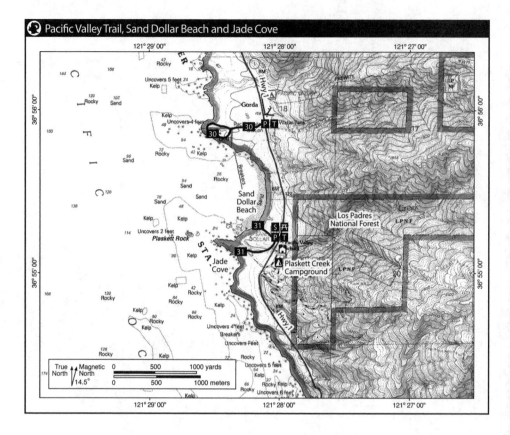

Pacific Valley Trail, Sand Dollar Beach and Jade Cove

table, fire ring, and pedestal grill. Drinking water is available. For more information call Reserve America at (800) 444-7275 or visit ReserveAmerica.com.

INFORMATION: Open 8 a.m.–sunset. There's a $10 parking fee at Sand Dollar Beach. If you're willing to hike 0.3 mile, you'll find free parking at turnouts on Highway 1 north and south of Sand Dollar Beach. Dogs must be leashed. No camping or fires permitted in Pacific Valley, Sand Dollar Beach, or Jade Cove.

WEBSITE: parksman.com

PHONE: USFS Pacific Valley Station: (805) 927-4211; USFS Monterey District Headquarters: (831) 385-5434

Trip 30

PACIFIC VALLEY TRAIL

LENGTH AND TYPE: 0.7-mile out-and-back

RATING: Easy

TRAIL CONDITION: Clear, poison oak

HIGHLIGHTS: Dramatic views of eroding coastal cliffs, jagged outcrops, and sculpted arches

TO REACH THE TRAILHEAD: The trail starts from a free turnout on the west side of Highway 1, directly across from the Pacific Valley Station (see Visitor Center, page 128).

TRIP SUMMARY: Despite its name, this is not a valley, but 3 miles of gently sloping marine terrace. The flat coastal expanse represents a dramatic change from the Big Sur's trademark steep topography and offers some of the easiest hiking and beach access in the area. Bluff trails lead to daunting cliffs and promontories with spectacular views of the boulder-strewn coastline. Keep watch for passing whales, as well as seals and otters amid the nearshore kelp forests.

Trip Description

From the Highway 1 turnout, you'll step up and over a cattle gate onto a broad flat terrace. The US Forest Service manages this land, which has been extensively grazed for decades. At any time, you may share the trail with roaming livestock.

The trail traverses the terrace past waste-high coyote brush amid an open meadow. In spring these grasslands are speckled with buttercups, lupines, and poppies that have survived the intense grazing pressure.

Continuing toward the ocean, the trail leads to another cattle gate up and over the fence. Beyond it, the vegetation shifts from open grasslands to native lupine, poison oak, sagebrush, coyote brush, and sticky monkeyflower, easily identified by its narrow leaves and bright orange flowers. You'll soon wander past small, wind-sculpted dunes stabilized by low-lying sand verbena, lupine, lizard tail, and more poison oak.

Past the dunes, the trail veers north and gently climbs the scalloped cliffs to a dramatic **rocky promontory** (0.5 mile, 40'). Behind you to the northeast, the rocky ridges above **Limekiln** and **Hare Creeks** climb toward **Cone Peak,** comprising the steepest coastal slope in the Lower 48. To the west, **Plaskett Rock** thrusts above the surf amid natural arches carved by the Pacific. Watch for sea otters, which float on their backs to crack open shellfish. Resting otters are often mistaken for floating logs, as they wrap themselves in kelp in order to hold position on the surface.

You'll eventually circle back to the main trail, recrossing the coastal bluffs toward the turnout.

Trip 31

SAND DOLLAR BEACH & JADE COVE

LENGTH AND TYPE: 1-mile out-and-back

RATING: Easy

TRAIL CONDITION: Clear, poison oak

HIGHLIGHTS: Rugged cliffs overlook wave-washed coves speckled with veins of jade

TO REACH THE TRAILHEAD: The Sand Dollar Beach Day-Use Area is on Highway 1, 32.5 miles south of Big Sur Station, 63 miles south of Carmel, 0.1 mile north of Plaskett Creek Campground, and 15.1 miles north of Ragged Point ($10 day-use fee). There are restrooms and water at the trailhead.

TRIP SUMMARY: This hike begins along open bluffs blanketed in fragrant coastal scrub and heads south to cliffs overlooking Jade Cove. A steep 100-foot spur descends to a beach brimming with jade that has been sculpted smooth by the pounding surf. The trail then doubles back north toward the horseshoe cove at Sand Dollar Beach.

Trip Description

From the west side of the parking lot (90'), clamber up and over a cattle gate in the fence, then head south beside the planted Monterey cypress trees that shade the lot. The trail soon

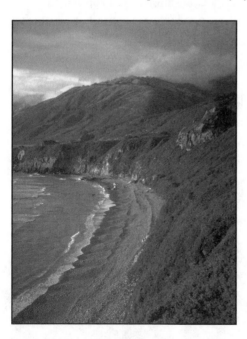

turns west toward the south end of **Sand Dollar Beach.** You'll stroll past open grasslands and low-lying coastal scrub to the dramatic cliffs above **Jade Cove** (0.2 mile, 60'). A short but steep and unstable spur leads down to the cove. Be aware of poison oak as you scurry down this spur.

Large green jade boulders and coarse gravel extend beyond the pounding surf into deep water. Just offshore is 100-foot **Cave Rock,** whose jade inner walls are continuously smoothed and polished by breaking waves.

A sweeping crescent of coarse white sand is home to one of Big Sur's most consistent surf breaks.

STONE OF HEAVEN ■

Ranging in size from pebbles to large stones, jade lies scattered throughout Jade Cove, atop the sand, beneath overhangs, and just off the beach, accessible to both beach-combers and divers. The USFS prohibits jade collection above the mean high tide line.

Chinese consider jade the stone of heaven, and artisans have carved the gem into tools and art objects for thousands of years. The type of jade found here is the mineral nephrite. Pure nephrite is white, but impurities lend the local jade a range of brilliant shades, from light turquoise to deep emerald green. Jade is strong and durable, harder than some types of steel, and the most difficult gem to polish.

Jade Cove comprises a jumble of rocks known as the Franciscan complex, formed millions of years ago when a massive tectonic plate was driven beneath the continent. Colliding plates crushed the rocks, which were then sheared off by the massive Sur-Nacimiento Fault and squeezed upward to form the rocky cove. Cov-ered by ocean sediments for millennia, jade formed as minerals in the sedimentary rock (probably sandstone). Buried deep in the earth, these minerals were exposed to high pressure at low temperatures, metamorphosing them into jade.

■ ■

Head back past the parking lot a few feet north to a trail **junction** (0.5 mile, 40') on the left that leads toward the beach. You'll soon reach a fork. The right branch leads to an overlook, an excellent spot to watch for migrating gray whales. In spring, mothers escort their calves close to shore for protection from such predators as great white sharks and orcas. This is also an excellent spot to bird-watch. Boasting black bodies and bright orange beaks, oystercatchers perch along the rocks, while plovers scurry through the surf, and pelicans skim nearshore waves.

The left branch leads down to Sand Dollar Beach, the longest contiguous stretch of sand along the Big Sur coast. At low tide, it's an ideal spot for a barefoot stroll, surf casting, or surfing. Winter surge strips sand from the beach and replaces it with small granite rubble.

Ragged Point

RAGGED POINT lies midway between LA and San Francisco, where the vast Pacific meets the towering Santa Lucia Range. Here, a private parcel welcomes tourists with a short, sheer trail that skirts Big Sur's tallest waterfall, plunging 300 feet to a black sand beach. Those willing to brave the trail are rewarded with exquisite views. In wet weather, the trail is often closed, while the owner may restrict access anytime.

DIRECTIONS: Ragged Point lies off the west side of Highway 1, 15 miles north of Hearst Castle and 44 miles south of Big Sur.

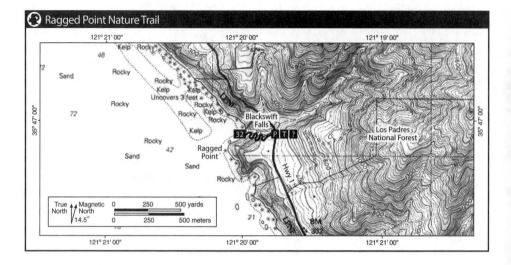

VISITOR CENTERS: Pacific Valley Station: (805) 927-4211. Open daily 8 a.m.–5 p.m. The station is on the east side of Highway 1, 16 miles north of Ragged Point. Hearst San Simeon State Historical Monument (Hearst Castle): (805) 927-2010. Open daily 8 a.m.–6 p.m. The visitor center is off Highway 1, 14 miles south of Ragged Point.

NEAREST CAMPGROUND: The nearest campground to the north is Plaskett Creek, while the nearest campgrounds to the south are in San Simeon State Park.

INFORMATION: This trail is on private land, and the owner may deny access at any time.

WEBSITE: raggedpointinn.com | **PHONE:** (805) 927-4502

Trip 32

RAGGED POINT NATURE TRAIL

LENGTH AND TYPE: 1-mile out-and-back

RATING: Moderate to strenuous

TRAIL CONDITION: Passable to difficult, poison oak

HIGHLIGHTS: In winter this tallest tiered waterfall in Big Sur cascades 300 feet into the surf off Ragged Point.

TO REACH THE TRAILHEAD: Ragged Point is off Highway 1, 23 miles north of Cambria and 44 miles south of Big Sur. Turn west into the Ragged Point Inn & Restaurant parking lot. The trail begins at the gazebo, just past the coffee shop and gift shop.

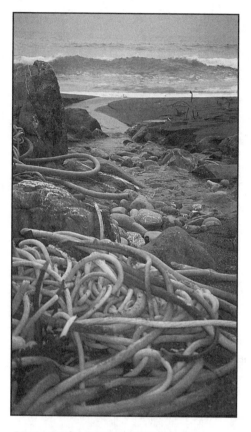

Blackswift Creek plunges 300 feet before disappearing into the surging tide.

TRIP SUMMARY: This hike descends the steep canyon beside Blackswift Falls, which plunges hundreds of feet onto the soft black sand of a secluded cove at the edge of the Pacific. This short, steep hike is subject to washouts each winter and is moderately overgrown with coastal brush in the spring. Watch for poison oak and ticks, which cling to trailside plants.

Trip Description

From the trailhead (380'), you'll switch-back along the steep, eroding canyon walls beside **Blackswift Creek**. Views from the top bear witness to a dramatic topo-graphical change, from gentle slopes and broad marine terraces south of the point to Big Sur's trademark rocky bluffs north of the point.

The trail drops 0.2 mile to a small wooden bridge at the base of **Blackswift Falls.** Stop on the bridge to admire the 300-foot tiered waterfall as it tumbles to the beach and mingles with the churning surf. Wander amid the granite boulders atop black sand before returning up the trail.

Piedras Blancas

TRUE TO ITS NAME, *Piedras Blancas* (Spanish for white stones) is named for a trio of treacherous white rocks just off the point. In 1875, a lighthouse was built to guide mariners along this lonely, fogbound coast. Today, the lighthouse is automated, and the only residents are thousands of noisy, boisterous seals, including massive elephant seals, which beach just south of the light.

The Bureau of Land Management (BLM) manages Piedras Blancas and is restoring the site. Guided tours offer insight into a bygone era of maritime travel. For tour information, see page 138.

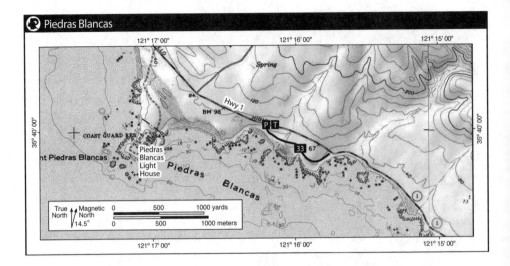

DIRECTIONS: Piedras Blancas is off Highway 1, 7.7 miles north of San Simeon.

VISITOR CENTER: Hearst San Simeon State Historical Monument (Hearst Castle): (805) 927-2010. The visitor center is a mile west of Highway 1, 5 miles north of San Simeon State Park, directly across the street from W.R. Hearst Memorial State Beach. Open daily 8 a.m.–sunset.

NEAREST CAMPGROUND: See San Simeon State Park (page 142).

INFORMATION: The BLM prohibits entry to the access roads, grounds, or lighthouse outside of designated times unless you're part of a scheduled tour. For information about docent-led guided tours visit piedrasblancas.org or call (805) 927-7361.

WEBSITE: blm.gov, piedrasblancas.org, or hearstcastle.org

PHONE: BLM, Piedras Blancas Light Station: (805) 927-7361.

Trip 33

PIEDRAS BLANCAS

LENGTH AND TYPE: 0.8-mile out-and-back

RATING: Easy

TRAIL CONDITION: Well maintained, good for kids

HIGHLIGHTS: Thousands of elephant seals spar for dominance, mate and give birth, or merely bask in the sun, flip sand on their backs, and snort at gaping tourists.

TO REACH THE TRAILHEAD: The Piedras Blancas elephant seal rookery is on the west side of Highway 1, 7.7 miles north of San Simeon. The parking lot is at Vista Point. There are no facilities or water at the trailhead.

TRIP SUMMARY: This short, easy trail skirts a broad marine terrace to a small sandy cove inhabited by thousands of noisy northern elephant seals.

BASKING & BARKING & BELCHING, OH MY! ■ ■ ■ ■ ■ ■ ■ ■ ■

The best time to view Piedras Blancas's elephant seals is December through March. Arriving in early December, enormous bulls wage violent, often-bloody battles to establish dominance. The successful bull becomes the alpha male and has the best chance of mating. When females arrive in late December, this bull establishes and guards his harem.

Days after the females arrive, they give birth and produce thick, rich milk that is 55% fat. Newborn pups suckle for a month, growing from about 70 pounds at birth up to 300 pounds. Weaned pups are lovingly nicknamed "weaners." By late March most of the adult females have mated with either the alpha male or competing beta bulls.

Females soon return to the ocean alone, leaving weaners to fend for themselves and learn how to swim and feed. They remain on the beach until the end of April, wading in tide pools, snorting at tourists, molting their black baby fur, and growing shiny new silver coats.

All elephant seals return to shore to molt in spring and summer. Females and juveniles land in April and May, subadult males in May and June, and enormous males in July and August. You'll recognize adult males by their enormous size (more than twice the weight of adult females) and large proboscis (reminiscent of an elephant's trunk).

■ ■

These weaned elephant seals will snort at tourists, molt their black fur, and wade in the tidepools before venturing for months alone in the open ocean.

Trip Description

From the parking lot, follow the raucous barking sounds south. You'll skirt the open bluffs 0.1 mile, enjoying sweeping views of the sea and rocky shore. The trail quickly reaches a small cove packed flipper to flipper with elephant seals.

Turn your attention from the rookery to the **Piedras Blancas lighthouse**, built in 1875 to guide ships between the lights at Point Conception to the south and Point Piños to the north. The original tower was 115 feet tall and housed a first-order Fresnel lens. Today, technology has eased navigation and the light is now automated. The original Fresnel lens is on display at the Veterans Building on Main Street in Cambria, 13 miles south.

Guided tours of the lighthouse are offered Tuesday, Thursday, and Saturday September 1–June 14 and Monday–Saturday June 15–August 31 ($10/adults, $5 children ages 6–17, free/children age 5 and under). Contact the Piedras Blancas Light Station for further information: (805) 927-7361, piedrasblancas.org.

Hearst Memorial State Beach

THIS SANDY COVE was once part of the 24,000-acre Hearst property at San Simeon, a playground for the family, friends, and guests of media tycoon William Randolph Hearst. In 1953 the Hearst Corporation, which owns Hearst Castle and the surrounding acreage, donated the park grounds in memory of its founder.

San Simeon remains a popular year-round destination for visitors interested in hiking, swimming, fishing, kayaking, picnicking, and whale- and bird-watching. In May the park hosts "A Day in Old San Simeon," a celebration of the area's 19th-century heyday.

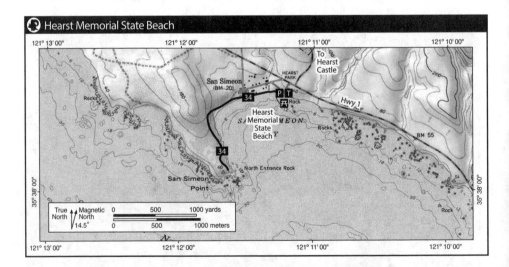

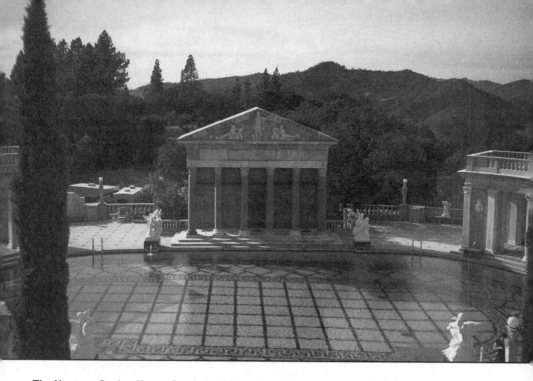

The Neptune Pool at Hearst Castle is 104 feet by 58 feet and holds 345,000 gallons of water.

ONE MAN'S CASTLE ■ ■ ■ ■ ■ ■ ■ ■ ■ ■ ■ ■ ■ ■ ■ ■ ■ ■ ■

Perched high atop the San Simeon hills, Hearst Castle was the collaborative vision of eccentric news baron William Randolph Hearst and architect Julia Morgan. Transformation of the ranch and campsite into the lavish 165-room castle began in 1919 and dragged on nearly 30 years. It remains unfinished. A showcase for Hearst's international collection of antiques and art pieces, the 250,000-acre estate also included guesthouses, elaborate gardens and pools, tennis courts, and a zoo. Famous guests through the years included President Calvin Coolidge, Winston Churchill, Charlie Chaplin, and myriad other bigwigs and Hollywood celebs.

On most Friday and Saturday evenings from September through December, Hearst Castle offers two-hour living history tours ($30/adults, $15/children ages 6–17) that capture the bygone lifestyle of this great estate. Docents dress in elegant vintage clothing, discuss the social life of Hearst's guests, and lead visitors on enchanting strolls around La Cuesta Encantanda (The Enchanted Hill). For more information, visit hearstcastle.org.

■ ■

DIRECTIONS: Hearst Memorial State Beach is directly across Highway 1 from the Hearst Castle entrance, 8 miles north of Cambria and 60 miles south of Big Sur. Turn west on San Simeon Road and continue 0.2 mile to the large parking area.

VISITOR CENTER: Hearst San Simeon State Historical Monument (Hearst Castle): (805) 927-2010. The visitor center is a mile west of Highway 1, 5 miles north of San Simeon State Park, directly across the street from W.R. Hearst Memorial State Beach. Open daily 8 a.m.–sunset.

NEAREST CAMPGROUND: San Simeon Creek Campground, within San Simeon State Park, is 5 miles south of San Simeon (134 sites, $35/night; reservations recommended in summer and first come, first served October 1–March 14). On a plateau overlooking the Pacific, this campground includes showers and RV sites (no hookups). For more information call (800) 444-7275 or visit parks.ca.gov. Washburn Campground, within San Simeon State Park, 5 miles south of San Simeon (68 sites, $22/night; reservations recommended in summer; no showers), is a mile inland on a plateau overlooking the Santa Lucia Range. For more information call (800) 444-7275 or visit parks.ca.gov.

INFORMATION: The beach is open until sunset. There is no entrance fee. The day-use area offers 150 parking spaces, restrooms, water faucets, 24 picnic tables, barbecue grill stands, and a concession stand. Dogs must be on a leash. No overnight camping. Easy beach access makes this a great spot for fishing, beachcombing, swimming, and boat launching. In summer the concession stand sells bait and rents fishing poles, kayaks, and boogie boards. Licenses are not required when fishing from the pier, but limits are enforced.

WEBSITE: parks.ca.gov | **PHONE:** (805) 927-2020

Trip 34

HEARST MEMORIAL STATE BEACH

LENGTH AND TYPE: 2.5-mile out-and-back

RATING: Easy

TRAIL CONDITION: Clear, poison oak

HIGHLIGHTS: Soothing views of the Pacific from atop open bluffs

TO REACH THE TRAILHEAD: The trail begins from the north side of the main parking lot.

TRIP SUMMARY: This hike explores the half-mile coastal crescent that curls toward San Simeon Point. You'll stroll the soft white sand above open bluffs of coastal scrub, through forests of eucalyptus, pine, and cypress to tide pools teeming with life. Foxes, coyotes, and bobcats slink along the bluffs, while red- and white-tailed hawks and northern harriers scour the brush for the rabbits, mice, and voles. Watch nearshore kelp beds to spot sea otters, harbor seals, and sea lions as they frolic, feed, or happily float by.

Trip Description

From the parking lot, walk toward the beach through a stately eucalyptus grove to a small picnic area. Heading west, the route crosses **Arroyo del Puerto Creek** (0.1 mile, 10'), an ankle-deep wade in all but the wettest months.

CONTENDER FROM DOWN UNDER ■ ■ ■ ■ ■ ■ ■ ■ ■ ■ ■ ■ ■ ■

Early California settlers planted introduced Australian bluegum eucalyptus trees as windbreaks, ornamentals, and for firewood. The species adapted so well to woodland areas along the central coast, that it quickly outcompeted native plants. Turns out, the trees secrete certain pathogens that inhibit the growth of native plants and discourage wildlife. As a result, the eucalyptus stands have little to no understory and are considered extremely invasive.

■ ■

The path curves south to a **junction** (0.5 mile, 20'), where you'll bear right on a distinct trail toward the eroding bluffs. Atop the bluffs, you'll stroll past eucalypti and brief glimpses of glistening **San Simeon Bay**. The trail soon merges with a dirt road to **San Simeon Point** that passes numerous coastal overlooks. Pause at the point (1.2 miles, 20') to appreciate this pristine coastline before returning the way you came.

If you wish to hike farther, the trail leads west through a dense cypress forest to emerge on windswept dunes west of the point.

William Randolph Hearst bought out his coast-side neighbors to secure his private beach to host family, friends, and guests.

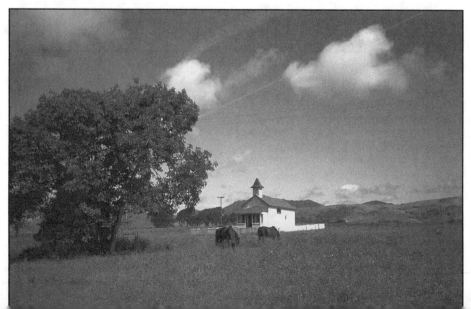

San Simeon State Park

OFFERING EXCEPTIONAL BEAUTY and respite from the everyday bustle, San Simeon was the perfect location for William Randolph Hearst to build his 165-room castle. It began as a rancheria during the mission era, serving as a coastal access point for supplies shipped to and from Monterey's Mission San Antonio. The park's Washburn Day-Use Area served as a gravel quarry through the late 1920s.

Set aside in 1932, San Simeon State Park is one of California's oldest reserves. Its 541 acres comprise miles of sandy beaches and rocky shorelines, as well as Monterey pine forests, rolling grasslands, and seasonal wetlands, creeks, and bogs.

DIRECTIONS: The park is off Highway 1, 35 miles north of San Luis Obispo and 65 miles south of Big Sur. Turn east on San Simeon Creek Road, drive a quarter mile, then turn right at the park entrance.

VISITOR CENTER: Hearst San Simeon State Historical Monument (Hearst Castle): (805) 927-2010. The visitor center is a mile west of Highway 1, 5 miles north of San Simeon State Park, directly across the street from W.R. Hearst Memorial State Beach. Open daily 8 a.m.–sunset.

NEAREST CAMPGROUNDS: Both the Washburn and San Simeon Creek Campgrounds lie within the park. San Simeon Creek Campground (134 sites, $35/night) provides a picnic table and fire ring at each site, restrooms with flush toilets and showers, pay phones, and a dump station and water fill-up for RVs. The adjoining Washburn Campground (68 sites, $22/night) provides a picnic table and fire ring at each site and vault toilets. Reservations are required between March 14 and September 30. For more

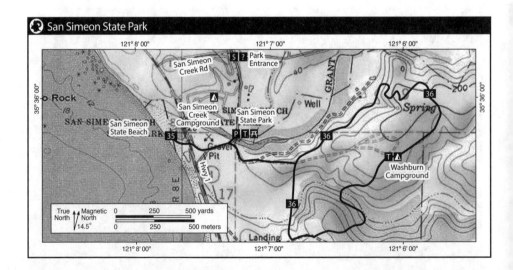

information call Reserve America at (800) 444-7275 or visit ReserveAmerica.com. The rest of the year, sites are available on a first-come, first-serve basis.

INFORMATION: San Simeon State Beach is open from sunrise to sunset. No dogs or bikes allowed on park trails. The San Simeon Nature Trail is wheelchair-accessible from the footbridge crossing San Simeon Creek to the beach and along the seasonal wetlands.

WEBSITE: parks.ca.gov | **PHONE:** (805) 927-2020

Trip 35

SAN SIMEON STATE BEACH

LENGTH AND TYPE: 1-mile out-and-back

RATING: Easy

TRAIL CONDITION: Well maintained, poison oak, good for kids

HIGHLIGHTS: Follow San Simeon Creek through seasonal wetlands to the beach and watch for elephant seals, sea otters, and gray whales.

TO REACH THE TRAILHEAD: The trailhead is adjacent to the Washburn Day-Use Area off Highway 1, immediately past the small bridge over San Simeon Creek. Head east on San Simeon Creek Road, drive a quarter mile, then turn right into the park. Water and restrooms are available.

Follow San Simeon Creek through seasonal wetlands as it deposits fine sand and gnarled driftwood along San Simeon State Beach.

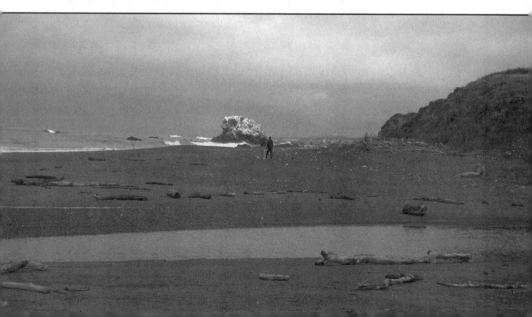

TRIP SUMMARY: This easy hike begins on an elevated boardwalk through San Simeon Creek's unique seasonal wetland and riparian habitat. From the end of the boardwalk, stroll the beach barefoot in either direction. Bring binoculars for a chance at spotting migrating gray whales.

Trip Description

From the parking area, head north along the raised wooden boardwalk toward the mouth of **San Simeon Creek** (20'), which shelters a healthy population of turtles, frogs, snakes, and fish. This boardwalk shields the surrounding seasonal wetlands, which offer habitat to several endangered species. Winter rains fill the wetlands with 1 to 2 feet of nutrient-rich water, nourishing a multitude of small organisms waiting in the mud. As you stroll, listen to the chorus of chirping frogs and watch ducks, egrets, and herons descend on the marsh to feed.

Wheelchair access ends where the boardwalk stops, while the trail continues west under Highway 1 (0.1 mile, 10') to **San Simeon Beach.** Endangered snowy plovers nest along the south end of the beach directly west of the bridge, leading to seasonal closures between February and September. If the beach is closed, head north toward the creek to watch the tides roll in and out. Return the way you came.

POND TURTLE PRIMER ■ ■ ■ ■ ■ ■ ■ ■ ■ ■ ■ ■ ■ ■ ■ ■ ■ ■

By late spring, female Southwestern pond turtles leave San Simeon Creek in search of nesting sites on nearby hills. After digging a hole, they deposit several eggs and return to the creek. When the rainy season arrives, turtle hatchlings instinctively make their way to the creek, where they feed, grow, and spawn, renewing the life cycle. The creek is home to some 50 Southwestern pond turtles. Try to spot them basking on logs or swimming and diving in the shallows.

■ ■

Trip 36

SAN SIMEON NATURE TRAIL

LENGTH AND TYPE: 3.2-mile loop

RATING: Easy

TRAIL CONDITION: Well maintained, poison oak, good for kids

HIGHLIGHTS: A rural landscape wedged between the sheer Santa Lucia Range and the mighty Pacific

TO REACH THE TRAILHEAD: Choose between two trailheads. The northern trailhead is in Washburn Campground, across from Site 213 at the end of Washburn Campground Road. The southern trailhead is 0.1 mile east of the Washburn Day-Use Area, beside a footbridge over San Simeon Creek. Water and restrooms are available at both trailheads.

TRIP SUMMARY: San Simeon Creek ripples through a rolling landscape that's lush green after winter rains, blanketed with wildflowers in spring, and studded with gnarled coast live oaks and wind-sculpted Monterey pines year-round. Diverse habitats shelter a range of wildlife, including woodpeckers, elusive bobcats, coyotes, wintering golden eagles, and wild turkeys. Interpretive signs describe the seasonal wetlands, vernal pools, an 1800s ranch site, and prehistoric cultural sites of the Chumash and Salinian peoples.

Trip Description

From the southern trailhead at the **Washburn Day-Use Area** (30'), a raised wooden boardwalk leads east amid seasonal wetlands, home to endangered Southwestern pond turtles and red-legged frogs. You'll soon cross **Washburn Campground Road** (0.1 mile, 40') and skirt the road for 0.4 mile before reaching an unmarked junction (0.5 mile, 80'). Turn left and hike past eucalyptus trees to the **Whitaker Homesite** (0.8 mile, 40'), an 1800s ranch. A spur to your right leads 0.2 mile to **Washburn Campground.**

Instead, bear left along the trail, which gradually descends to **Whitaker Flats** through introduced Australian bluegum eucalypti amid a thick understory of German ivy from South Africa. These exotic plants invade woodlands throughout California and choke out native plants, threatening the natural ecosystem.

A mature forest of gnarled live oaks and wind-sculpted Monterey pines shades the trail along San Simeon Creek.

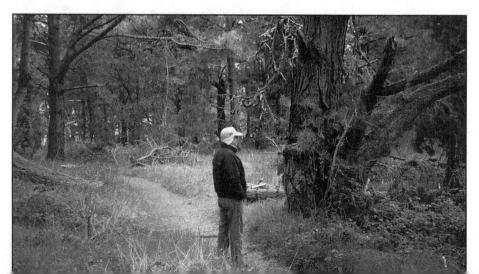

Your only major climb begins and ends in 0.2 mile at the next unmarked junction (1 mile, 180'). The right branch leads 0.3 mile to an open grassy knoll that offers views of the shore inland to the **Santa Lucia Range**. Your route continues along the left branch, descending 100 feet and then climbing 120 feet to a bench and overlook adjacent to the **vernal pools** and **mima mounds**.

VERNAL POOLS & MIMA MOUNDS ■ ■ ■ ■ ■ ■ ■ ■ ■ ■ ■ ■

The uplands of San Simeon State Park contain small puddles called vernal pools amid scattered humps of soil called mima mounds—one of few places they occur together. At first glance, these pools and mounds may look like little more than stagnant water in a muddy field. But this landscape teems with life in winter and supports rings of brilliant wildflowers in spring.

When rain falls, the ground absorbs some water, while the rest flows overland as runoff. In a vernal pool grassland, this runoff accumulates in shallow depressions atop the hardpan, a layer of impermeable clay or minerals. The hardpan contains the water like a bathtub. The only way for vernal pools to empty is by evaporation, a process that can take days, weeks, or months, depending on rainfall, temperature, and the size of the pool.

Exactly how mima mounds form is a subject of debate. One of the more interesting theories is that the mounds are a byproduct of generations of industrious pocket gophers. Gophers prefer to build nests in deep soil. If the soil is shallow, gophers will carry in dirt from surrounding slopes, thereby creating mounds.

■ ■

From the pools and mounds, descend toward **Fern Gully**. Just past a wire fence, you'll reach a junction with the westbound and southbound **Nature Trail** (1.5 miles, 180'). Turn left on the southbound route past **Huff & Puff Hill** and cross Fern Gully on slotted wooden **Willow Bridge** (2.2 miles, 40'). Pause here to listen to warblers, thrushes, winter wrens, and dozens of other songbirds in the surrounding riparian woodland.

Leaving the bridge, you'll climb **Pine Ridge,** where wildlife includes bobcats, coyotes, deer, skunks, and foxes, as evidenced by plentiful scat. Though wind hushes through the open pines, calling to mind the Sierra Nevada, the glistening Pacific is in sight less than a mile west.

Continue through the pine and oak woodland and descend to a long **wooden bridge** (2.9 miles, 40') amid the wetlands. From this bridge, wheelchair-accessible platforms return 0.3 mile to the trailhead beside the footbridge, 0.1 mile east of the Washburn Day-Use Area.

PART TWO

■　■　■　■　■　■　■　■　■　■　■　■　■

Ventana & Silver Peak Wildernesses

E NCOMPASSING MORE THAN 200,000 acres, the Ventana and Silver Peak Wildernesses lie within Los Padres National Forest, a place of exquisite beauty and profound isolation. Here rugged coastal ranges offer hikers unparalleled opportunities to explore more than 300 miles of trails and closed roads. Here, just a few miles from the vast Pacific, you'll find fog-shrouded redwoods, oak-studded grasslands, jagged marble peaks, waterfalls, thermal pools, and brisk swimming holes—a rejuvenating escape from the confinements of city life.

Bottchers Gap

■ ■ ■ ■ ■ ■ ■ ■ ■ ■ ■ ■ ■

P ERCHED AMID THE HIGHEST PEAKS of the northern Ventana Wilderness, Bottchers Gap is a 2050-foot ridge saddle created by the Palo Colorado Fault. Following the uplift of the Santa Lucia Range, this northwest-trending fault carved the bed of the Little Sur River. The main fork of the Little Sur flows west for most of its course, until it meets the fault, which forces it into a sharp northwest turn to join the South Fork Little Sur River.

The gap welcomes almost year-round hiking and camping, except during severe winter storms and prolonged summer droughts. It features two trails that lead through dramatically different environments. The eastern Skinner Ridge Trail climbs one of the region's highest viewpoints, while the Little Sur Trail descends deep into the riparian forests and mystical redwoods along the Little Sur River.

DIRECTIONS: To reach Bottchers Gap from Highway 1, turn east on narrow, paved Palo Colorado Road. The junction lies 2 miles north of Bixby Creek Bridge and 11.4 miles south of the Carmel Valley Road (County Road G16) junction in Carmel. *Palo Colorado* (Spanish for red wood) winds through a redwood-lined canyon, climbs through oak woodlands and chaparral, and ends at Bottchers Gap, 7.7 miles inland.

VISITOR CENTER: Big Sur Station: (831) 667-2315. The station is on Highway 1, a half mile south of Pfeiffer Big Sur State Park. Open daily 8 a.m.–6 p.m. Memorial Day through Labor Day, 8 a.m.–4:30 p.m. the rest of the year.

NEAREST CAMPGROUND: Bottchers Gap Campground (12 sites, $12/night) provides a picnic table, fire ring, and pedestal grill at each site. There's a maximum of eight people per site, and sites are granted on a first-come, first-serve basis. No water is available. For more information call Parks Management Co. at (805) 434-1996 or (805) 434-9199, or visit campone.com.

INFORMATION: Fire permits (available from the campground host) are required for all stoves. Dogs are permitted and allowed off leash, except in designated camp-grounds, where a 6-foot or shorter leash is required. There's a $5 day-use fee to park your car at the trailhead.

WEBSITE: www.fs.usda.gov/lpnf | **PHONE:** Los Padres National Forest Head-quarters: (805) 968-6640; Parks Management Company: (805) 995-1976

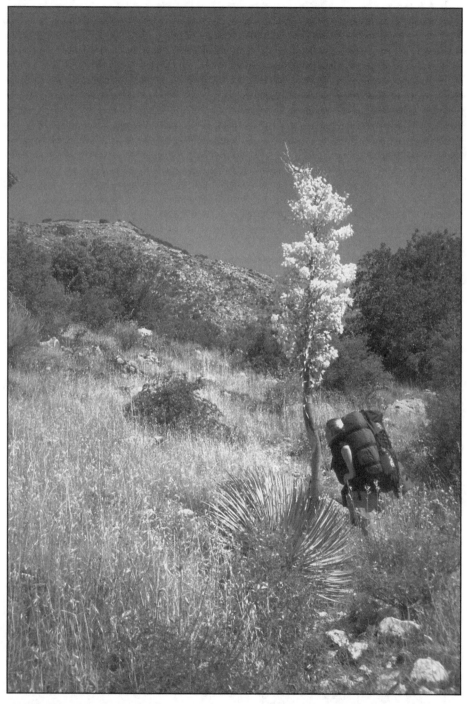

On Pico Blanco, lush redwood canyons are adjacent to desert-like settings with succulents such as Our Lord's candle.

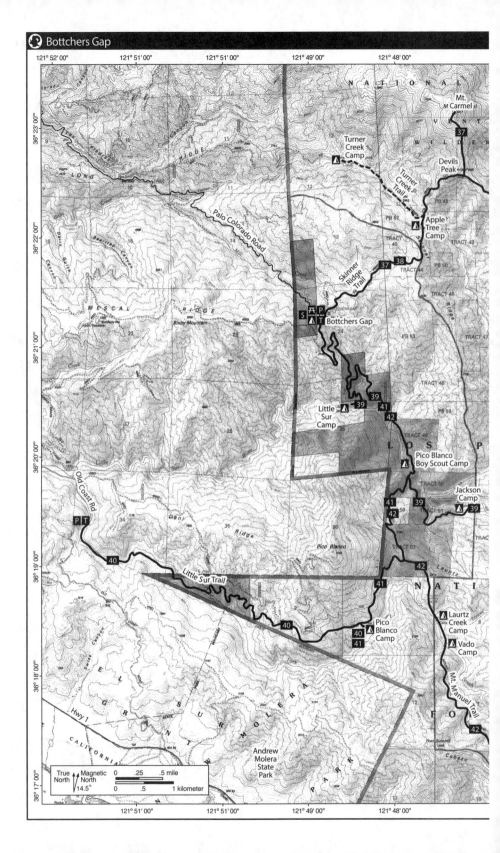

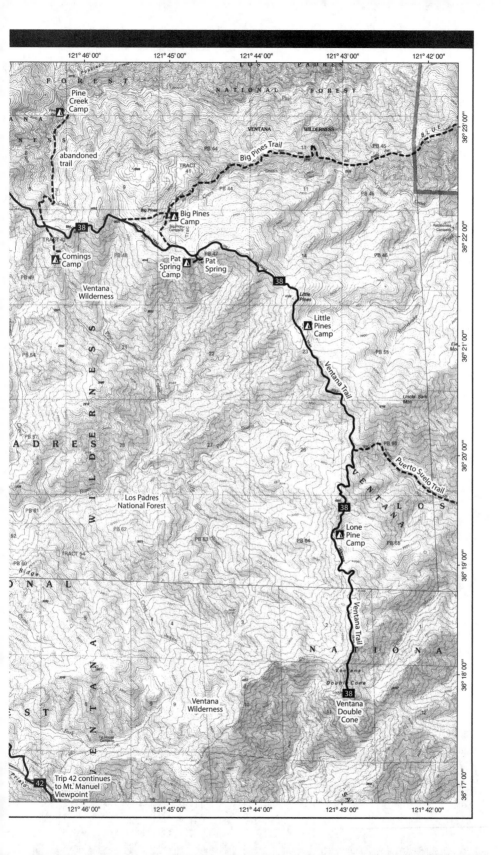

Trip 37

DEVILS PEAK & MT. CARMEL

LENGTH AND TYPE: 9.4-mile out-and-back

RATING: Strenuous

TRAIL CONDITION: Passable, poison oak

HIGHLIGHTS: Spectacular vistas atop Devils Peak and Mt. Carmel stretch from Monterey Bay to Big Sur.

TO REACH THE TRAILHEAD: The Skinner Ridge Trail begins at the trailhead sign on the northeast corner of the parking lot.

TRIP SUMMARY: You can approach this as either moderate to strenuous day hikes or an overnight trip to Apple Tree or Turner Creek Camps.

Day hikes to Devils Peak and Mt. Carmel are rewarding ascents that overlook the entire rim of the Little Sur watershed. To the north, peaks of the Santa Lucia Range fold in on themselves as they meet the Carmel and Salinas Valleys. Clear days promise views of Monterey Bay and the Santa Cruz Mountains, more than 40 miles away. The best times to

Challenging ascents lead to spectacular vistas atop Skinner Ridge.

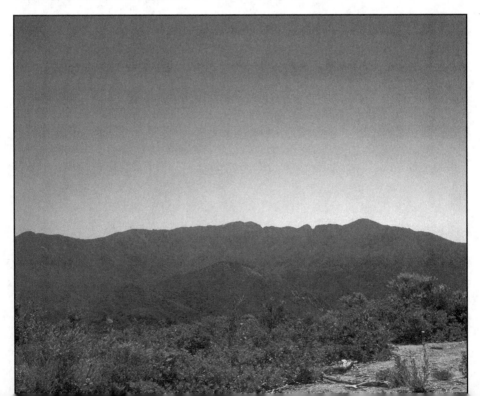

hike are clear days in spring, fall, or between winter storms. Fog often shrouds the coast in summer, obscuring most views.

If you're willing to haul gear, you'll find two camps just off Skinner Ridge Trail. The closest is Apple Tree Camp (3.2 miles from Bottchers Gap), a pleasant spot in all but the driest months (July–October) and perfect for novice backpackers seeking solitude but not a strenuous hike. Just 1.5 miles farther, Turner Creek Camp lies alongside the wildflower-strewn banks of Turner Creek, a gorgeous spot in spring.

Trip Description

The **Skinner Ridge Trail** begins along a singletrack path (2080') and quickly climbs north above **Bottchers Gap**'s oaks, madrones, and bays to a mosaic of chaparral. As you climb, look north to pick out the **Palo Colorado Fault**, which forms the **Little Sur River** drainage to the north and the **Mill Creek** drainage to the south. The gap is a saddle where the fault crosses a ridge separating the two drainages. West of the fault lie metamorphic rocks such as schist, marble, and gneiss, while quartz diorite lies to the east.

There's no mistaking **Pico Blanco** to the south, an enormous marble outcrop that towers over the Little Sur like a great pyramid, separating the north and south forks. *Pico Blanco* (Spanish for white peak) holds one of the West Coast's largest remaining deposits of pure limestone and marble. Some 525 feet thick and 2.5 miles long and containing an estimated 640 million tons of limestone, the deposit is privately owned. Fortunately, there's strong opposition to any attempts to quarry here, due to the adverse environmental impact it would have on adjacent national forest and state park lands.

As the trail climbs toward **Skinner Ridge,** it roller coasters through minor gullies, crossing three small seasonal springs in the Mill Creek drainage. The first is the largest, and if you're not bound for **Apple Tree** or **Turner Creek Camps,** this is the last water you'll see for at least 5 miles in summer and fall. The route from here is shady and viewless due to dense, 10- to 15-foot-high thickets of brush, dominated by different species of ceanothus.

After 2 miles of steep ascents and descents, the dense growth abruptly gives way to an open grassy knoll atop Skinner Ridge, highlighted by bracken ferns and seasonal wildflowers. The **Skinner Ridge viewpoint** (2.1 miles, 3370') lies just off the trail to the left. Vibrant wildflowers and green budding plants explode from the hillsides following winter rains. In summer, sprawling oaks and madrones offer a shady spot to rest. Some of the largest madrones in Big Sur grow along this ridge.

All too soon you must leave the ridge and begin a steep, 280-foot drop in less than a quarter mile to a saddle and the **Turner Creek Trail junction** (2.8 miles, 3180').

SIDE TRIP ■

Turner Creek Trail descends into a broad gully that closely follows the **Church Creek Fault.** A dense canopy of madrones shelters a sparse understory, except for the poison oak that grows aggressively alongside and sometimes on the trail. A quarter mile farther you'll arrive at **Apple Tree Camp** (3.1 miles, 2920'), which offers two small sites. To the right, the first site lies amid the shade of bays and white alders a few yards from **Turner Creek**'s seasonal headwater stream. The second site is nestled alongside the stream, and in wet season, the water gurgles along small mossy pools. Out of season, this creek may run dry, and to find water, you must continue down to **Turner Creek Camp** (4.8 miles, 2790').

Unfortunately, the trail from Apple Tree to Turner Creek is heavily overgrown. Just past Apple Tree's second campsite, you'll cross the creek and battle through a dense understory of blackberries, cow parsnip, thimbleberries, and tangles of poison oak. The gradual 1.5-mile descent crosses the creek three more times, then follows the north bank to the camp. The first site lies in the shade of white alders and an atypical walnut tree. The lush understory boasts spectacular spring wildflowers and bountiful berries by late summer. Also beware the mosquitoes and flies that flourish this time of year.

■ ■

From the Turner Creek Trail junction, the main route heads northeast along the **Big Pines Trail.** This trail is well cleared of brush, though that could change in the future. The route skirts the ridgetop, crossing a firebreak that was bulldozed during fires in the late 1990s. The subsequent passage of many hikers has created a clear trail that climbs **Devils Peak** through open oak woodlands. Live and black oaks offer well-deserved shade to hikers on this sunny stretch through chamise and manzanita.

Continue uphill to a switchback labeled simply TRAIL, pointing north toward the summit. An unofficial campsite lies a few yards past this sign, atop an exposed ridge with expansive views of rolling grasslands, forested canyons, ravines, and beaches that are typically shrouded in fog in summer. Devils Peak viewpoint is only a few hundred feet past this switchback.

To reach the summit, veer left at the unmarked **Mt. Carmel–Devils Peak Trail junction** (3.8 miles, 4130') that branches north off the Big Pines Trail. Along this trail, another unmarked trail veers left to the summit of **Mt. Carmel,** just past a notable sprawling black oak. If you miss this junction, you'll continue southeast to an unofficial **campsite** (3.9 miles, 4154'). Although void of water, this site boasts magnificent views of the Little Sur watershed.

If you're headed to Mt. Carmel, veer left on the aforementioned unmarked trail less than 100 feet past the Big Pines Trail–Devils Peak junction. You'll clearly see Mt. Carmel just to the north, well worth the 20- to 30-minute uphill hike. The trail descends to a minor saddle topped by a few large fallen black oaks before climbing toward the summit. Consider wearing a long shirt and pants, as the narrow trail scrapes past encroaching manzanita, scrub oak, and coyote brush. Fortunately, the trail is virtually devoid of poison oak.

At the **summit** (4.7 miles, 4417'), a telephone pole that was lugged in and erected for enhanced views is now split in two and leaning precariously. Were it not for the existence of a large granite outcrop, you might never see above the chaparral. Once you climb these boulders, the panorama comes into view.

About 20 miles southeast of Carmel, this is one of the northernmost summits in the Ventana Wilderness. On a clear day, you can see the sparkling blue **Pacific** and all of **Monterey Bay**. Moss Landing lies due north, just above the tip of the Monterey Peninsula, 19 miles away. Flat-topped **Palo Escrito Peak** (4465') lies some 16.5 miles to the east, rising amid the **Sierra de Salinas** (Salt Marsh Mountains), an eastern component of the Santa Lucia Range that flanks the west side of Salinas Valley. Just east of Palo Escrito is the city of Salinas itself, about 21 miles away, named for salt marshes at the mouth of the Salinas River, from which the Spanish commercially extracted salt. On a day with excellent visibility, you may be able to spot Santa Cruz, some 43 miles away on the north shore of Monterey Bay.

As at most peaks along this dramatic coast, the best times to hike are between mid-November and April, taking advantage of cooler temperatures, fogless days, and fewer pesky mosquitoes and flies. Be prepared for rain and snow if you hike in winter, when snow levels can drop to 2000 feet. Take in the view and return the way you came. If you're hiking farther, skip to the following trip.

Trip 38

VENTANA DOUBLE CONE VIA VENTANA TRAIL

LENGTH AND TYPE: 29.8-mile out-and-back

RATING: Challenging

TRAIL CONDITION: Passable (with brush, poison oak, and deadfalls), tread evident

HIGHLIGHTS: Unobstructed views from wildflower-strewn oak woodlands, golden grassland ridges, and atop nearly mile-high Ventana Double Cone

TO REACH THE TRAILHEAD: See TRIP 37 Devils Peak & Mt. Carmel (page 152) for the first 3.8 miles of this route to the unmarked Mt. Carmel–Devils Peak trail junction.

TRIP SUMMARY: This book describes several routes to the remote 4853-foot summit of Ventana Double Cone, in the heart of Ventana Wilderness. The most popular options

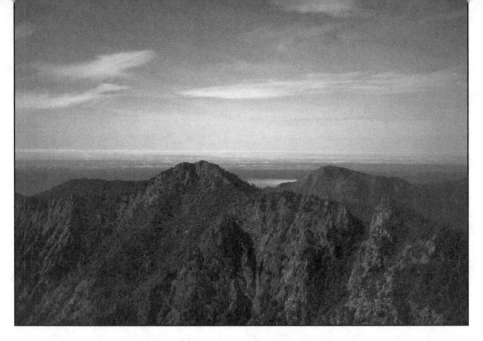

Views west toward Pico Blanco at the summit of Ventana Double Cone

include this route from Bottchers Gap, as well as routes from Los Padres Dam along the Carmel River Trail (page 185) and the Big Pines Trail (page 187), and from China Camp via Pine Valley (page 205). Each route has its advantages and disadvantages. Read on for general details, but see each trip description for specifics.

No matter which way you approach Ventana Double Cone, expect a long hike with ample opportunities to commune peacefully with nature—that is, if the flies, ticks, encroaching brush, and poison oak don't wear you down! Rising nearly a mile above the Pacific some 6 miles distant, the summit offers unobstructed 360-degree views of deep gorges, diverse ecosystems, and isolated peaks along the northern Santa Lucia Range.

This route promises incredible ridgetop views (particularly in winter and spring) and the shortest hike, but it also involves the greatest elevation gain. Although the Ventana Trail junction is just 6.3 miles from Bottchers Gap (versus 9.1 miles from Los Padres Dam), this route requires an additional 1000 feet of climbing as it roller coasters along Skinner Ridge and Devils Peak.

If you can arrange a shuttle vehicle, consider combining trips for an excellent point-to-point backcountry excursion. Begin from Bottchers Gap and tackle the 14.9 miles to Ventana Double Cone, then hike out 15.5 miles to Los Padres Dam via the Puerto Suelo and Carmel River Trails (see TRIP 46 Ventana Double Cone via Carmel River Trail, page 185).

As at most peaks along this dramatic coast, the best times to hike are between mid-November and April, taking advantage of cooler temperatures, fogless days, and fewer pesky mosquitoes and flies. Be prepared for rain and snow if you hike in winter, when snow levels can drop to 2000 feet. During the driest months (August through November), you may not find water until Big Pines Camp (upper Danish Creek) or Pat Spring. In drought years there's even a chance these two water sources could run dry. In such conditions, consider one of the alternative routes.

Trip Description

From the unmarked **Mt. Carmel–Devils Peak Trail junction** (3.8 miles, 4130'), you'll continue southeast along the **Big Pines Trail** on a gentle descent across meadows dotted with sprawling oaks and madrones. This stretch promises fantastic views of the **Little Sur River** drainage, including its headwaters below **Ventana Double Cone** (4853'). Notice the different colors and textures that distinguish each ecological community. Velvety light and dark green chaparral line the dry south-facing slopes, golden grasslands dotted with oaks and pines cap the knolls and ridges, dark green hardwood forests flourish on cool north-facing slopes, and emerald redwood canopies shelter the deepest valleys and narrow stream courses.

The trail descends a yucca-flecked slope, followed by a 500-foot drop to a clearing atop a minor saddle. Pause here to picnic beneath impressive black oaks and madrones, the latter identified by peeling paper-thin bark. The trail rises to round a small summit (3682'), then descends to two smaller saddles. At the second saddle, you'll reach the **Big Pines Trail junction** (5.1 miles, 3500'), which connects the southbound **Comings Camp Trail** and northbound **San Clemente Trail** and leads to the eastbound **Ventana Trail**.

SIDE TRIP ■

> From the Big Pines Trail junction, the **Comings Camp Trail** descends southeast for half a mile into a mature forest dominated by oaks, madrones, and the occasional massive ponderosa pine. This shady, viewless trail reaches a minor gully before the final descent to **Comings Camp** (5.6 miles, 3200'). Nestled beneath several enormous trees, the first campsite is big enough to accommodate a large group, perhaps as many as 10 tents. A smaller second site lies about 100 yards down the trail alongside willows and a large black oak. The camp offers little other than stone fire rings. Water is not provided, though in wet months, a small creeklet may trickle past the willows at the second site.
>
> For a second side trip: From the Big Pines Trail junction, the faint **San Clemente Trail** branches left and descends 1.5 miles northwest to **Pine Creek Camp**. This trail is so overgrown with poison oak and brush, you'd be better off skipping it altogether.

■ ■

From this four-way junction with the San Clemente and Comings Camp Trails, the Big Pines Trail continues straight, climbing east to a minor ridge, then descending to a saddle with impressive views north across the **Carmel** and **Salinas Valleys**. Passing live oaks and a few massive black oaks, the trail emerges amid ponderosa pines and an open grassy knoll atop a 4052-foot ridge. From here steep switchbacks drop to a major saddle and the **Ventana Trail junction** (6.3 miles, 3620').

You'll veer right onto the Ventana Trail along a well-graded slope past tanoaks, madrones, and lone ponderosa pines to the headwaters of the south fork of **Danish Creek** (7 miles, 3560'). From here a spur darts left across the creek and returns downstream a half mile to the Big Pines Trail. Pass the spur and continue upstream 0.1 mile to a spacious, **unnamed camp** that many mistake for Pat Spring Camp. The first campsite lies beneath an impressive madrone amid scattered ponderosa pines and oaks. Another site sits across Danish Creek atop a flat saddle 50 yards northeast of the first site. In summer and fall the creek may run dry. To find water, head downstream a half mile toward **Big Pines Camp** or upstream toward **Pat Spring,** 0.3 mile past the divide.

Past the camp, the route rises 0.2 mile southeast to a prominent saddle and a four-way junction with the **Pat Spring Camp Trail** and **Pat Spring Trail** (7.3 miles, 3740'). Pay attention at this potentially confusing junction. The trail straight ahead leads 100 yards downslope to **Pat Spring**—but this is *not* the Ventana Trail. Many hikers mistakenly think Pat Spring is along the Ventana Trail, which is how it appears on US Forest Service maps. To continue on the Ventana Trail, you'll turn left past the junction and climb northeast toward a minor ridge. The trail to **Pat Spring Camp** branches right.

SIDE TRIP ■

Pat Spring Camp is among the most scenic in the Ventana Wilderness. From the Ventana Trail junction, turn right on the **Pat Spring Camp Trail** and climb west along a minor ridge. Within 50 feet you'll reach the first campsite on your left, while the second site (9.8 miles, 3880') lies atop a minor summit with views of marble-capped **Pico Blanco** and the Pacific. Past the second site, a narrow trail leads 0.1 mile farther to a dramatic outcrop overlooking the Little Sur watershed.

To obtain water, return to the Ventana Trail junction, turn right on the eastbound **Pat Spring Trail,** and continue downhill 100 yards to the spring—a reliable water source in all but the driest years.

■ ■

Fifteen feet past the four-way junction, the Ventana Trail veers left on a moderate climb to a **ridge** (7.6 miles, 4180') topped with ponderosa pines, madrones, and live oaks, where you'll catch glimpses north across Carmel Valley to the **Sierra de Salinas**. A gradual climb leads southeast to a **saddle** (8.4 miles, 3940') that offers views southwest across the Little Sur drainage to Pico Blanco, which splits the river's south and main forks. Beyond lies the broad Pacific.

It's a moderate climb from the saddle to **Little Pines** summit (9.1 miles, 4189'), beyond which lies the **Little Pines Camp Trail junction** (9.4 miles, 3970'). This easily missed unmarked spur branches left 100 feet to the camp, a dry, undesirable spot that's littered with multiple fallen snags.

Past this spur, you'll cross open pine, oak, and madrone woodland, then descend grassy slopes along the western flank of **Uncle Sam Mountain,** which boasts stunning views south toward Ventana Double Cone and its unnamed 4653-foot neighbor. Onward 0.3 mile, the trail crosses the first of four ephemeral creeklets (9.7 miles, 3720'), which typically only flow in wet season.

Past the fourth creeklet (10.3 miles, 3620'), the trail descends to the signed **Puerto Suelo Trail junction** (11.2 miles, 3520'). The only major saddle along this ridge, Puerto Suelo lies along the fractured path of **Church Creek Fault,** which runs northwest out to sea. The Puerto Suelo Trail descends southeast 2.6 miles to **Hiding Canyon Camp,** along the **Carmel River Trail.**

Continue along the Ventana Trail, which climbs 0.2 mile to a westbound switchback on your right. (If you miss the switchback, you'll wind up descending a granite-lined gully on a rapidly diminishing deer trail.) Beyond the switchback, the well-graded trail climbs a 4366-foot ridge, crosses a southeast ridge, and gradually descends to a saddle and the **Lone Pine Camp Trail junction** (12.6 miles, 4300'). A sign marked WATER points southeast along a spur on your left.

The spur descends a few feet past the remains of **Lone Pine Camp,** since reclaimed by overgrowth and large fallen snags. In winter you'll find water less than 0.1 mile down a shallow gully from the junction, while in summer you may have to descend cross-country several hundred feet to find the merest trickle. Don't expect to find water from late summer till the first winter rains.

Beyond the saddle, the Ventana Trail climbs a series of moderate switchbacks along exposed slopes blanketed in fragrant shoulder-high chaparral. Take in outstanding views south toward Ventana Double Cone, which separates the Carmel, Big Sur, and Little Sur River watersheds. Near the summit, vegetation switches to mature stands of live oaks, madrones, and lone Coulter pines, distinguished from ponderosas by their foot-long cones with hook-like scales.

Less than a mile from the peak, the narrow trail follows a granite ridge to a minor saddle, then bypasses the north summit. Here you'll find the rare Santa Lucia fir, endemic to the northern Santa Lucia Range.

SANTA LUCIA FIR ■ ■ ■ ■ ■ ■ ■ ■ ■ ■ ■ ■ ■ ■ ■ ■ ■ ■ ■

Found both in deep canyons and perched high atop the Santa Lucia Range lives the rarest and most narrowly distributed of all fir species, the endemic Santa Lucia fir. The species' seemingly disparate habitats share one attribute: Each is relatively fire resistant. For although the range is subject to periodic blazes, this fir has not developed resistance to fire.

Fossil evidence suggests that Santa Lucia firs were once widely distributed throughout western North America. The tree thrived during the Miocene epoch (24 million to 5 million years ago), as the climate was much warmer and wetter than today, including regular summer rainfall. But during the Pliocene epoch (5 million to 1.6 million years ago), the climate began to cool, ushering in the ice ages of the Pleistocene (1.6 million to 11,000 years ago). The fir could not withstand the colder, drier conditions and thus retreated to milder climates amid the coastal mountains.

Ventana Double Cone supports a small, isolated grove of Santa Lucia firs, easily identified by droopy, densely foliated crowns that extend from the base of the tree with lower branches that nearly touch the ground.

■ ■

From a saddle (14.8 miles, 4640') between the two summits, hike the remaining 0.1 mile to the main **summit** (14.9 miles, 4853'), capped by the foundation of a fire lookout station and a logbook filled with the musings of fellow hikers.

On clear, fogless days, the views encompass all major peaks and watersheds along the northern Santa Lucia Range. To the northwest, the Little Sur River drainage crouches beneath the sheer marble cliffs of Pico Blanco. The Carmel River drainage lies northeast, its headwaters due east. Off to the south, the Big Sur River drainage leads west to Highway 1, joined by small tributaries all along the way.

Notice how Ventana Double Cone is connected to its sister peaks by steep, narrow ridgelines. One conspicuous ridge extends 2 miles southeast from this summit to 4727-foot **Ventana Cone,** while to the left and just above Ventana Cone, another ridge continues 2.5 miles east-southeast to 4965-foot **South Ventana Cone.**

Scratching the horizon to the right of Ventana Cone is 5862-foot **Junipero Serra Peak,** the highest mountain in central California's Coast Ranges. Though nearly 20 miles distant, it towers higher than any neighboring summit or cone. To its right rises 5155-foot **Cone Peak,** 21 miles away and only 3.2 miles from the Pacific. Its rise from shore represents the steepest gradient in the continental United States.

Celebrate your accomplishment before heading back down the trail.

Trip 39

LITTLE SUR & JACKSON CAMPS

LENGTH AND TYPE: 10.2-mile out-and-back

RATING: Moderate

TRAIL CONDITION: Passable (with brush, poison oak, and deadfalls), tread evident

HIGHLIGHTS: Enjoy mountain views en route to camps nestled amid redwoods beside the Little Sur River.

TO REACH THE TRAILHEAD: At Bottchers Gap, the trail begins 30 feet west of the parking lot at the gated dirt Pico Blanco Road.

SACRED MOUNTAIN ■

The region's native Esselen people revered Pico Blanco as a sacred mountain from which all life originated. According to Esselen legend, three creatures—eagle, coyote, and hummingbird—rode out the great flood atop this mountain and went on to recreate the world.

The present owners value the peak in a less sacred light. The Granite Rock Company of Watsonville bought Pico Blanco in the late 1960s, intending to mine the peak for limestone, an essential ingredient in concrete. Fortunately, their plans to lop off the top several hundred feet of the mountain were met with a groundswell of opposition. The resulting environmental lawsuits went all the way to the U.S. Supreme Court and put an end to mining plans on Pico Blanco.

■ ■

TRIP SUMMARY: You can approach this as either a moderate day hike or an overnight backpacking trip. Little Sur Camp lies 2.6 miles from Bottchers Gap, while Jackson Camp is 5.1 miles from the trailhead. The hike takes you from redwood-lined gullies along Pico Blanco Road into dry mountainous terrain that overlooks marble-capped Pico Blanco. The road winds along the Little Sur River through Pico Blanco Boy Scout Camp, on land donated to the scouts in 1948 by William Randolph Hearst. Hearst first purchased the land in 1921 in order to preserve the redwoods from intense logging pressure. Scouts descend on the camp between mid-June and mid-August, thwarting any plans for a wilderness escape. Crossing the river, the Little Sur Trail heads east toward Jackson Camp, home to two riverside sites.

Trip Description

From the west side of the parking lot at **Bottchers Gap** (2080'), head south along the gated dirt road toward **Pico Blanco Boy Scout Camp.** After a gradual quarter-mile descent, you'll reach the first switchback and views of **Pico Blanco, Marble Peak,** and **Ventana Double Cone.** You'll also see evidence of the 1977 Marble–Cone Fire, which consumed thousands of acres. Covered in chaparral, the dry south-facing slopes burned more completely than the damp, tree-lined north-facing slopes.

Past the first switchback, the trail leads north into a stand of redwoods, hairpins south, then reaches another switchback and the **Little Sur Camp Trail junction** (1.8 miles, 1230'), on the east side of the road. Pause for views of the **Little Sur River** drainage and 3709-foot **Pico Blanco,** the largest single mass of limestone west of the Rocky Mountains.

SIDE TRIP ■

To reach **Little Sur Camp,** take the 0.8-mile spur on your right, which leads south along a shady ridge, plunging nearly 600 feet to the banks of the Little Sur. As you meander past live oaks and Douglas firs, keep an eye on the trail for encroaching poison oak. A series of moderate to steep switchbacks drop east into a dense forest of bays, oaks, and madrones. Consider bringing protective head netting once temperatures rise above 70°F, as flies make their presence known. After descending west on an easier grade, you'll arrive in camp (2.6 miles, 670'), which provides two small riverside sites.

Use caution when scrambling over a couple of large fallen trees across the trail. Due to the camp's proximity to both Bottchers Gap and Pico Blanco Boy Scout Camp, these sites fill up quickly during spring vacation and between mid-June and mid-August when the scouts arrive.

■ ■

Past the Little Sur Camp Trail junction, the main route descends north 0.3 mile, returning to the welcome shade of a redwood forest. The next switchback crosses a fault-line creek beside a small waterfall and weaves through several gullies past welcoming signs for the Pico Blanco Boy Scout Camp. The camp's **ranger station** is on the west side of the trail, 100 yards past the first sign. Follow signs toward the main camp, as spur roads and trails only lead to camp structures and sites. The road gently roller coasters down to the Little Sur, then crosses it on a wooden footbridge into Pico Blanco Boy Scout Camp proper (3.6 miles, 820').

Just past the bridge and quartermaster's store, the road forks into three branches. The left branch leads to **Camp Geronimo,** where it parallels the river upstream to a crossing. The right branch leads through camp to a gravel beach with a refreshing waist- to chest-high wading pool. Instead, follow the middle branch, which soon passes the central kitchen and quickly climbs, passing a small sign for the start of the **Los Padres National Forest Trails** and a spur on the right marked simply TRAIL (3.7 miles, 950').

You may either follow this spur or continue on the road—both climb roughly 250 feet in 0.3 mile. The road makes a hairpin turn right and then snakes steeply westward, passing a ruin marked by a lonely chimney. The spur climbs more gradually, veering west and then looping around to join the road. From that point, you'll ascend 25 yards farther to the **Little Sur Trail junction** (4 miles, 1080').

The eastbound **Little Sur Trail** to **Jackson Camp** is essentially a viewless trail that leads south-southeast 200 feet above the Little Sur River in the shade of tanoaks and redwoods. Half a mile from the junction, you'll reach a seasonal spring that's little more than a mud puddle in summer. A few hundred yards farther the trail narrows at a small washout. Be especially careful if you're lugging heavy gear, as this section could erode further over time.

Past the washout, the trail makes a hairpin turn east across a creeklet in a redwood-lined gully blanketed in sword ferns, redwood sorrel, and trillium (4.6 miles, 1120'). Here the trail leaves Boy Scout territory and enters the Ventana Wilderness. You'll climb another 100 yards, then make the final half-mile descent into **Jackson Camp** (5.1 miles, 930'), whose two sites lie along the south bank of the Little Sur.

You'll literally emerge at the first site, while the second site lies just 20 yards downstream. Enjoy the serene backcountry and return when you're rested. A trail from the Boy Scout camp climbs the river to Jackson Camp, so expect badge-carrying visitors in July and August.

Trip 40

COAST ROAD TO PICO BLANCO CAMP

LENGTH AND TYPE: 12-mile out-and-back or 12.4-mile point-to-point

RATING: Strenuous

TRAIL CONDITION: Passable (some brush and/or deadfalls), tread evident to faint along the private property boundary

HIGHLIGHTS: Stroll along the redwood-flanked Little Sur River to a crystal clear swimming hole near Pico Blanco Camp.

TO REACH THE TRAILHEAD: The south end of Coast Road emerges on Highway 1 opposite the entrance to Andrew Molera State Park, 4.5 miles north of Pfeiffer Big Sur State Park and 22 miles south of Carmel. The north end of Coast Road emerges on Highway 1 at the north end of the Bixby Creek Bridge, 2 miles south of the Palo Colorado Road junction, and 13.4 miles south of the Carmel Valley Road (County Road G16) junction. In wet months the 10.3-mile road may be impassable for two-wheel-drive vehicles.

The best route to the trailhead is via the south end of Coast Road, as this stretch is shorter than the north end (3.8 miles versus 6.5 miles), usually in better condition, and the grade is more consistent. You'll find mileage markers at half-mile intervals along Coast Road. The trail begins at a gate on the east side of the road, 100 feet north of Mile 6.5. Watch for the fire warning sign. Unlatch and close the gate behind you to begin the descent to the Little Sur's South Fork.

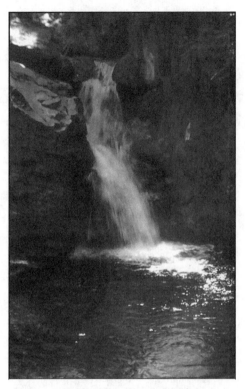

After a strenuous hike, the respite of the refreshing emerald swimming pool at the end of Pico Blanco Camp is not to be missed.

TRIP SUMMARY: You can approach this as either a strenuous day hike or an overnight trip. The camp is also accessible from Bottchers Gap via the Little Sur Trail (see TRIP 41 Pico Blanco, page 167). Although this trail is the shorter route (6 miles versus 7.4 miles), tangled overgrowth, persistent poison oak, and dangerous washouts make it tough going. If you have time, choose the overnight option, as you'll want time to enjoy the swimming hole at trail's end.

The camp lies amid redwood groves and open oak woodlands along the sun-drenched south-facing canyon walls of the Little Sur. Just upstream, the South Fork has carved into Pico Blanco's marble flanks, creating a redwood-shaded grotto highlighted by a waterfall and swimming hole.

The 12.4-mile point-to-point trip from Bottchers Gap to Coast Road is an ideal weekend trip (see TRIP 41 Pico Blanco, page 167). Watch for ticks in spring, when brush encroaches on the trail, particularly beneath Pico Blanco on the last 3 miles of the route.

Trip Description

From the trailhead gate (290'), descend the lightly used **Little Sur Trail** through redwood groves to the **South Fork** of the **Little Sur River**. You'll follow its banks upstream 1.5 miles past small unofficial campsites nestled beneath the lush riparian and redwood forest. During the wet season (November through April), fragile wildflower blooms paint the trail. Redwood sorrel, western starflower, Douglas' iris, and Solomon's seal thrive in the cool, damp understory and continue to bloom through June. A vigorous secondary forest rises above the stumps of redwoods that inhabited these banks for thousands of years.

You may also notice several downed and dying tanbark oaks, victims of sudden oak death. Hikers toting heavy packs will find these fallen oaks a particular nuisance, as they must clamber over or crouch to get through the tangle.

TREE KILLER ■

Responsible for killing California oaks in epidemic proportions, sudden oak death is caused by the fungus-like pathogen *Phytophthora ramorum*. Since it first appeared in 1995, the disease has killed hundreds of thousands of tanoaks, coast live, black, and Shreve oaks in Northern California. Though left unharmed, neighboring species such as Douglas fir, rhododendron, buckeye, madrone, manzanita, bigleaf maple, bay laurel, and evergreen huckleberry may serve as "carriers" of the pathogen, which may then spread aerially via windblown rain. Mortality is most common where oaks and these carriers grow side by side.

Until the disease is better understood, researchers ask hikers to help prevent the spread of *P. ramorum*. Before leaving the area, thoroughly clean your tires, shoes, and your pets' feet.

■ ■

You'll soon leave **Los Padres National Forest** and cross private property, skirting the river 0.3 mile farther upstream to a **campsite** for one to two tents (1.8 miles, 425'). From

Nestled along the edge of a redwood-forested gorge, Pico Blanco Camp is just a short walk upstream from one of Big Sur's most magnificent swimming pools.

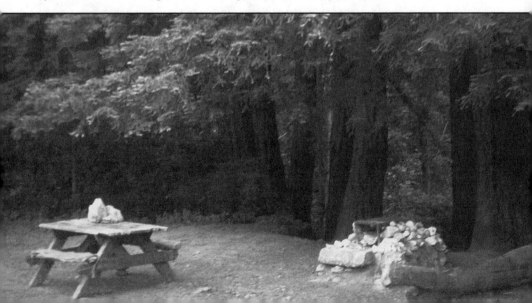

here the Little Sur Trail fords the South Fork and crosses a creek. This is usually an easy boulder-to-boulder hop, except during winter storms, when a knee- to waist-high wade is inevitable. During intense rainfall, the river may be too swift and deep to cross.

Onward, the route begins its first major ascent, climbing from the cool redwood canopy into fragrant coastal scrub. Trail conditions deteriorate from this point, largely due to aggressive brush. A crew from the Ventana Wilderness Alliance restored some of the trail but reported many sections still in need of work.

You'll continue climbing east amid dense northern and southern coastal scrub and chaparral species. South-facing slopes allow the southern species to tolerate hot, dry summers, while ocean fog creeps up the canyon, providing moisture to the northern scrub. The trail leads through a fragrant tapestry of black sage, bush lupine, coyote brush, sagebrush, and poison oak to a seeping spring that supports a small grove of redwoods. From here the trail meanders 150 feet to a switchback across the private dirt **Granite Rock Road** (2.2 miles, 760').

Continue east, ducking through two minor gullies that host seasonal creeks. Though passable, the trail is narrow and slippery with several brush-covered washouts. Past the second gully, the trail parallels Granite Rock Road for 0.6 mile to another **switchback** (2.8 miles, 840'). This marks the start of a steep climb of more than 1000 feet in 2 miles.

The trail first climbs north, then switchbacks, reentering the US Forest Service land along the south flanks of **Pico Blanco**. Hardwoods and redwoods are limited to the ravines, while the scrub-clad slopes and grassy ridgelines are studded with such drought-tolerant species as Our Lord's candle, a yucca that shoots forth a large stalk of cream-colored blossoms.

Among the oldest known rocks along the Coast Ranges, Pico Blanco's limestone and marble outcrops create dramatic vegetation zones. Though the area often receives more than 60 inches of rainfall per year, the runoff drains into the marble and limestone rather than remaining in the overlying soil. Thus the slopes are dominated by drought-tolerant species.

Past these blinding outcrops, the trail meanders through hardwood-lined ravines, crosses a broad meadow, and climbs to an oak-clad **ridge** (4.8 miles, 1840') with views up and down the South Fork drainage. Beyond the ridge, you'll begin the descent into camp.

The trail crosses open slopes and a series of shallow gullies. Past the third gully, home to a small seasonal tributary, you'll reach the **Pico Blanco Camp Trail junction** (5.9 miles, 1385'). Descend this 0.1-mile trail past sprawling oaks and a grassy slope into **Pico Blanco Camp** (6 miles, 1300'). The camp offers four sites with fire rings. Three lie on the perimeter of a sun-drenched grassy slope, while the fourth lies 20 yards south of the first site you reach along the trail. Be on your guard for poison oak.

A quick 100-foot stroll upstream from camp lies a **waterfall oasis**, widely considered one of the most beautiful spots in the Ventana Wilderness. You'll arrive at a deeply eroded marble gorge that enfolds a deep emerald swimming hole. At best, the water reaches the mid-50s Fahrenheit, making your swim brisk, refreshing, and likely brief. The midday to early afternoon sun warms the pool and adjacent boulders, though this may not be sufficient heat following your chilly swim. Return to camp to warm up.

If you're venturing farther along the Little Sur Trail to **Bottchers Gap** or the **Manuel Peak Trail,** refer to the following trip description. To reach the **Manuel Peak Trail junction,** continue 1.2 miles past the camp along the Little Sur Trail (see TRIP 42 Manuel Peak & Pfeiffer Big Sur State Park, page 169).

Trip 41

PICO BLANCO

LENGTH AND TYPE: 14.8-mile out-and-back or 12.4-mile point-to-point

RATING: Strenuous

TRAIL CONDITION: Passable (with brush and poison oak encroachment and deadfalls), tread evident

HIGHLIGHTS: Follow a magnificent, steep-sided canyon through redwood groves to a perfect swimming hole at Pico Blanco Camp.

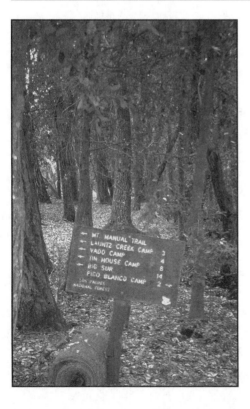

TO REACH THE TRAILHEAD: At Bottchers Gap the trail begins 30 feet west of the parking lot at the gated dirt Pico Blanco Road.

TRIP SUMMARY: This route leads 7.4 miles to Pico Blanco Camp. You can approach it as a strenuous day hike, a one- to three-night out-and-back, or a point-to-point trip. On a two- to three-night trip, consider staying at Little Sur Camp (2.6 miles from Bottchers Gap) or Jackson Camp (5.2 miles from Bottchers Gap), then hiking on to Pico Blanco Camp (see TRIP 39 Little Sur & Jackson Camps, page 161). For a rewarding 12.4-mile

The Manuel Peak Trail junction leads to remote and isolated areas of Ventana Wilderness.

point-to-point passage, leave a shuttle vehicle at the trailhead along Coast Road (see TRIP 40 Coast Road to Pico Blanco Camp, page 163).

The hike descends into the Little Sur drainage via Pico Blanco Road, promising panoramic views of Pico Blanco, the largest marble and limestone deposit in the Lower 48. The road follows the banks of the Little Sur into Pico Blanco Boy Scout Camp. Scouts descend en masse between mid-June and mid-August, thwarting any plans for a wilderness escape. Past the camp, you'll join the Little Sur Trail, which leads east 1.2 miles to Jackson Camp and west 2.6 miles to Pico Blanco Camp. Pico Blanco is nestled along the edge of a redwood-lined gorge. Just upstream, a waterfall oasis harbors a deep emerald swimming hole.

Trip Description

See TRIP 39 Little Sur & Jackson Camps (page 161) for the first 4 miles of this route to the **Little Sur Trail junction.**

Assuming you're not headed to Jackson Camp, you'll turn right and head westbound on the **Little Sur Trail,** climbing through a dense forest dominated by tanoaks, madrones, and redwoods. Fondly referred to as "Cardiac Hill," the following steep 1350-foot ascent to the top of **Launtz Ridge** over less than a mile ends at a minor 2194-foot crest. Pause to rest and take in impressive views of the Little Sur drainage.

From here the trail forks. The faint trail to the right leads to an unofficial campsite atop a grassy knoll. Branch left on the Little Sur Trail, which descends gradually from the crest into dense woodland. You'll soon arrive at the signed **Manuel Peak Trail junction** (5.3 miles, 2090').

Branch right at this junction and continue west on the Little Sur Trail. The next 0.3 mile drops steeply into **Duveneck's Hole,** a dilapidated group of hunting huts amid a shady redwood canyon. Skirt the north edge of the canyon beyond the shacks for your first foreboding glimpse of **Pico Blanco**'s marble-strewn south face. The cool redwood and tanoak canopy abruptly changes to dry scrubby oaks and chaparral, which is replaced in turn by arid, yucca-studded grassy slopes—a stark contrast brought on by the peak's mineral composition. **Pico Blanco**'s marble and limestone slopes drain water quickly, leaving only plants adapted to such dry conditions.

The trail switchbacks three times across the lower slopes before turning southwest for a quarter-mile descent. Consider wearing long pants for this stretch, as the narrow trail is choked with poison oak, coyote brush, and yucca. Stop every few hundred feet and check for ticks, a factor in all but the driest months.

The trail forks again at the **Pico Blanco Camp Trail junction** (7.3 miles, 1385'). The right branch leads 5.9 miles west to **Coast Road** (see TRIP 40 Coast Road to Pico Blanco Camp, page 163). Head down the left branch 0.1 mile southeast to **Pico Blanco Camp** (7.4 miles, 1300'). Just upstream from camp is a scenic waterfall oasis and swimming hole, the perfect spot for a refreshing dip. (For details about the camp and swimming hole, see TRIP 40 Coast Road to Pico Blanco Camp, page 163.)

Trip 42

MANUEL PEAK & PFEIFFER BIG SUR STATE PARK

LENGTH AND TYPE: 25.4-mile out-and-back (Manuel Peak)

RATING: Challenging

TRAIL CONDITION: Passable to Vado Camp, difficult to impassable to Pfeiffer Big Sur State Park; poison oak, trail washouts, faint tread, trail closure as of 2008 Basin Complex Fire eastbound on Mt. Manuel Trail from Pfeiffer Big Sur State Park.

HIGHLIGHTS: This route follows the redwood-lined Little Sur River gorge past marble-capped Pico Blanco to the Manuel Peak summit for glorious coastal and inland views.

TO REACH THE TRAILHEAD: At Bottchers Gap the trail begins 30 feet west of the parking lot at the gated dirt Pico Blanco Road.

TRIP SUMMARY: Approach this as an out-and-back hike rather than a point-to-point trek since the Mt. Manuel Trail is closed westbound from Pfeiffer Big Sur State Park. Seriously consider curtailing your hike, however, as sections between Vado Camp and Manuel Peak

The region's native Esselen people revered Pico Blanco as a sacred mountain from which all life originated.

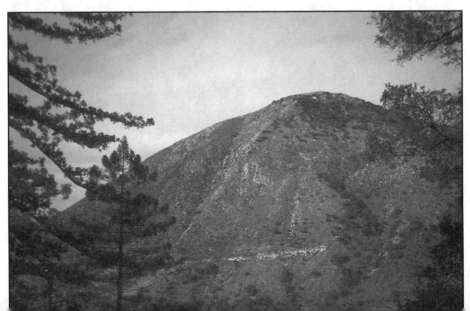

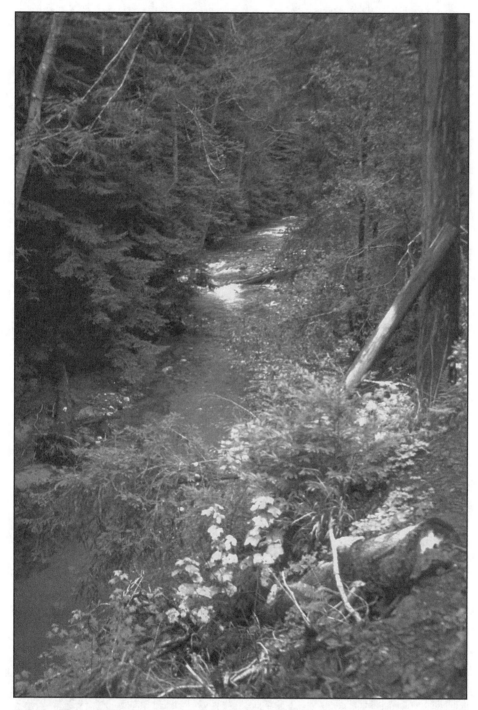

Expect solitude under the shade of towering redwoods along the South Fork Little Sur River.

are considered impassable due to trail washouts, deadfalls, and brush encroachment. From Vado Camp (ruined in 2003 by downed trees), the route switchbacks to a major ridge, where the trail practically vanishes, then summits Manuel Peak. Washouts, overgrowth, and the lack of water and trail markings make this strenuous stretch very hard to follow. In addition, during the dry season (June through November), you may not find water between Vado Camp and Pfeiffer Big Sur State Park, a grueling 11 miles on hot summer days.

Instead, plan an out-and-back overnight deep into the heart of the Little Sur drainage. Camp at Launtz Creek or Pico Blanco, then day hike the steep climb from Vado Camp to Manuel Peak. The point-to-point passage from Bottchers Gap to Pfeiffer Big Sur State Park is a two- to four-day, 18.1-mile haul along strenuous and dangerous trails due to 2008 fire damage and lack of trail restoration efforts.

As in most of the Ventana Wilderness, flies are often a nuisance, particularly in warmer months (May through October), while ticks are prevalent during the wet season (November through April). Poison oak is a year-round concern.

Trip Description

See TRIP 41 Pico Blanco (page 167) for the first 5.3 miles of this route to the **Manuel Peak Trail junction** (2090').

At the signed junction, branch left and climb past oak- and madrone-filtered views down the **South Fork Little Sur** canyon, framed by **Pico Blanco** to the west and **Post Summit** to the south. The trail crosses several minor gullies as it climbs past shady tanoak, live oak, and madrone forests into chaparral, chamise, and manzanita brush. You'll soon descend into a cool, damp redwood forest highlighted by sprawling tanoaks.

The trail drops north past a major gully, then briefly south along the north bank of **Launtz Creek** to **Launtz Creek Camp** (6.9 miles, 1920'), a favorite stop along the **Manuel Peak Trail**. Though more spacious than the recently damaged **Vado Camp,** there's only room for about three tents on its sloping creekside sites. You'll find year-round water.

Beyond camp the trail crosses the creek, turns upstream 100 yards, then climbs southwest along a few short switchbacks to the minor ridge that divides Launtz Creek and the South Fork Little Sur. You'll descend this minor ridge along a well-graded trail to the South Fork canyon floor. The trail follows the river upstream, crossing it three times over a quarter mile.

Just past the third crossing, look for several large downed trees. Provided the Forest Service or another crew has not cut or moved these trees, they mark the **Vado Camp Trail junction** (7.8 miles, 1790'). This 100-foot spur crosses the South Fork to a small east-sloping gully, the site of camp. In 2003 a major windstorm toppled several large trees directly onto the site. What remains amid the tangle would at best accommodate one or two tents along a bench on the south side of the gully. In summer and fall the South Fork often runs dry, requiring a short hike downstream for water.

Most hikers hang up their boots at Vado Camp, as the trail to **Manuel Peak** is overgrown and often difficult to follow. Between Manuel Peak and **Pfeiffer Big Sur State Park**, the trail is clearly marked, but washouts make the steep descent dangerous, especially for those lugging heavy packs. Nevertheless, as some of you have your hearts set on the summit, the trail description follows. Respect your limits and tread carefully.

From camp you'll cross the South Fork and climb west along a series of switchbacks. The trail continues its steady ascent south, dipping in and out of minor redwood-lined gullies. At the fourth **gully** (9.4 miles, 2280'), a small creeklet flows during the wet season (November through April), your last chance for water for another 8.5 miles.

Continue climbing past redwood-shaded gullies, sprawling oaks, and dense ceanothus thickets. From the first major gully, the steadily deteriorating route climbs a series of well-graded switchbacks, rising 900 feet in the next 1.1 miles on a trail that more closely resembles a deer path. Overgrown brush obscures views of **Cabezo Prieto** ridge and allows only occasional brief glimpses of Post Summit and Manuel Peak. You'll climb almost to the top of Cabezo Prieto (3554'), then battle through 0.1 mile of heavily overgrown sections to a narrow crest that offers the first of several spectacular 360-degree views.

Head south along the crest for a mile past dense stands of ceanothus, scrub oak, manzanita, and yerba santa. Check your clothing for ticks during the wet season (November through April). Also watch for poison oak. The trail crosses several bulldozed sections that make passage difficult. Just past the first saddle, the trail widens and the brush thins out somewhat.

You'll climb to a minor point, then descend to a minor saddle near a dense stand of Coulter pines, which offer welcome shade. Just past a conspicuous, yet camouflaged reflector is the spur to the **Manuel Peak viewpoint** (12.7 miles, 3379'). See TRIP 20 Manuel Peak Trail (page 105) for a description of the summit and the remaining 5.4 miles to Pfeiffer Big Sur State Park.

Los Padres Dam

■　■　■　■　■　■　■　■　■　■　■　■

M OST OF THE NORTHERN SANTA LUCIA RANGE drains into the Carmel River. Above Los Padres Dam, the river flows as a small creek from the Church Creek Divide into Pine Valley, where it joins the waters from Pine Ridge, Ventana Cone, Uncle Sam Mountain, and Elephant Mountain. Before the dam was built, steelhead trout would migrate upstream from the Pacific to spawn. Landlocked rainbow trout still inhabit deep pools upstream. Two routes lead from the dam into the Carmel River watershed, each geared toward different seasons.

The Carmel River Trail offers a gentle descent south into the lush canyon, skirting the riverbanks and crossing several times. This popular route is ideal between May and October, when temperatures can soar into the 90s Fahrenheit. Sheltered beneath a shady riparian forest, the river offers drinking water and several refreshing swimming holes. In fall the colors are spectacular, low water makes for easier boulder hopping, and the fly, tick, and mosquito populations have diminished. Don't attempt this route after periods of heavy rain, as the river may be swift and dangerous to cross.

When the river is swelled, opt for the westbound Big Pines Trail, which leads to winter camps. Ambitious hikers can continue south toward Ventana Double Cone or west toward Bottchers Gap for a ridgetop circuit of the northern Ventana Wilderness. Breathtaking views abound.

DIRECTIONS: To reach the Los Padres Dam Trailhead from the north, drive 5.2 miles south of Carmel on Highway 1, then turn left and head eastbound on Carmel Valley Road (County Road G16). In 11.7 miles you'll reach the heart of Carmel Valley Village, your last opportunity for gas, food, and supplies. Continue through the village another 4.3 miles to the junction with the north end of Cachagua Road. Turn right and take this narrow paved road 5.9 miles to Nason Road. Turn right and drive 0.6 mile, passing the USFS Carmel River Station on your right. Park at the lot a minute farther on the right beside a locked gate.

From Southern California and the central Salinas Valley, leave Highway 101 at Greenfield and take Elm Avenue (County Road G16) 5.8 miles southwest to Arroyo Seco Road (County Road G17). The two roads merge for the next 6.5 miles until you

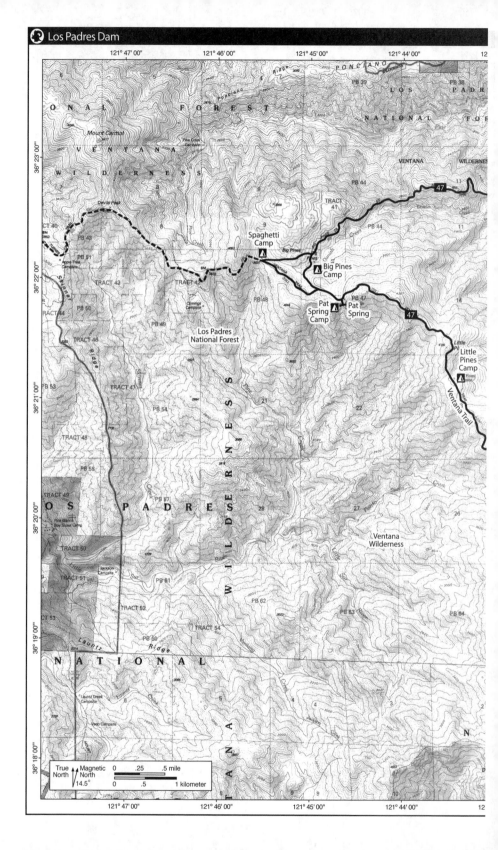

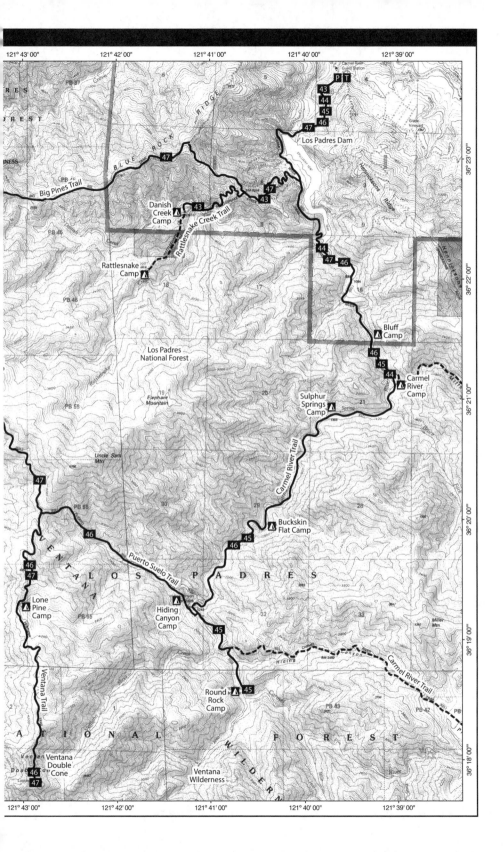

reach a fork. Take the right branch onto Carmel Valley Road (County Road G16) and drive 17 miles to the south end of Cachagua Road. Turn left, drive 1.3 miles to a junction with Tassajara Road, and then continue straight 4.5 miles to Nason Road. Turn left on Nason and drive 0.6 mile to the parking lot on the right just past the USFS Carmel River Station. There is no fee. There are no facilities or water at the station.

VISITOR CENTER: Big Sur Station: (831) 667-2315. The station is on Highway 1, a half mile south of Pfeiffer Big Sur State Park. Open daily 8 a.m.–6 p.m. Memorial Day through Labor Day, 8 a.m.–4:30 p.m. the rest of the year.

NEAREST CAMPGROUNDS: White Oaks Campground (7.9 miles along Tassajara Road) and China Camp (10.7 miles along Tassajara Road) are small USFS campgrounds open year-round on a first-come, first-serve basis. Both charge a $5 parking fee. Facilities include vault toilets, fire rings, and picnic tables. For more information contact the USFS Monterey District Headquarters at (831) 385-5434.

INFORMATION: No swimming allowed in Los Padres Reservoir. Fire permits required for all stoves. Dogs permitted and allowed off leash, except in designated campgrounds, where a 6-foot or shorter leash is required.

WEBSITE: www.fs.usda.gov/lpnf

PHONE: Los Padres National Forest Headquarters: (805) 968-6640

Trip 43

DANISH CREEK CAMP

LENGTH AND TYPE: 7.6-mile out-and-back

RATING: Moderate

TRAIL CONDITION: Passable, with narrow tread, poison oak, brush, and deadfalls

HIGHLIGHTS: Outstanding views of the Carmel River and Danish Creek watershed

TO REACH THE TRAILHEAD: This hike begins at the Los Padres Dam Trailhead.

TRIP SUMMARY: The Big Pines Trail ascends the ridge crest above Danish Creek, offering views deep into the Carmel River watershed. Beware of profuse low-lying poison oak along this stretch. From this ridge, the Danish Creek Camp Trail descends densely forested northern slopes to the canyon floor. Sites are nestled alongside the year-round creek. This spacious plot is the most easily reached camp from Los Padres Dam.

Trip Description

Pass through the gate at the end of the parking lot (1050'), where a trail sign points the way southwest toward **Los Padres Dam**. You'll hike a half mile along the one-lane dirt road, passing through an open grove of impressive lichen-draped valley and live oaks.

On a gentle ascent southeast, the trail reaches open ground with views west toward prominent **Blue Rock Ridge,** which parallels the **Big Pines Trail** above the reservoir. As the spillway and dam come into view (0.4 mile, 1180'), the trail branches left across the spillway, then leads toward the dam along the main road.

Pause atop **Los Padres Dam** (0.5 mile, 1120') to gaze south across the reservoir toward the **Carmel River** watershed. Skirting the lake, the road heads south, crossing a steep-walled gully lined with sycamore trees, easily identified by mottled cream-and-white bark that resembles a jigsaw puzzle. For 0.3 mile you'll climb steadily above the reservoir.

Equestrians should note the steep, narrow **spur road** (1.3 miles, 1090') that branches right from the main road and rejoins the Big Pines Trail. Used primarily as a horse trail, this 1.2-mile road does lead toward **Big Pines Camp** and cuts 0.7 mile off your route, but it presents a much steeper and more strenuous gradient.

A quarter mile farther you'll pass a road that branches left toward the reservoir and loops back to the main road. Continue straight ahead to a fork and veer right. The road soon narrows, becoming the **Carmel River Trail.** Keep watch for abundant poison oak along this narrow path. You'll climb 100 yards to the signed **Big Pines Trail junction** (1.8 miles, 1170').

Those bound for **Danish Creek, Rattlesnake Creek,** or **Big Pines/Bottchers Gap/Ventana Double Cone** will branch right (see TRIP 47 Ventana Double Cone via Big Pines Trail, page 187). While the tread is clear, the trail is severely overgrown with poison oak as it climbs switchbacks high above the western half of the reservoir to a chaparral-cloaked **ridge** (2.8 miles, 1920').

The Los Padres Dam prevents steelhead from migrating farther upstream.

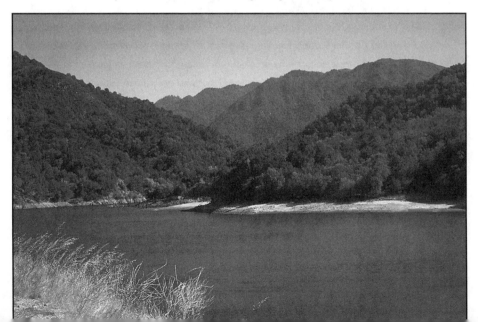

Atop the open ridge, you'll arrive at a marked junction with the **Danish Creek Trail** (3 miles, 2050'). Here the trail branches left and descends toward **Danish Creek**. Though it's been a dry hike to this point, take heart, as the creek flows year-round.

Your descent begins on a gentle grade west through scrubby thickets, then turns south down a steep gully. In winter and early spring, a seasonal stream tumbles alongside the trail toward Danish Creek. After a 0.8-mile descent you'll reach **Danish Creek Camp** (3.8 miles, 1430'), set in a broad meadow amid creekside granite boulders.

Boasting colorful spring wildflowers and a canopy of oaks, madrones, and sycamores, the meadow is large enough to hold groups of up to a dozen tents. You'll find a timeworn table and cooking grate beneath a sprawling live oak, whose bark seems to be engulfing a granite boulder at its base. Be forewarned that mosquitoes and flies are thick in summer.

In colder months the south-facing campsites get a fair amount of sun. Watch for lizards and snakes, which slither amid the leaf litter to bask in the warm rays. Frequenting the creek's sunny banks are juvenile western skinks that flash bright blue tails, an adaptation that fools predators into attacking the detachable tail, allowing the skink to escape.

A few yards upstream a faint trail traces the creek's north bank. This unmaintained, heavily overgrown trail follows the creek, then scales the northwest walls of **Rattlesnake Creek** canyon on a nearly impassable route to **Rattlesnake Camp**.

DAM FIGHT ■

In 1995, California American Water, which owns the Los Padres Dam, reservoir, and adjacent lands, proposed construction of a new concrete dam to replace the current earthen dam. Critics argued that the $127 million project would mar the picturesque Carmel River Valley.

The proposed 28-story dam would drown 266 acres of habitat along Danish Creek and the Carmel River (including 24 acres in Ventana Wilderness), as well as 27 cultural and historic sites, many of which are sacred to the native Esselen tribe. It would also impact the migration of steelhead trout and destroy an estimated 90,000 trees and shrubs.

Fortunately, the Monterey Peninsula electorate voted down the project, though the fight will likely continue, as water—or the lack of it—has always driven state and local governments to quench the thirst of an ever-growing population.

■ ■

Trip 44

BLUFF & CARMEL RIVER CAMPS

LENGTH AND TYPE: 9.8-mile out-and-back

RATING: Easy to moderate

TRAIL CONDITION: Clear, poison oak, good for kids

HIGHLIGHTS: Experience wilderness solitude amid brilliant autumn colors, the gurgling Carmel River, and crystal clear wading pools.

TO REACH THE TRAILHEAD: This hike begins at the Los Padres Dam Trailhead.

TRIP SUMMARY: This route meanders through Carmel River canyon, lush with ferns and shaded by colorful deciduous trees. Those on day hikes or short weekend trips visit the riverside Bluff Camp, only 4.1 miles from the trailhead and big enough to hold a large group. Just 0.8 mile farther along the trail, the smaller Carmel River Camp lies at the confluence of Miller Creek and the Carmel River.

While summer temperatures and accompanying low water levels are best for hiking and swimming, flies are a constant annoyance, often swarming your eyes and ears. The wet sea-

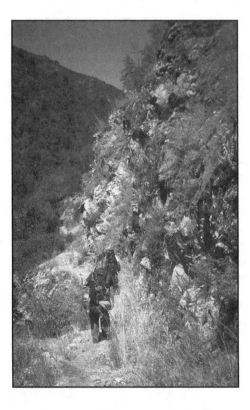

son (November through April) brings an onslaught of ticks, which exploit the overgrown trail to hitchhike on unsuspecting hikers. Wet months also mean high water, which may end your hike at Bluff Camp, where a waist- to chest-high wade could be dangerous. Heavy storms can also rapidly swell the Carmel River and its tributaries, making the fords impassable.

Trip Description

See TRIP 43 Danish Creek Camp (page 176) for the first 1.8 miles of this route to the signed **Big Pines Trail junction** (1170'). Those bound for **Danish Creek Camp, Rattlesnake Creek,** or **Big Pines/Bottchers Gap/Ventana Double Cone** will branch

Poison oak is common on the narrow spurs off the Carmel River Trail.

right here (see TRIP 43 Danish Creek Camp and TRIP 47 Ventana Double Cone via Big Pines Trail, page 187).

Instead, continue on the **Carmel River Trail,** which climbs high above the south end of the reservoir, emerging from dense forest dominated by live oak into drier brushy cover. A short descent on switchbacks leads down to **Danish Creek** (2.8 miles, 1050'), which flows east into the reservoir. In wet season you'll face a risky ford through high water. Although California American Water prohibits camping along the creek, there is an unofficial site along the south bank.

Crossing the creek, you'll soon reach a smaller perennial creek that cascades over a small granite-faced waterfall. One hundred yards past this creek a trail sign points south, 1 mile to **Bluff Camp** and 2 miles to **Miller Canyon** and **Carmel River Camp.** You'll climb above the river to a sharp turn cleared of vegetation, offering impressive views up the canyon to **Miller Mountain,** origin of the Carmel River's Bruce Fork.

The final 0.1 mile to Bluff Camp is entirely downhill. Less than 100 feet from camp you'll reach a junction. Though both paths descend into camp, the one that plunges straight ahead is steeper and only saves a few extra steps. The path on your left is a better choice, especially in late summer and fall when slippery dry leaves blanket the ground.

Bluff Camp (4.1 miles, 1150') is the only legal option on California American Water's private land. This delightful camp on the Carmel River offers three sites and a convenient swimming hole for a refreshing dunk. The first site lies along the west bank, adjacent to large granite boulders that border the swimming hole (3 to 4 feet deep in late spring and summer). Across the river lie the other two sites, which share a spacious bench on the east bank, large enough to accommodate a half dozen tents. An open canopy of alders and sycamores filters the sun.

Crossing the river can be a challenge. In summer and fall you can simply boulder-hop a small rock dam upstream. But in wetter months a wade is inevitable. During or after a rainstorm, crossing could involve a risky 2- to 5-foot ford across a swiftly rising river. Don't attempt to cross in such conditions.

Across the river, the trail climbs the narrow canyon to a minor ridge, leaving private land for the **Ventana Wilderness** (4.4 miles, 1430'). As you traverse the canyon's steep granite walls, the trail narrows due to washouts and erosion, requiring careful footing.

You'll soon wind back down to the signed **Miller Canyon Trail junction** (4.8 miles, 1220'), at the confluence of Miller Creek and the Carmel River. (For a description of the Miller Canyon Trail, see TRIP 48 Miller Canyon & Pine Valley Loop, page 195). Turn right at the junction and continue on the Carmel River Trail across the river to beautiful **Carmel River Camp** (4.5 miles, 1220').

Many hikers prefer this idyllic riverside camp over Sulphur Springs Camp and Buckskin Camp, farther along the Carmel River Trail. Depending on the season, you'll find a waist- to head-high swimming hole, especially welcome on hot summer days. The first two sites lie along the south bank beneath live oaks just past the confluence with Miller Creek. Each can accommodate two to three tents. Across the river lies the camp's main site, marked by a table, fire ring, and cooking grate. Just upstream from the main camp, the trail crosses the river again and follows a bend west to a smaller site beneath a filtering canopy of maples, sycamores, and alders.

Few people venture farther than Carmel River Camp, and poison oak encroaches on the little-used trail beyond. If you're continuing farther, refer to the following trip description.

ANGLER'S DELIGHT ■

Fishing season along the Carmel River centers on two species: steelhead in the lower sections in winter, and trout in the upper sections from spring through fall. From the last Saturday in April to November 15, only trout fishing is allowed from Los Padres Dam upstream. Resident rainbow and brown trout thrive at the confluence at Carmel River Camp. Your odds will improve the farther upstream you're willing to go.

You are restricted to artificial lures and barbless hooks. Anglers can keep up to five trout, though only two of those may be rainbows more than 10 inches in total length. There is no size restriction for brown trout. Visit the California Department of Fish & Game website for details: dfg.ca.gov.

■ ■

Trip 45

HIDING CANYON & ROUND ROCK CAMPS

LENGTH AND TYPE: 20.4-mile out-and-back, loop, or point-to-point

RATING: Strenuous

TRAIL CONDITION: Potentially impassable due to high water crossing along the Carmel River during the wet season, abundant poison oak, trail washouts, and faint tread

HIGHLIGHTS: Hike backcountry trails through narrow gorges, past waterfalls and deep swimming holes, to remote, peaceful camps.

TO REACH THE TRAILHEAD: This hike begins at the Los Padres Dam Trailhead.

TRIP SUMMARY: The Carmel River Trail offers numerous day-hiking and backpacking opportunities. Highlights along this 15.2-mile trail include Bluff, Carmel River, and Hiding

Canyon Camps, the gorge below Round Rock Camp, Pine Valley, and Pine Falls. (For a description of the upper Carmel River Trail, see TRIP 49 Pine Valley, page 199.)

The well-established yet overgrown trail meanders through the Carmel River canyon, carpeted with ferns and shaded by deciduous trees. The best time to hike this route is in fall, as temperatures are mild, water levels are low, ticks and flies have diminished, and autumn colors burst forth from mature sycamores, maples, oaks, and alders that line the river. Heavy rainfall may end your hike at Bluff Camp, as the Carmel River and its tributaries can rise a few feet, making passage hazardous. Be aware of changing weather conditions before entering the narrow canyon. If you're headed to Hiding Canyon Camp, regardless of the season, expect to forge or boulder-hop the river more than two dozen times. Walking sticks and river shoes are a big help.

Trip Description

See TRIP 44 Bluff & Carmel River Camps (page 179) for the first 4.5 miles of this route to **Carmel River Camp.**

Just upstream from the main site at Carmel River Camp (1220') the trail crosses the river and follows a bend west beneath a filtering canopy of maples, sycamores, and alders. Few people venture beyond the camp, and poison oak encroaches on the little-used trail beyond. At times, you may find yourself waist high in this highly toxic plant. Watch for the plant's distinctive three-leaf cluster. Hungry ticks also lay in wait for unsuspecting hikers. Wear long pants and check every few minutes for hitchhiking pests.

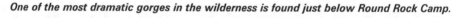

One of the most dramatic gorges in the wilderness is found just below Round Rock Camp.

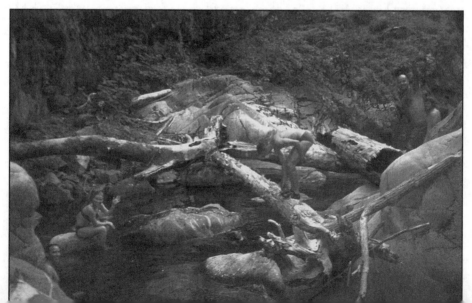

For the most part, the tread is well established and easy to follow, except at a few of the numerous river fords. If you find yourself on anything other than an obvious trail, you've likely wandered off course. Simply backtrack until you rejoin the official trail.

After two more river crossings, you may catch whiffs of sulfur (similar to the smell of rotten eggs), your pungent introduction to **Sulphur Springs Camp** (5.8 miles, 1350'). Unfortunately, these hot springs rich in hydrogen sulfide are not large enough to soak in. One site is equipped with a table and cooking grate. This camp and Buckskin Flat Camp are the smallest and least attractive of the camps along the **Carmel River.** You're better off staying at Carmel River Camp or venturing farther to idyllic **Hiding Canyon Camp.** The latter lies just 3.4 miles from the trailhead but requires more than two dozen river crossings, which, depending on water levels, poison oak, flies, and ticks, can be an arduous trek.

From Sulphur Springs, the trail crosses a year-round creek that originates from the east slope of **Elephant Mountain,** which forms the granite southwest wall of the Carmel River drainage 4020 feet above. Upstream, you'll cross five more times amid riparian woodlands dominated by bigleaf maples, black oaks, sycamores, and alders before arriving in **Buckskin Flat Camp** (7.4 miles, 1580'). Marked by a sign, the riverside site sits atop a grassy flat. There is no table or cooking grate.

In fall, leaves bearing deep hues of yellow, orange, and red blanket the forest floor and surface pools. It's the perfect season to hike the river, as water levels remain low and you can boulder-hop its course with ease.

AUTUMN COLORS EXPLAINED ■ ■ ■ ■ ■ ■ ■ ■ ■ ■ ■ ■ ■ ■

Every autumn, brilliant hues paint the canyon floor along the Carmel River. Many changes occur in the leaf of a deciduous tree before it falls from the branch. The process begins in the abscission layer, where the leaf and stem connect.

In fall, plant hormones respond to diminished daylight, swelling the cells of the abscission layer and forming a cork-like material that gradually cuts off flow between the leaf and the tree. Deprived of water and nutrients, the leaves stop producing green-hued chlorophyll and other colors become visible. Oranges come from carotene, yellows from xanthophyll, bright reds and purples from anthocyanin, and browns from tannins. As the abscission layer continues to swell, the cells disintegrate until the leaf either falls or is blown from the tree.

The process is an energy-saving strategy. Without their leaves, trees are able to go dormant in the winter. Other than limited root growth, their biological processes come to a temporary halt.

■ ■

SIDE TRIP ▪

Although Round Rock Camp is not the most ideal backcountry camp, the gorge in which it rests is among the most beautiful in the Santa Lucia Range. The 0.6-mile Round Rock Camp Trail leads to the canyon floor, where the swift river plunges from pool to pool, carving its deep path between massive smooth granite walls.

From the junction, descend 0.2 mile to the river and make your way downstream 50 feet. Be mindful of slippery boulders and poison oak, which recoils in the fissures. The sounds of cascading water echo up from the gorge below. Enjoy the solitude as you take a bracing dip in the headwaters of the Carmel River.

You'll cross the river to a small grassy terrace and unofficial campsite—actually, more picturesque than camp proper. The trail climbs 0.2 mile, then descends south past riverside tangles of blackberry and poison oak. The overgrown yet established trail crosses the river just downstream from an enormous boulder, perhaps Round Rock itself, which looms over a shallow wading pool. A couple hundred feet later you'll reach Round Rock Camp (10.2 miles, 1920'), with a table and room enough for up to a dozen small tents atop a grassy terrace.

▪ ▪

Past Buckskin Flat Camp, you'll climb 0.3 mile to a small ridge, then return to the river's edge for a gradual ascent that at times feels more like a continual wade. The trail launches into another series of river fords, crisscrossing through mats of blackberries, thimbleberries, and ubiquitous poison oak. Head-high chain ferns shade still pools, while horsetail rushes and mosses grow in spongy clumps between granite boulders.

Past the tenth ford, the trail passes a significant canyon and tributary that stem from **Uncle Sam Mountain,** the massive granite ridge looming more than 4750 feet overhead. Swift runoff from this major peak follows the **Church Creek Fault,** among the largest fault systems in the **Ventana Wilderness,** whose shattered course provides a natural channel. If you're on your way to **Round Rock Camp,** you'll observe this northwest-trending fault in deep channels and waterfall basins along the Carmel River.

The twelfth crossing skirts a moss-covered granite wall—be aware that both the USGS and USFS maps inaccurately label this site of Hiding Canyon Camp, which lies 0.2 mile farther upstream. Expect to get your feet wet in all but the driest months, as the trail is often submerged by high water.

True to its name, **Hiding Canyon Camp** (9.2 miles, 1740') is easy to miss. You'll reach the turnoff just as the trail leaves the river's edge to climb the canyon. Just across the river, the camp offers two large sites, each with a table and cooking grate. The first site sits atop a narrow terrace along the west bank. The larger, preferred site is just a few feet upstream near an enormous ponderosa pine with a 6-foot-plus diameter. You'll recognize ponderosas by their golden puzzle-piece bark and pine needles bunched in threes.

If you're willing to hike upriver off trail for 0.4 mile, you'll pass through a narrow sandstone gorge and arrive at **Ventana Mesa Creek Falls,** which tumbles into a swimming hole. Farther upriver, the canyon widens and turns south, entering a second gorge at the confluence with **Ventana Mesa Creek.** A few feet farther upstream the creek cascades into a deep granite-lined pool. If the water level is low enough in late summer and fall, you can press on for 200 feet to a larger swimming hole and waterfall within a mossy, fern-lined grotto. The refreshingly cold water is a welcome escape on a hot summer day.

From Hiding Canyon Camp, the Carmel River Trail continues across the river and ascends the east-facing canyon wall. Climb 0.1 mile to a stunning overlook of the narrow river gorge. The trail leads up a minor ridge to the easily missed unmarked **Round Rock Camp Trail junction** (9.6 miles, 2030'). If you're continuing on the Carmel River Trail, refer to TRIP 50 Hiding Canyon & Round Rock Camps (page 202) and follow that trail description in reverse.

Trip 46

VENTANA DOUBLE CONE VIA CARMEL RIVER TRAIL

LENGTH AND TYPE: 31-mile out-and-back, loop, or point-to-point

RATING: Challenging

TRAIL CONDITION: Potentially impassable due to high water crossing along the Carmel River Trail during the wet season, with abundant poison oak. Passable yet difficult with deadfalls, washouts, and brush encroachment along Ventana Double Cone Trail.

HIGHLIGHTS: Find solitude atop 4853-foot Ventana Double Cone as you soak up panoramic views of the furrowed Santa Lucia Range and broad Pacific.

TO REACH THE TRAILHEAD: This hike begins at the Los Padres Dam Trailhead.

TRIP SUMMARY: This book describes several routes to the remote summit of Ventana Double Cone, in the heart of Ventana Wilderness. For general information on the Ventana Trail, see the summary for TRIP 38 Ventana Double Cone via Ventana Trail (page 155).

From Los Padres Dam, this route ascends the cool Carmel River canyon along year-round sections of the river to Hiding Canyon Camp, where it begins a steep 3113-foot climb over 6.3 miles to the summit. Watch for poison oak.

As at most peaks along this dramatic coast, the best times to hike are between mid-November and April, taking advantage of cooler temperatures, fogless days, and fewer pesky mosquitoes and flies. This route is also a good choice in summer heat and fall drought, as from Hiding Canyon Camp you can reach the summit with a daypack and plenty of water.

Be prepared for rain and snow if you hike in winter, when snow levels can drop to 2000 feet and the river may be impassable.

Trip Description

See TRIP 44 Bluff & Carmel River Camps (page 179) for the first 4.9 miles of this route to **Carmel River Camp.**

Just upstream from the main site at Carmel River Camp (1220') the trail crosses the river and follows a bend west beneath a filtering canopy of maples, sycamores, and alders. Few people venture beyond the camp, and poison oak encroaches on the little-used trail beyond. Hungry ticks also lay in wait—wear long pants and check every few minutes for hitchhikers.

After two more river crossings, you'll reach **Sulphur Springs Camp** (5.8 miles, 1350'). This and Buckskin Flat Camp are the smallest and least attractive of the camps along the **Carmel River.** Instead, stay at Carmel River Camp or **Hiding Canyon Camp.** The latter lies just 3.4 miles from the trailhead but requires more than two dozen river crossings, which, depending on the season, can be an arduous trek.

From Sulphur Springs, the trail crosses a year-round creek that originates from the east slope of **Elephant Mountain.** Heading upstream, you'll cross five more times before arriving in **Buckskin Flat Camp** (7.4 miles, 1580'), atop a grassy flat. There is no table or cooking grate.

Past camp, you'll climb 0.3 mile to a small ridge, then return to the river's edge for a gradual ascent. The trail launches into another series of river fords, crisscrossing through mats of blackberries, thimbleberries, and ubiquitous poison oak. Past the tenth ford, the trail passes a significant canyon and tributary that stem from **Uncle Sam Mountain,** the massive granite ridge towering more than 4750 feet overhead.

The twelfth crossing skirts a moss-covered granite wall—be aware that both the USGS and USFS maps inaccurately label this the site of Hiding Canyon Camp, which lies 0.2 mile farther upstream. Expect to get your feet wet in all but the driest months, as the trail is often submerged by high water.

The spur to Hiding Canyon Camp (9.2 miles, 1740') is easy to miss. You'll reach the turnoff just as the trail leaves the river's edge to climb the canyon. Just across the river, you'll find two large sites with a table and cooking grate. The first site sits atop a narrow terrace along the west bank, while the second, larger site is just a few feet upstream near an enormous ponderosa pine.

If you're willing to hike upriver off trail for 0.4 mile, you'll pass through a narrow sandstone gorge and arrive at **Ventana Mesa Creek Falls,** which tumbles into a swimming hole. Farther upriver, the canyon widens and turns south, entering a second gorge at the confluence with **Ventana Mesa Creek**. A few feet farther upstream the creek cascades into a deep granite-lined pool. If the water level is low enough in late summer and fall, you can press on for 200 feet to a larger swimming hole and waterfall within a mossy, fern-lined grotto.

The **Puerto Suelo Trail** (9.2 miles, 1740') begins atop a flat bench on the west bank just downstream from Hiding Canyon Camp. Those bound for **Ventana Double Cone** or **Bottchers Gap** will climb this trail to the **Ventana Trail junction**. In drought years it's best to fill water bottles here.

You'll begin a steep climb west through a minor gully and across a small creek, then wander through several other minor gullies, dry practically year-round. In half a mile the trail begins a series of switchbacks, ascending a brushy slope to a minor saddle. Continue past fragrant stands of bays and tanoaks and across small tributaries to **Uncle Sam Creek**. The trail crosses and then recrosses the creek, which may be your last opportunity for water between here and the summit.

Continue climbing northwest through overgrown ceanothus thickets. The last 0.3 mile of the Puerto Suelo Trail ascends very steep, short switchbacks. Just 0.1 mile from the saddle, clear water bubbles up from two neighboring springs, reliable in all but the driest months.

Climb the final 200 feet to the Puerto Suelo saddle and Ventana Trail junction (11.8 miles, 3530'). See TRIP 38 Ventana Double Cone via Ventana Trail (page 155) for the final 3.7 miles to the summit (15.5 miles, 4853').

Trip 47

VENTANA DOUBLE CONE VIA BIG PINES TRAIL

LENGTH AND TYPE: 35.4-mile out-and-back, loop, or point-to-point

RATING: Strenuous to challenging

TRAIL CONDITION: Difficult with deadfalls, washouts, and brush encroachment

HIGHLIGHTS: Find serenity atop this summit with breathtaking views of a vast wilderness.

TO REACH THE TRAILHEAD: This hike begins at the Los Padres Dam Trailhead.

TRIP SUMMARY: This book describes several routes to the remote 4853-foot summit of Ventana Double Cone, in the heart of Ventana Wilderness. For general information on the Ventana Trail, see the summary for TRIP 38 Ventana Double Cone via Ventana Trail.

This route offers a consistent grade and spectacular views, particularly in winter and spring. Be aware that the first 4 miles are overrun with poison oak, and developed trails along the fire break make the trail difficult and confusing to follow.

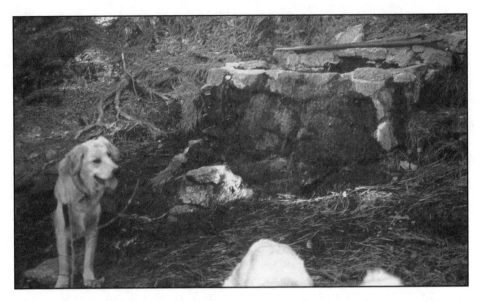

Although Ventana Wilderness offers hundreds of dog-friendly hiking trails, be aware that poison oak can also be carried on animals' fur.

As at most peaks along this dramatic coast, the best times to hike are between mid-November and April, taking advantage of cooler temperatures, fogless days, and fewer pesky mosquitoes and flies. Be prepared for rain and snow if you hike in winter, when snow levels can drop to 2000 feet and the river may be impassable.

During the driest months (August through November), you may not find water until Big Pines Camp (upper Danish Creek) or Pat Spring. In drought years there's even a chance these two water sources could run dry. In such conditions, consider one of the alternative routes.

Trip Description

See TRIP 43 Danish Creek Camp (page 176) for the first 3 miles of this route to the signed **Danish Creek Trail junction** (2050').

From this junction, the **Danish Creek Trail** branches left and descends to **Danish Creek Camp** (3.8 miles, 1430'), set in a broad meadow beside year-round **Danish Creek** (see TRIP 43 Danish Creek Camp). You'll continue straight through this junction on the **Big Pines Trail,** skirt a minor summit, and follow the ridgeline on a narrow overgrown trail for the next 0.3 mile.

You'll soon cross a steep overgrown **jeep road** (3.3 miles, 2110'), more commonly used as a horse trail, which angles right and descends 2.6 miles to **Los Padres Dam.** A few paces past the road you'll reach an oak-rimmed grassy ridge. In spring the black oaks sprout vibrant foliage amid a brilliant blanket of flowering poppies, lupines, shooting stars, and deer vetches.

The trail widens and follows an old road that climbs the Danish Creek watershed from saddle to ridge. For the most part, you'll have to scrape past encroaching chamise, sage, and broom, so check often for ticks, particularly during the wet season.

You'll quickly pass another old **jeep road junction** (3.4 miles, 2500') on your left. Also used as a horse trail, this road leads southwest to Danish Creek, 0.3 mile upstream from Danish Creek Camp. Onward 0.3 mile, you'll reach a third **spur road** (3.7 miles, 2650'), which doglegs right and heads first north-northeast through dense madrone and oak forests, then northwest on a gravel road to **Blue Rock Ridge**.

Bypassing these spurs, the Big Pines Trail continues west across forested slopes and exposed brush-covered ridges. After a moderate climb that almost tops a 2778-foot ridge, the trail switchbacks and descends to a minor **saddle** (4.9 miles, 2640') capped by a bare outcrop of pale-green serpentine, California's state rock. The unobstructed views from this open ridge are outstanding, stretching northwest across **Monterey Bay** and the **Santa Lucia Range,** which rise abruptly from the wave-washed Pacific. A short climb from the saddle you'll reach the signed **Ventana Wilderness Boundary** (5 miles, 2680').

CALIFORNIA'S STATE ROCK

Rare elsewhere on Earth, serpentine is common in California, scattered across some 2200 square miles. Originally part of the ocean floor, serpentine was thrust to the surface during ancient shifts in the Earth's crust. Intense heat and pressure metamorphosed the rock into a smooth, sometimes soapy green stone.

Due to its unique chemical composition, serpentine supports equally unusual plant species. In addition to a low water-holding capacity, soil derived from serpentine is low in calcium, phosphorous, and nitrogen and high in such toxic heavy metals as magnesium, chromium, and nickel. Most plants simply cannot tolerate these conditions.

Regardless, certain "serpentine endemics" have adapted to this soil and thrive on these shallow rocky outcrops. The rare vegetation in turn attracts birds, reptiles, amphibians, and mammals that may otherwise not be in the area. Slowly stroll across these barrens for glimpses of a rare ecosystem.

Following the ridge up a gentle grade, you'll soon begin a steep half-mile descent south to a minor **saddle** (5.8 miles, 2250'). The route crosses forested slopes of oaks, pines, and madrones, the latter distinguished by deep red flaky bark that peels back to expose a smooth orange trunk. Past the saddle, the trail skirts waist-high brush, ascends 0.2 mile west to a 2525-foot ridge summit, then quickly descends to a saddle within earshot of Danish Creek.

From here you'll begin the second largest climb on the Big Pines Trail, first across dry slopes covered in thickets of manzanita, ceanothus, and chamise and then beneath dense madrone canopies. Again, watch for profuse amounts of poison oak—thankfully, the last concentration of this toxic trailside companion en route to **Ventana Double Cone**. The steep ascent ends after a few switchbacks, emerging amid chaparral brush atop a 3097-foot **ridge summit** (7.2 miles).

From the summit, the trail begins a gentle descent that branches away from the road-bed within 0.1 mile (7.3 miles, 3020'). While orange flagging marked this turn on my hike, it remains an easily overlooked left turn through a narrow stretch of scrub oak, bay, and ceanothus thickets. If you miss the turn and continue along the roadbed 50 feet, you'll reach a maze of narrow overgrown deer trails that lack the packed tread of the well-established Big Pines Trail.

From the turnoff, you'll descend south past steep slopes with numerous deadfalls and encroaching brush to a minor saddle, then descend farther to another minor saddle (7.8 miles, 2980'). From here the trail ascends through shady hardwood forests past scattered young pines a few hundred yards above Danish Creek's gurgling headwaters.

Over the next 0.2 mile the trail narrows between fire-scarred pine snags, a target of industrious woodpeckers, which excavate their nests in spring in large snags. You'll follow the contour to a nearby **gully** (8 miles, 3220'), home to a small granite-lined creek between December and March. A few yards farther you'll cross another seasonal tributary and clam-ber across a tangle of downed debris. The trail passes a third seasonal creek (8.1 miles, 3260'), climbs beneath the remnants of a pre–Basin Complex pine forest, crosses a grassy bowl, and in 50 yards reaches the **Big Pines Camp Trail junction** (8.8 miles, 3350'). After the 2008 Basin Complex Fire, little remains of the camp, and the trail is deemed challenging at best. From this junction, the main trail continues straight and contours southwest 0.1 mile to another junction (8.9 miles, 3340'). Here you'll find a shortcut spur toward **Pat Spring Camp**. Fire destroyed trail signage, but with a watchful eye you can spot carved into the sign assurance of Pat Spring and the Ventana Trail.

If you skip the recommended shortcut, you'll continue west on the Big Pines Trail, climb briefly, then cross a seasonal tributary, the nearest water source to **Spaghetti Camp** (expect water from first rains through March). After a moderate 0.1-mile ascent beneath shady oaks, madrones, and pines, you'll arrive in camp.

Spaghetti Camp (9.1 miles, 3620') also marks the junction with the **Skinner Ridge Trail** (which leads west 6.3 miles to **Bottchers Gap**) and the Ventana Trail (which leads south 8.4 miles to Ventana Double Cone). Camp is flat and can easily accommodate two tents. The nearest reliable water source between December and March is upper Danish Creek, 0.1 mile along the Big Pines Trail, while during dry months (May through November) you may have to hike as far as Pat Spring, a mile along the Ventana Trail.

From camp the Ventana Trail crosses oak- and pine-clad slopes, skirting mounds of fallen snags and woody debris. You may surprise quail, woodpeckers, and band-tailed pigeons along this little-used trail. Half a mile later you'll reach an unmarked junction with the previously described shortcut spur from the Big Pines Trail.

Continue half a mile farther past the unofficial camp to a major saddle and four-way **junction** (10.1 miles, 3770') with the westbound Pat Spring Camp Trail and eastbound Pat Spring Trail.

See TRIP 38 Ventana Double Cone via Ventana Trail (page 155) for a description of the remaining 7.6 miles from this junction to the summit of Ventana Double Cone.

SIDE TRIP ■

You can save yourself time and energy by taking the shortcut toward **Pat Spring Camp** (8.9 miles, 3340'), which leads 0.4 mile to the **Pat Spring Trail.** The shortcut spur is on your left, 20 feet from the Big Pines Trail sign. It begins as a narrow trail that descends southwest 0.1 mile across the creek's upper headwaters (9 miles, 3290'). Fifty feet farther the trail climbs from the gully to the **Ventana Trail junction.** Look for the inconspicuous VENTANA LOOKOUT TRAIL sign posted on a tree trunk and turn left.

One hundred yards eastbound on the **Ventana Trail,** you'll reach an **unofficial camp,** just off the trail on your left. Shaded by large pines and madrones, the first site is perched alongside the south branch of Danish Creek, though it's often dry by late spring. The second site lies just above the creek on the opposite bank. Together the sites can accommodate a half dozen tents. If this stretch is dry, you can either head back to the last creek crossing or continue on the Ventana Trail and camp closer to **Pat Spring.**

Onward, you'll make a gentle 0.1-mile-ascent to a minor saddle and the easily missed four-way junction with westbound **Pat Spring Camp Trail** and eastbound Pat Spring Trail (9.7 miles, 3770').

■ ■

China Camp

■ ■ ■ ■ ■ ■ ■ ■ ■ ■ ■ ■ ■

N ESTLED AT 4270 FEET in a prominent saddle beneath a dense canopy of oaks and madrones, China Camp offers one of the easiest access points to Ventana's high country. This chapter also describes lower-elevation routes off Tassajara Road, along the Church Creek, Horse Pasture, and Tony Trails. Tassajara Road may be closed during storms due to fallen trees or small mudslides. Two routes extend from China Camp: the westbound Pine Ridge Trail and the northwest-bound Miller Canyon Trail.

Although the Pine Ridge Trail is the most heavily used path in the backcountry, most people begin from Big Sur and never reach Pine Ridge. This eastern section of the trail is remote, challenging, and strenuous, offering a trek across diverse terrain with sweeping panoramas of the vast wilderness. The route from China Camp suffers from encroaching brush, and few people hike farther than Pine Valley, whose dramatic sandstone cliffs shelter a spectacular waterfall and pine-studded meadow. This is the most direct route to the Black Cone Trail, but be prepared for a heavily overgrown path from Divide Camp to the north end of the Black Cone Trail atop Pine Ridge. Much of this terrain is intolerable in summer, when nagging flies swarm and temperatures soar into the upper 90s Fahrenheit.

From spring through fall, the Carmel River and Miller Canyon Trails offer pleasant routes downriver, though both trails are cloaked with poison oak. The trailhead for the Church Creek Trail lies in the heart of the wilderness, 5 miles beyond China Camp along Tassajara Road. The only trail that ascends the Church Creek drainage, it takes in some of Ventana's most dramatic sandstone outcrops.

DIRECTIONS: Heading south on Highway 1 from Monterey, turn left on Carmel Valley Road (County Road G16) in Carmel and head eastbound. In 11.7 miles you'll reach Carmel Valley Village, your last opportunity for gas, food, and supplies. Drive through the village and continue another 11.3 miles to the Tassajara Road junction.

Heading north on Highway 101 from Southern California, turn off on Route 101 Business, Greenfield's southernmost exit. In half a mile you'll turn left on Elm Avenue (County Road G16) and head southwest 5.8 miles to Arroyo Seco Road (County Road

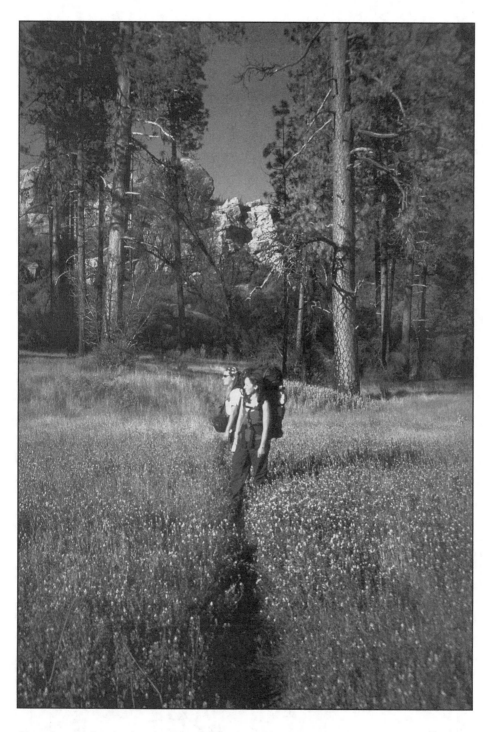

Towering ponderosa pines in the open meadow of Pine Valley.

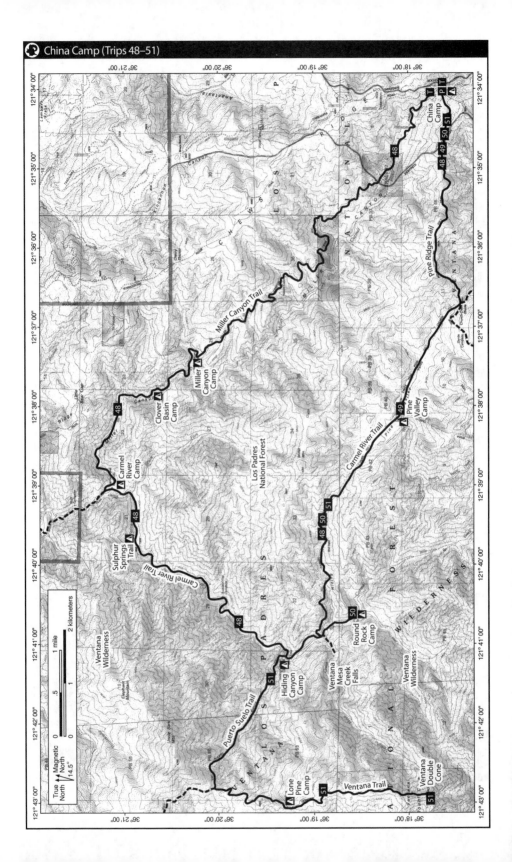

G17). The two roads merge for 6.5 miles and then fork. Take the right branch and continue 17 miles northwest on Carmel Valley Road to the Tassajara Road junction.

From the Tassajara Road junction, turn southwest and drive 1.3 miles to a fork with Cachagua Road. Take the left branch and continue 10.7 miles along Tassajara Road to the China Camp entrance. The pavement ends 1.8 miles from the junction, and 7.6 miles farther you'll pass White Oaks Campground (for details see Nearest Campground below). From there it's 1.3 miles to the entrance road at China Camp.

To reach the campground, hang a sharp right off Tassajara Road and drive 200 feet. If you're not camping, park in the small lot across Tassajara Road from the camp entrance.

VISITOR CENTER: Big Sur Station: (831) 667-2315. The station is on Highway 1, 4.2 miles south of Andrew Molera State Park and just south of Pfeiffer Big Sur State Park. Open daily 8 a.m.–6 p.m. Memorial Day through Labor Day, 8 a.m.–4:30 p.m. the rest of the year. USFS Monterey District Headquarters, King City: (831) 385-5434.

NEAREST CAMPGROUNDS: Two small USFS campgrounds, White Oaks Campground (7.9 miles along Tassajara Road) and China Camp (10.7 miles along Tassajara Road), are open year-round on a first-come, first-serve basis (6 sites; free). Facilities include vault toilets, fire rings, and picnic tables. There is no water available at the campgrounds.

INFORMATION: There's no fee if you park at the turnout on Tassajara Road directly across from the China Camp entrance. Fire permits are required for all stoves. Dogs are permitted and allowed off leash, except in designated camp-grounds, where a 6-foot or shorter leash is required.

WEBSITE: www.fs.usda.gov/lpnf

PHONE: Los Padres National Forest Headquarters: (805) 968-6640

Trip 48

MILLER CANYON & PINE VALLEY LOOP

LENGTH AND TYPE: 24.1-mile loop

RATING: Strenuous

TRAIL CONDITION: Difficult to impassable, poison oak, faint tread, trail washouts

HIGHLIGHTS: This loop takes in deep narrow river gorges rich in ferns and lined with colorful hardwoods where you'll find waterfall oases and pristine swimming holes.

TO REACH THE TRAILHEAD: Park at the large turnout on Tassajara Road across from China Camp, then stroll to the end of the entrance road. The trailhead is at the junction with gated Jeffery Road. There is no water at the trailhead.

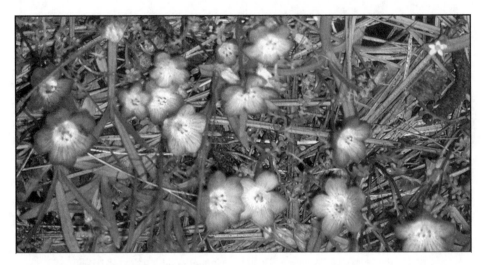

The recently charred landscape within Miller Canyon brought nutrients back into the soil to allow forest succession to begin anew.

TRIP SUMMARY: This route offers several loop, out-and-back, and point-to-point options. The following description comprises a loop through Miller Canyon to the Carmel River confluence, up Pine Valley to the river's headwaters at Church Creek Divide, then back to China Camp via the Pine Ridge Trail. This order assumes hikers will spend the final night in scenic Pine Valley, followed by a 2000-foot climb over the remaining 5.3 miles. Taking the reverse route would mean spending the last night at less scenic Miller Canyon Camp, followed by a nearly 3000-foot climb over the final 7.1 miles to the trailhead.

If you can arrange a shuttle vehicle, an excellent 15-mile point-to-point hike leads from China Camp along Miller Canyon and the Carmel River to Los Padres Dam. Highlights include scenic views from golden oak savannas and stays at the riverside Carmel River and Bluff Camps.

Miller and Carmel River Canyons are most pleasant in fall, when the lush hardwood forests turn brilliant hues of yellow, orange, and crimson. In late summer and fall, ticks, flies, and mosquitoes have diminished and temperatures are ideal for wading the creeks and rivers. After heavy winter storms, easy boulder-hopping crossings can turn swift and dangerous. In spring the broad meadows and open savannas are blanketed in wildflowers and vibrant new growth. Unfortunately, regardless of the season, the bottomland trails are heavily overgrown with poison oak.

Trip Description

Head northwest along gated **Jeffery Road** (4270') past sprawling oaks, peeling red madrones, and towering Coulter pines. The latter boast the world's heaviest cones. After a moderate mile-long descent, the road reaches a seasonal stretch of the **Miller Fork,** usually dry from May until the first winter rains. In a quarter mile you'll enter private property, posted by the Tanoak homeowners association. Follow the road past several private driveways, another seasonal branch of the Miller Fork, and the Tamarack homes' pond, then descend 0.1 mile to a second gate (1.8 miles, 3400'). Beyond this gate the route enters the **Ventana Wilderness.**

Continue 0.1 mile along the road until it doglegs sharply right and begins a steep climb east. The trail begins at this sharp turn, leading 0.1 mile to a junction with another road. Fifty feet down this road, you'll reach a fork. Take the left branch. The road ends at the **Miller Canyon Trail junction** (2 miles, 3360').

Miller Canyon Trail branches right 150 feet to another gate. Pass through the gate for a gentle descent toward a minor gorge that parallels **Miller Canyon.** The trail closely follows the Miller Canyon Fault northwest. Contouring above the minor canyon, the trail returns to private property along the banks of an alder-lined creek (3 miles, 2880'), where you'll find a few unofficial camps. Don't expect to find water during the dry season (May through October).

From the creek, the trail climbs to a series of minor saddles offering fine views. Atop the third saddle, the trail descends 0.3 mile to a more dependable creek that usually flows through early summer. Here you'll find the **Nason Cabin site** (4.3 miles, 3090'), featuring scattered homestead relics along a small creekside clearing. The site also hosts an unofficial camp. Beyond this point the already narrow trail suffers from overgrown brush and destructive washouts. In wet season, hitchhiking ticks are prolific.

The trail climbs to a fourth saddle for oak-filtered views along the **Carmel River** and Miller Fork, featuring fire-scarred ridges and cleft gullies that shelter rare Santa Lucia firs. A range of textures and hues distinguish the distinct plant communities. Along the canyon floors, lush deciduous forests flash vibrant green in the spring and deep orange, red, and yellow in the fall.

From the fourth saddle (4.9 miles, 3070'), the trail steadily descends 2.2 miles to **Miller Canyon Camp,** leading past a sixth saddle and through a minor gully. In wet months the trail crosses a nettle-lined seasonal creek beneath a small waterfall. Continue 150 feet to the **Hennickson Trail junction** (6.4 miles, 2420').

Although the US Forest Service has abandoned the **Hennickson Trail** to the elements, hikers still pass this way. The route rockets up 900 feet in 2 miles along a brushy waterless trail to the **Tin House** on **Hennickson Ridge.**

Past the junction, the Miller Canyon Trail continues past endemic stands of Santa Lucia firs, easily identified by densely foliated crowns that extend from the base of the tree and lower branches that nearly touch the ground. The trail descends 0.4 mile past talus slopes to a small seasonal tributary and a 20-foot waterfall that flows from the first winter rains until summer.

The trail follows this small tributary through its narrow gorge, crossing it a second time through shoulder-high thickets of stinging nettles. This invasive nonnative plant features clusters of small white flowers that bloom from the base of stinging pubescent leaves.

A few hundred yards past the stinging nettles, the trail approaches the Miller Fork for the first of 20 crossings. After heavy winter storms, these fords become increasingly swift and dangerous downstream. In all other seasons it's an easy boulder-hop across to **Miller Canyon Camp** (7.1 miles, 2000').

This is the larger of two official camps along the Miller Canyon Trail. The first site is perched atop the east end of a creekside bench a few yards from the crossing, marked by a dilapidated LOS PADRES NATIONAL FOREST sign, a table, and a fire ring. A hundred feet farther, the second site sits atop the west end of the bench and is large enough to accommodate up to two tents.

Beyond camp the trail leads 0.1 mile to the first major river bend and your second boulder-hop across the Miller Fork. You'll follow an old roadbed heavily overgrown with poison oak and cross the river three more times before arriving in **Clover Basin Camp** (7.7 miles, 1870').

This camp occupies a large meadow amid a marshy basin near the banks of the Miller Fork. Equipped with a fire ring and tree stump seating, the camp can accommodate up to four tents. Mosquitoes and flies can be a nuisance in all but the driest months. American Indians roamed this watershed for thousands of years, as evidenced by mortar holes in rocks adjacent to camp. Here the Esselen tribe hunted a wide variety of birds, fish, and mammals and gathered a variety of acorns to leach and grind into flour.

Past camp, you'll closely follow the Miller Fork, occasionally picking your way through unavoidable thickets of poison oak. The trail meanders along the deep, narrow river gorge blanketed in ferns, mugwort, and blackberries, as well as colorful alders, maples, buckeyes, and bays. You'll cross the river 16 more times before reaching the **Carmel River Trail junction** (10.2 miles, 1220').

From this junction, the trail crosses the Miller Fork just above its confluence and returns upstream to China Camp along the **Carmel River** and **Pine Ridge Trails.** See TRIP 45 Hiding Canyon & Round Rock Camps (page 181) for the route description to **Hiding Canyon Camp** and TRIP 50 Hiding Canyon & Round Rock Camps (page 202) for the route from Hiding Canyon to China Camp (follow the latter in reverse). If you're on a point-to-point trip from China Camp to **Los Padres Dam,** continue downstream along the Carmel River Trail 4.8 miles below the confluence to the Los Padres Dam Trailhead. Refer to TRIP 44 Bluff & Carmel River Camps (page 179) and follow that trail description in reverse.

Trip 49

PINE VALLEY

LENGTH AND TYPE: 12-mile out-and-back

RATING: Moderate

TRAIL CONDITION: Passable to difficult, poison oak

HIGHLIGHTS: Tall ponderosas amid an open meadow, ancient sandstone cliffs, buttes, and boulders, and Pine Falls, which cascades 50 feet into an emerald swimming hole

TO REACH THE TRAILHEAD: Park at the large turnout on Tassajara Road across from China Camp. The trailhead is on the camp side of the road, 100 feet south of the parking lot and 150 feet south of the camp entrance. The trail begins on a saddle above China Camp. It is marked, though encroaching brush often obscures the sign. There's no water at the trailhead.

TRIP SUMMARY: This trail leads past old-growth pine forests, waterfall oases that shelter deep swimming holes, and wildflower-strewn meadows that remind one of the Sierras. Naturally, this is a popular year-round day hike, so it's best to avoid it during major holidays. Though the valley lies within day-hike range, allow at least six hours for the round-trip to enjoy the scenery or visit Pine Falls for a refreshing swim. The route is ideal in spring and fall,

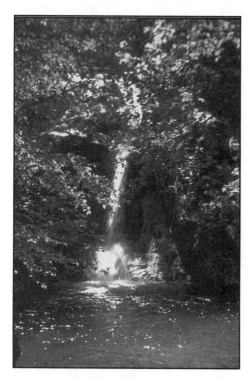

as temperatures are moderate and storms infrequent. Summer temps can reach the upper 90s Fahrenheit, and flies and mosquitoes pose a nuisance. Winter temps can dip below freezing, and snow is common above 4000 feet. If your timing is perfect, however, between winter storms the valley can hit the upper 60s Fahrenheit, and you'll likely have the valley all to yourself.

Trip Description

The route begins at a marked trailhead on a major saddle above **China Camp** (4350'), 6 miles from **Pine Valley** and 24 from **Big Sur.** Like most trails in the **Ventana Wilderness,** this one is not regularly maintained.

Pine Falls cascades 50 feet into an emerald swimming hole below Pine Valley.

In 1999 fire scorched the area, allowing fire-adapted species to thrive. As a result, trail sections over the first 1.2 miles are heavily overgrown. You'll gradually climb 400 feet, then descend the same elevation through shoulder-high brush dominated by ceanothus and tanoak.

In 0.6 mile you'll emerge from the worst of the overgrown sections at the route's high point (4750'). Views stretch south to the **Black Cone Trail** ridgelines and the **Church Creek** and **Tassajara Creek** drainages, west along the **Coast Ridge,** and southeast toward **Cone and Junipero Serra Peaks.** Rising nearly a mile above the Pacific, Cone Peak is perched atop the farthest visible ridge, 17 miles south. Dominating the horizon, 5862-foot Junipero Serra rises high above the unseen **Salinas Valley.**

The trail gradually descends a scenic ridge across golden grasslands and past thickets of new growth sprouting from the remains of a charred forest. The ridge separates the **Miller Creek** drainage and the Church Creek drainage. You'll continue through oak woodlands and grasslands speckled with stalks of Our Lord's candle, top a minor saddle, and climb the ridge to a prominent saddle. Views vanish briefly as the trail switchbacks southwest and then climbs north to the second highest point along the route (2.1 miles, 4740'). From here the route is all downhill to Pine Valley.

Pause for glimpses through the bare branches of burned snags. Look west to spot the sandstone formation that parallels Church Creek Fault. The trail turns southwest on a steep grade, dropping 850 feet through open oak woodlands carpeted with vibrant wildflowers in spring. After 1.5 miles the trail switchbacks down to **Church Creek Divide** (3.6 miles, 3650'). This divide marks the four-way junction of the westbound **Pine Ridge Trail,** the southeast-bound **Church Creek Trail,** and the northwest-bound **Carmel River Trail** to Pine Valley.

Forming a deep saddle between two west-trending ridges, the divide sits atop the 29-mile east-west **Church Creek Fault.** For millions of years the North American and Pacific plates have ground past one another, here creating Church Creek canyon. From the divide, the fault continues northwest, following the Carmel River Trail to **Hiding Canyon Camp,** ascending the **Puerto Suelo Trail** to the prominent **Puerto Suelo** saddle, and emerging at the Pacific near **Kaslar Point.** To the northwest lie the headwaters of the **Carmel River,** while to the southeast lie the headwaters of the **Salinas River** along Church Creek. Oddly enough, the latter winds some 80 miles north of the Carmel River before finding its way to sea.

From the divide, the Carmel River Trail turns right and leads 1.7 miles to the wildflower-strewn meadows and tall pines of Pine Valley. Over the first 0.3 mile you'll cross the typically dry headwaters of the Carmel River. As the grade levels off (4.5 miles, 3160'), you'll notice sandstone cliffs to your right and hear trickling water off to your left. The scene is reminiscent of the Sierras, with ponderosa pines rising from an open meadow beside steep sandstone cliffs.

You'll continue through mixed evergreen and riparian forests, highlighted by rare endemic Santa Lucia firs at the valley's east end. A large gate marks the official **Pine Valley entrance** (5.3 miles, 3140'), at a junction with the Pine Valley–Pine Ridge Trail and the cross-country trail to Pine Falls. The main trail leads to a year-round stretch of the Carmel River. If you have time, don't miss the side trip to the falls.

SIDE TRIP ■

The 0.7-mile trail to **Pine Falls** is narrow, overgrown, and washed out in a few precarious places. Your payoff is a scenic waterfall oasis and swimming hole, among Ventana's most spectacular sights.

From the Pine Valley–Pine Ridge Trail junction (5.3 miles, 3140'), turn left and cross the river, heading downstream a few yards before recrossing past the first of three small unofficial campsites. The trail closely follows the river, crisscrossing it multiple times on the way downstream past riparian forests and endemic Santa Lucia firs.

You'll emerge at an overlook directly above 50-foot Pine Falls (6 miles, 2700'). The descent to its base is hazardous, as you must clamber across slick boulders. Use the conveniently placed rope to negotiate the final 20 feet through a minor gully. The crystal clear pool is wide and deep enough for swimming, but as temperatures only reach the high 50s Fahrenheit at best, your swim will be a quick one. Enjoy the brisk plunge and return the way you came.

■ ■

If you're bound for the more spacious upper meadow, turn right at this junction onto the Carmel River Trail, following a decrepit sign marked BEAR BASIN. You'll pass through a gate toward a small cabin on private land. A longtime Pine Valley resident lives and gardens on the small plot to your right.

A hundred feet past the cabin you'll ascend a minor knoll, then descend into upper Pine Valley and the official **Pine Valley Camp** (5.4 miles, 3200'), equipped with a fire ring and room for up to three tents. Six or seven unofficial campsites also lie nestled amid the pine-studded meadow, each equipped with a fire ring and room for up to three tents. These fill up quickly on holiday weekends.

Scamper up the valley walls at dawn or dusk for spectacular pine-filtered views, highlighted by grazing deer and active woodpeckers. If the valley is deserted, you may even hear the cry of a lone coyote or happen across the tracks of an elusive bobcat along the riverbanks.

PINE VALLEY NATIVES ■ ■ ■ ■ ■ ■ ■ ■ ■ ■ ■ ■ ■ ■ ■ ■ ■ ■

For thousands of years, fertile Pine Valley was home to the Esselen people, providing them with excellent hunting, gathering, and living grounds. The Esselen may have used fire to clear underbrush and maintain the pine stands and broad meadow, where deer, rabbits, antelopes, and even bears once commonly grazed. In the adjacent forest, doves, quails, and other game birds flocked beneath the abundant canopy of oaks, bays, pines, and madrones. Wild roses grow in dense thickets on the east edge of the valley, perhaps cultivated by the Esselen for straight, strong arrow shafts. Beneath the sandstone cliffs, women took harvested acorns from the surrounding oak woodlands and ground the nutritious meat into flour. Their mortar holes still pepper sandstone outcrops just downstream from the Pine Valley–Pine Ridge Trail junction.

Today, few Esselen remain to answer the many questions one might have about their ancestors' lives in Pine Valley or elsewhere along the Santa Lucia Range. Most of their people were decimated by disease brought by Spanish missionaries. Those who survived were often captured and sent to work in the Spanish missions. Others were killed without mercy. Sadly, much of their culture, language, mythology, and religion was also lost.

■ ■

Trip 50

HIDING CANYON & ROUND ROCK CAMPS

LENGTH AND TYPE: 18.8-mile point-to-point

RATING: Strenuous

TRAIL CONDITION: Difficult to impassable, poison oak, steep faint tread

HIGHLIGHTS: This peaceful wilderness escape leads through steep, narrow gorges to cascading waterfalls, deep emerald pools, and remote camps.

TO REACH THE TRAILHEAD: Park at the large turnout on Tassajara Road across from China Camp. The trailhead is on the camp side of the road, 100 feet south of the parking lot and 150 feet south of the camp entrance. The trail begins on a saddle above China Camp. It is marked, though encroaching brush often obscures the sign. There's no water at the trailhead.

TRIP SUMMARY: This trip offers hikers overnight excursions within the rugged northern Santa Lucia Range. If you can arrange a shuttle vehicle, the 18.8-mile one-way route takes you from China Camp to Los Padres Dam past pine-studded meadows, lush forests, secluded canyons, narrow gorges, waterfalls, and swimming holes. Highlights include Pine

Valley, Pine Falls, the pools and waterfalls below Round Rock, Ventana Mesa Creek Falls above Hiding Canyon Camp, Carmel River Camp, and Bluff Camp.

You can also arrange two- to four-night out-and-back trips, spending at least one night in Pine Valley and the other night(s) at Round Rock or Hiding Canyon Camps. Or you can take the 24.1-mile loop that leaves China Camp on the Miller Canyon Trail and returns through Pine Valley (see TRIP 48 Miller Canyon & Pine Valley Loop, page 195).

These trails are ideal in spring and fall, as temperatures are moderate and storms infrequent. Summer temps can reach the upper 90s Fahrenheit, and flies and mosquitoes pose a nuisance. Winter temps can dip below freezing, and snow is common above 4000 feet. Poison oak is a year-round problem on the lower Carmel River Trail.

Trip Description

See TRIP 49 Pine Valley (page 199) for the first 5.3 miles of this route to **Pine Valley**.

The **Carmel River Trail** crosses Pine Valley's broad meadow to a four-way junction with the **Pine Falls spur** and **Pine Valley–Pine Ridge Trail** (3140'). Consult TRIP 49 Pine Valley for the route to **Pine Falls** and TRIP 52 Pine Ridge, Sykes Hot Springs, & Big Sur (page 207) for a description of the Pine Valley–Pine Ridge Trail. This route leads northwest along the Carmel River Trail.

You'll pass through a wooden gate on your right and cross private property in sight of the owner's small cabin. The trail ascends a minor knoll and enters a large open meadow. In a scene reminiscent of the Sierras, deer graze beside towering pines amid grasslands blanketed in spring wildflowers.

The Carmel River Trail leads past Jack English's cabin in the heart of Pine Valley.

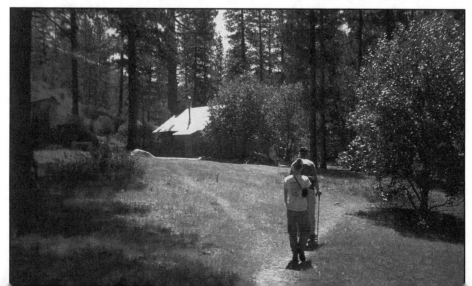

Offering pine-filtered views of the surrounding sandstone cliffs, the trail ascends northwest 200 feet in half a mile to a saddle (6.2 miles, 3414') that divides the **Carmel River and Hiding Canyon Creek drainages.** From this saddle, the route drops past four shallow gullies, then switchbacks across the seasonal headwaters of **Hiding Canyon Creek** (6.7 miles, 2950'). Continue downslope, following the path of the Church Creek Fault.

Crossing the headwaters eight more times, the route passes from exposed south-facing slopes to a shady creekside route past sycamores, bays, alders, and oaks. Expect to find year-round water by the eighth crossing (8.1 miles, 2140').

Past this crossing you'll leave the creek and ascend through dense overgrowth. During the wet season (November through April), ticks lie in wait amid the chamise- and broom-clad slopes. Wear light-colored pants to protect your legs and easily spot these hitchhikers. The trail switchbacks high above Hiding Canyon Creek for far-reaching vistas of the Carmel River drainage.

Leaving the canyon behind, you'll cross a minor ridge, switchback, and descend 0.1 mile southwest to the **Round Rock Camp Trail junction** (9.2 miles, 2030'). This easily missed unmarked junction leads to a spectacular overhanging gorge.

SIDE TRIP ■

From the **Round Rock Camp Trail junction,** hike 0.2 mile downslope to the headwaters of the **Carmel River,** then meander downstream 50 feet cross-country. The swift river plunges from pool to pool, carving a deep path through smooth massive granite walls. Be mindful of slick boulders and poison oak that shelters in the crevices. Pause for a refreshing dip in the brisk water.

Cross the river on the main trail past an unofficial campsite atop a small grassy terrace. The trail gradually ascends the canyon for 0.2 mile, then descends south along the riverbanks amid thickets of blackberry and poison oak. Make your way through this tangle and cross the river just downstream from an enormous boulder—perhaps Round Rock—which overlooks a shallow swimming hole.

Follow the trail 200 feet farther to **Round Rock Camp** (10.2 miles, 1920'), set atop a small grassy terrace. Marked by a table and a sign, the camp is roomy enough for up to a dozen small tents.

■ ■

From the Round Rock Camp Trail junction, the Carmel River Trail steeply descends the east-facing canyon wall. Pause to enjoy views on the way down. In a few minutes you'll reach the Carmel River's east bank. Expect to get your feet wet in all but the driest months—during heavy rainfall the river actually floods the trail.

Just across the river lies **Hiding Canyon Camp** (9.2 miles, 1740') and the nearby **Puerto Suelo Trail junction.** True to its name, the camp is easy to miss. The turnoff lies just downstream from the first crossing. You'll find two large sites, each with a table and cooking grate. The first site sits atop a narrow terrace along the west bank, while the larger, preferred site lies a few feet upstream near an enormous ponderosa pine with a 6-foot-plus diameter. You'll recognize ponderosas by their golden puzzle-piece bark and pine needles bunched in threes.

SIDE TRIP ▪

If you're willing to hike upriver off trail for 0.4 mile, you'll pass through a narrow sandstone gorge and arrive at **Ventana Mesa Creek Falls,** which tumbles into a swimming hole. Farther upriver, the canyon widens and turns south, entering a second gorge at the confluence with **Ventana Mesa Creek.** A few feet farther upstream the creek cascades into a deep granite-lined pool. If the water level is low enough in late summer and fall, you can press on for 200 feet to a larger swimming hole and waterfall within a mossy, fern-lined grotto. The refreshingly cold water is a welcome escape on a hot summer day.

▪ ▪

Refer to TRIP 45 Hiding Canyon & Round Rock Camps (page 181) and reverse that description for the remaining 9.2 miles of this route to the Los Padres Dam Trailhead.

Trip 51

VENTANA DOUBLE CONE VIA PINE VALLEY

LENGTH AND TYPE: 31.8-mile out-and-back

RATING: Challenging, faint tread and overgrown along Puerto Suello Trail

TRAIL CONDITION: Passable to difficult, poison oak

HIGHLIGHTS: Stop at secluded waterfall oases on your way to 4853-foot Ventana Double Cone, which boasts panoramic views of the Santa Lucia Range.

TO REACH THE TRAILHEAD: Park at the large turnout on Tassajara Road across from China Camp. The trailhead is on the camp side of the road, 100 feet south of the parking lot and 150 feet south of the camp entrance. The trail begins on a saddle above China Camp. It is marked, though encroaching brush often obscures the sign. There's no water at the trailhead.

TRIP SUMMARY: This book describes several routes to the remote 4853-foot summit of Ventana Double Cone, in the heart of Ventana Wilderness. For general information on the Ventana Trail, see the summary for TRIP 38 Ventana Double Cone via Ventana Trail (page 155).

This route from 4270-foot China Camp leads 15.9 miles to the summit (4853'). Although the trailhead lies more than 2000 feet higher than the Bottchers Gap Trailhead and nearly 3400 feet above Los Padres Dam, it descends 2530 feet to Hiding Canyon Camp, then climbs 3113 feet in 6.3 miles to Ventana Double Cone. Highlights include the scenic waterfalls at Pine Falls, Round Rock, and Ventana Mesa Creek (see TRIPS 49 and 52). These short detours are well worth the extra mile, especially in summer, as the bracing water will revive you after a sweaty toil to the summit.

As at most peaks along this dramatic coast, the best times to hike are between mid-November and April, taking advantage of cooler temperatures, fogless days, and fewer pesky mosquitoes and flies. This route is also a good choice in summer heat and fall drought, as from Hiding Canyon Camp you can reach the summit with a daypack and plenty of water. Be prepared for rain and snow if you hike in winter, when snow levels can drop to 2000 feet and the river may be impassable. Also watch for poison oak.

If you can arrange a shuttle vehicle, consider combining trips for an excellent point-to-point backcountry excursion. From China Camp, you'll summit Ventana Double Cone, then descend the Carmel River Trail to Los Padres Dam (see TRIP 46 Ventana Double Cone via Carmel River Trail, page 185) for a 31.4-mile grand tour of the wilderness.

Trip Description

See TRIP 50 Hiding Canyon & Round Rock Camps (page 202) for the first 9.2 miles of this route to **Hiding Canyon Camp**.

The **Puerto Suelo Trail** (9.6 miles, 1740') begins atop a flat bench on the west bank just downstream from camp. Those bound for **Ventana Double Cone** will climb this trail toward the **Puerto Suelo** saddle and the **Ventana Trail junction**. In drought years it's best to fill water bottles here.

You'll begin a steep climb west through a minor gully and across a small creek, then wander through several other minor gullies, dry practically year-round. In half a mile the trail begins a series of

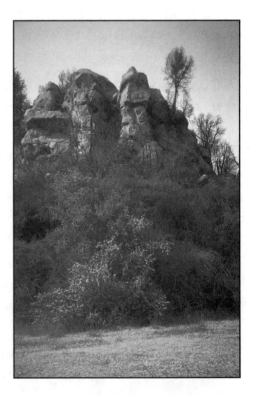

Sandstone cliffs rise above the broad pine-studded meadow at Pine Valley.

switchbacks, ascending a brushy slope to a minor saddle. Continue past fragrant stands of bays and tanoaks and across small tributaries to **Uncle Sam Creek**. The trail crosses and then recrosses the creek, which may be your last opportunity for water between here and the summit.

Continue climbing northwest through overgrown ceanothus thickets. The last 0.3 mile of the Puerto Suelo Trail ascends very steep, short switchbacks. Just 0.1 mile from the saddle, clear water bubbles up from two neighboring springs, reliable in all but the driest months.

Climb the final 200 feet to the Puerto Suelo saddle and **Ventana Trail junction** (12.2 miles, 3530'). The Ventana Trail branches left at this junction and climbs above the saddle toward Ventana Double Cone.

See TRIP 38 Ventana Double Cone via Ventana Trail (page 155) for the final 3.7 miles to the summit (15.9 miles, 4853').

WINDOW ON THE WILDERNESS ■ ■ ■ ■ ■ ■ ■ ■ ■ ■ ■ ■ ■ ■

Ventana Wilderness owes its name to the rugged twin peaks of 4853-foot Ventana Double Cone. Legend relates that a rock arch once spanned the deep cleft between the peak's sister spires, forming a natural window on the wilderness. Arriving in the area in the late 1700s, early Spanish inhabitants named the double summit *Ventana* (Spanish for window).

Descendents of the native Esselen people believe the legendary arch served as a gateway for the souls of all native people as they left their earthly existence. Others claim it was the portal through which the Great Spirit heard humankind's collective prayers.

The magnificent double summit still dominates the Ventana Wilderness skyline, inspiring newfound reverence among modern-day visitors.

■ ■

Trip 52

PINE RIDGE, SYKES HOT SPRINGS, & BIG SUR

LENGTH AND TYPE: 23.1-mile point-to-point

RATING: Challenging

TRAIL CONDITION: Passable to difficult, poison oak

HIGHLIGHTS: This arduous hike takes in rugged ridges, steep canyons, and exposed hillsides, rewarding the faithful with waterfalls, hot springs, and swimming holes.

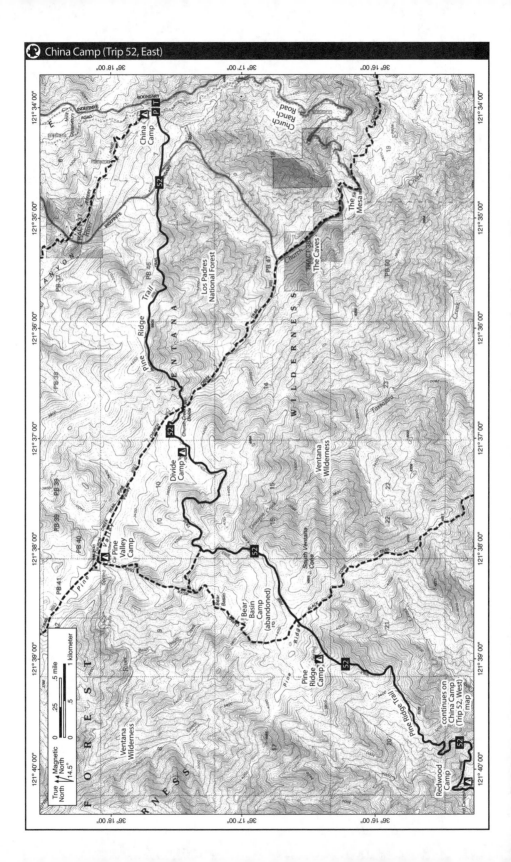

TO REACH THE TRAILHEAD: Park at the large turnout on Tassajara Road across from China Camp. The trailhead is on the camp side of the road, 100 feet south of the parking lot and 150 feet south of the camp entrance. The trail begins on a saddle above China Camp. It is marked, though encroaching brush often obscures the sign. There's no water at the trailhead. The first 1.2 miles of the trail are heavily overgrown yet passable.

TRIP SUMMARY: This trip offers hikers several overnight itineraries within the rugged northern Santa Lucia Range. If you can arrange a shuttle vehicle, consider two point-to-point routes that cross the Ventana Wilderness: (1) the Pine Ridge Trail from China Camp to Big Sur, and (2) the Pine Ridge Trail, Black Cone Trail, and Marble Peak Trail from China Camp to Arroyo Seco. Highlights on the route to Big Sur include massive ponderosa pines atop ridges and large meadows, ancient redwood groves along the Big Sur River, and oak-dotted golden hillsides blanketed in spring wildflowers.

If you can't arrange a shuttle, consider the following out-and-back destinations:

Accessed via China Camp, Pine Valley is well worth a 1.7-mile detour along the Carmel River Trail. From there a 0.7-mile downstream trek leads to Pine Falls, a 50-foot cascade that fills a deep swimming hole.

Past Pine Valley, the Pine Ridge Trail leads to spectacular views atop Pine Ridge, reminiscent of a Sierra crest. Expect snow above 4000 feet in the winter and profuse wildflowers in spring. The trail is lightly traveled between Pine Ridge and Sykes Camp. Several sections between the ridge and the Big Sur headwaters are heavily overgrown, and heavy winter rains spawn dangerous trail washouts. Trekking poles are a good idea.

Redwood Camp offers solitude deep within a redwood-lined canyon, while Sykes Camp is well-known for its three small 100°F hot springs, which are often crowded during spring break and on summer weekends.

Trip Description

See TRIP 49 Pine Valley (page 199) for the first 3.6 miles along the **Pine Ridge Trail** to **Church Creek Divide** (3.6 miles, 3650').

This divide marks the four-way junction of the westbound Pine Ridge Trail, the southeast-bound **Church Creek Trail,** and the northwest-bound **Carmel River Trail** to **Pine Valley.** If you plan to spend a night in Pine Valley, expect an easy 1.7-mile detour.

If you're not bound for Pine Valley, the route from Church Creek Divide continues straight, west along the Pine Ridge Trail. Immediately past the saddle the trail climbs past heavily overgrown madrones, manzanitas, and ceanothus, fire-adapted species that thrive on this fire-scarred hillside. You'll cross two small gullies laden with blackberries, horsetails, and fragrant hedge nettles. These seasonal creeks run dry by summer.

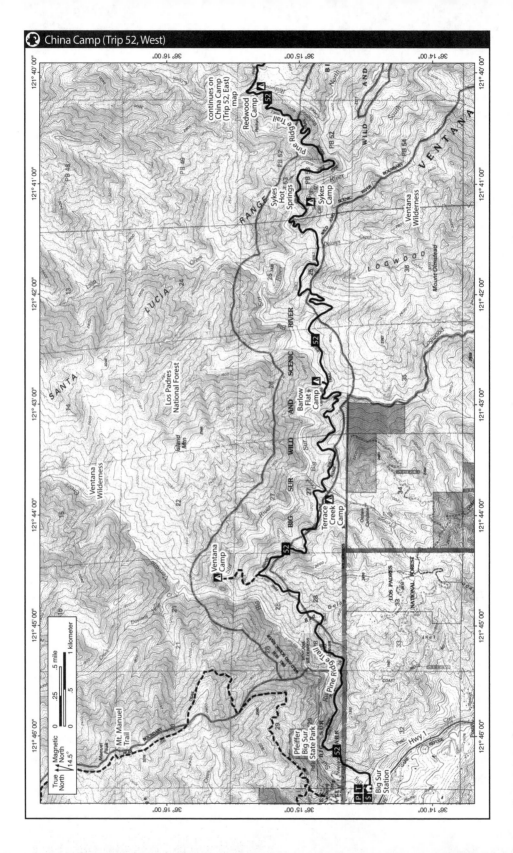

continues on China Camp (Trip 52, East) map

Redwood Camp

Pine Ridge Trail

Sykes Hot Springs

Sykes Camp

VENTANA

Ventana Wilderness

Mount Olmstead

LOGWOOD

RANGE

LUCIA

Los Padres National Forest

Island Mtn

Ventana Wilderness

SCENIC

AND

WILD

SUR

BIG

RIVER

Barlow Flat Camp

Big Sur

Terrace Creek Camp

Ventana Camp

Mt. Manuel Trail

Gulch

Pine Ridge Trail

Pfeiffer Big Sur State Park

Big Sur Station

LOS PADRES NATIONAL FOREST

Hwy 1

True North
Magnetic North
14.5°

0   .25   .5 mile
0   .5   1 kilometer

SIDE TRIP ■

If you do stay in Pine Valley and are westbound, consider taking the **Pine Valley–Pine Ridge Trail** onward to the Pine Ridge Trail instead of hiking back through Church Creek Divide. The 1.5-mile Pine Valley–Pine Ridge Trail leads onward to the Pine Ridge Trail, saving you 2.4 miles overall, though requiring an additional 500 feet of climbing through heavy overgrowth. You'll find the trailhead at the official **Pine Valley entrance** (5.3 miles, 3140'), at a junction with the Carmel River Trail and the cross-country trail to **Pine Falls.**

From this junction, the trail (marked BEAR BASIN) crosses the **Carmel River** past a campsite that can accommodate up to four tents. Passing the site, you'll climb steeply above Pine Valley. A passage through live oaks, tanoaks, and ceanothus gives way to views northwest toward flat-topped 4766-foot **Uncle Sam Mountain, Puerto Suelo** (the deep saddle left of Uncle Sam's base), and the rocky twin peaks of 4853-foot **Ventana Double Cone.**

You'll climb 800 feet in the first mile to a shallow saddle (6.3 miles, 3950'), at a junction with an abandoned spur to **Bear Basin.** This spur leads right 1.1 miles to spacious **Bear Basin Camp,** alongside reliable, spring-fed **Bear Basin Creek.** Directly upslope from camp another spur ascends southwest half a mile through dense overgrowth to the Pine Ridge Trail, though poor trail conditions make for extremely slow going.

If you intend to head west along the Pine Ridge Trail, continue from the shallow saddle (6.3 miles, 3950') on the Pine Valley–Pine Ridge Trail another half mile to the Pine Ridge Trail, although this section is also overgrown.

■ ■

Cool crystalline waters offer a respite from the brush-choked, sun-drenched slopes leading into the Big Sur River basin.

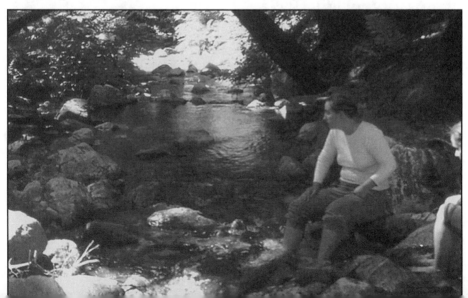

After half a mile past head-high brush and scattered black oaks, madrones, and ponderosa pines, you'll round a minor ridge and reach the **Divide Camp Trail junction** (4.1 miles, 3800'). The spur leads 200 feet to the first of two sites in the shade of large pines, oaks, and alders. Each can accommodate up to two tents. A hundred feet west of camp is a small spring that dwindles to a muddy seep by midsummer and early fall.

Past the spur junction, the Pine Ridge Trail climbs above camp, meanders southwest past two small seeps, and leads 100 feet farther to a larger spring-fed creeklet lined with enormous chain ferns. A large fallen oak blocks the trail, requiring careful footing, especially if you're carrying a heavy pack. Past the creeklet, trail conditions worsen, and you must forge through overhead thickets of ceanothus. Fortunately, there's very little poison oak, and the trail is well graded. In spots the brush clears, offering glimpses of Ventana's high peaks. Flat-topped Uncle Sam Mountain lies 6 miles northwest, rising above the Puerto Suelo saddle. A long ridge leads left from the saddle up to Ventana Double Cone.

Ascending toward Pine Ridge, you'll cross a small spring-fed creek (4.7 miles, 4000'), the most reliable water source in the 3.6 miles between Divide Camp and **Pine Ridge Camp**. The route contours past an unnamed 4751-foot peak to the south, then reaches the **Pine Valley–Pine Ridge Trail junction** (5.8 miles, 4230'). Westbound hikers who spend the night in Pine Valley rejoin the Pine Ridge Trail here (see side trip on the previous page for details).

Past the junction, the trail becomes increasingly overgrown with bay laurel, ceanothus, manzanita, and scrub oak, species that are thriving in the wake of numerous fires, particularly the 1999 Kirk Complex Fires. Press on through the encroaching brush to ascend a minor saddle (6.5 miles, 4410'). Pause here for views southeast along **Tassajara Creek** canyon to the highest point in the **Santa Lucia Range,** 5862-foot **Junipero Serra Peak.**

FIRE AS A SHAPING FORCE ■ ■ ■ ■ ■ ■ ■ ■ ■ ■ ■ ■ ■ ■ ■

Over just two days in fall 1999, the Ventana Wilderness was hit by some 1200 lightning strikes as a subtropical system from the Gulf of California unexpectedly formed into a massive electrical storm over the Santa Lucia Range. This awe-inspiring display ignited the Kirk Complex Fires, a series of 47 wildfires that swept across more than 90,000 acres of the wilderness over three months, sparing only the most protected canyons and barren ridges.

The region is no stranger to fire. Every acre of the wilderness has been scorched at least twice this century. As a result, many plants are well adapted to fire. Since the Kirk Complex Fires, aggressive brush has overrun the eastern section of the Pine Ridge Trail, rendering it impassable to many hikers' standards. Without maintenance, this section may be completely overgrown within the next couple of years.

■ ■

From the saddle, the trail gently ascends 200 feet, then quickly descends to Pine Ridge (7.3 miles, 4550'). Listen for woodpeckers at work on the enormous charred pine snags that stand like sentinels atop the ridge. This ridge separates the three major drainages of the northern Santa Lucia Range. The Carmel River headwaters of **Blue Creek** lie just north of the ridge, the **Big Sur River** headwaters of **Cienega Creek** flow southwest, and Tassajara Creek runs southeast into the **Arroyo Seco,** then north to the **Salinas River** and out to sea. From Pine Ridge, your major climbing is behind you. Unfortunately, your major bushwhacking is not.

A few minutes along the ridge you may notice a metal plaque nailed to a burnt snag with flagging tied around its base. This unofficial sign marks the north end of the **Black Cone Trail** (7.4 miles, 4540'). Though the trail has been officially abandoned, volunteers recently cleared its entire length (see TRIP 53 Black Cone Trail to Arroyo Seco, page 215). It offers an incredibly scenic, well-graded southeast passage across Ventana's major ridges.

From this junction, another abandoned spur strikes through the encroaching brush— easily overlooked were it not for an unofficial marking flag. If you're willing to tear through brush, this spur descends to Bear Basin Camp and then climbs 0.8 mile to a south-climbing ridge and a junction with the Pine Valley–Pine Ridge Trail.

Continue on the Pine Ridge Trail. As you leave the ridge, look southeast toward the Black Cone Trail, which crosses the flanks of 4965-foot **South Ventana Cone**. The 2800-foot descent into the Big Sur River canyon begins moderately at first, along a narrow gravel path that veers west and crosses three minor gullies. The vegetation changes and retreats somewhat from the trail. Thickets of chamise, yucca, manzanita, and wartleaf are only knee- to waist-high, allowing ocean views on clear days.

You'll pass large pine snags as you descend 300 feet in 0.3 mile to the signed **Pine Ridge Camp Trail junction** (7.7 miles, 4260').

SIDE TRIP ■

Pine Ridge Camp Trail descends 0.1 mile to a flat-topped ridge with incredible westward views. **Pine Ridge Camp** (7.8 miles, 4170') offers one large site in the sparse shade of madrones, pines, and tanoaks that survived 1999's ravaging fires. The site can accommodate up to five tents. Beyond camp, past a large burned madrone, a narrow trail leads northwest a few feet to a reliable spring-fed creeklet. Campers enjoy unparalleled views of the deep Big Sur drainage as it rises from the Pacific. This is also a spectacular place to watch a sunset and enjoy the solitude.

From the junction, the Pine Ridge Trail descends past scorched ponderosa snags. Pause to admire views southeast toward the Black Cone Trail, which slices a nearly level route from South Ventana Cone toward Black Cone. Continue your descent on a steep grade for the remaining 2500 vertical feet to the Big Sur River canyon. Although encroaching brush is less of a problem along this narrow section, the tread is loose and washed out in places. Use caution when carrying a large pack.

You will pass thickets of chamise, ceanothus, fragrant black sage, scattered yuccas, and sticky monkeyflowers, the latter bearing bright orange blossoms and predictably sticky leaves. The route reaches a long saddle with views northwest toward Ventana Double Cone, which rises some 2500 feet from **Redwood Creek** below. You will descend past a hillside covered in invasive broom to a small gully just below a major saddle. Cross the gully to the **Big Sur Trail junction** (10.3 miles, 2320').

The Pine Ridge Trail veers right at the junction for the final 500 vertical feet to Redwood Creek. After 0.3 mile the thick brush finally gives way to redwoods nestled along the steep ravines and canyon bottoms. The spectacular views are behind you, but so are the worst trail conditions, and poison oak makes its reappearance. After a series of switchbacks, temperatures dramatically drop, as the trail enters the cool, damp redwood microclimate.

On a level grade the trail crosses Redwood Creek and passes the first of four official sites at **Redwood Camp** (11.2 miles, 1800'). The first small site along the west bank can accommodate up to two tents. To reach the other sites, you will have to hike farther downstream along a spur.

SIDE TRIP ■

Ten feet past the first site in **Redwood Camp**, you'll reach a 0.1-mile spur to the other sites. Cross the creek on the large redwood log and hike 100 feet downstream to the second site. Though there's only room for one tent, the sloping site does include a fire ring. The third site lies 50 feet farther downstream, amid large boulders and old-growth redwoods along the east bank. This small, shady site can accommodate up to two tents. The fourth and largest site sits atop an open bench 100 feet farther along the east bank, 70 feet past a small seep. Redwoods, tanoaks, and bays ring the perimeter, while starflowers and wild strawberries carpet the forest floor. This site can accommodate up to 10 tents.

■ ■

From camp the Pine Ridge Trail heads south and climbs above the west bank of Redwood Creek. To continue westbound along the Pine Ridge Trail, refer to TRIP 59 Sykes & Redwood Camps (page 246) and follow that trail description in reverse.

Trip 53

BLACK CONE TRAIL TO ARROYO SECO

LENGTH AND TYPE: 26.2-mile point-to-point, 30.2-mile out-and-back, or 31.6-mile loop

RATING: Challenging

TRAIL CONDITION: Passable to difficult, poison oak, overgrown brush, faint tread

HIGHLIGHTS: Epic views from the flanks of mountains along the recently restored Black Cone Trail

TO REACH THE TRAILHEAD: Park at the large turnout on Tassajara Road across from China Camp. The trailhead is on the camp side of the road, 100 feet south of the parking lot and 150 feet south of the camp entrance. The trail begins on a saddle above China Camp. It is marked, though encroaching brush often obscures the sign. There's no water at the trailhead.

TRIP SUMMARY: Following the 1977 Marble-Cone Fire, the US Forest Service abandoned the Black Cone Trail, which was quickly reclaimed by dense thickets of chaparral. The 1999 Kirk Complex Fires raged along most of the trail, exposing its residual tread. Soon volunteers from the Ventana Wilderness Alliance hiked the area to see whether it would be feasible to reestablish the trail. In cooperation with the USFS, volunteers removed brush and debris and regraded the trail.

As is the case with most wilderness trails, it still suffers from overgrowth, washouts, and annoying ticks, flies, and mosquitoes. Fortunately, there's little poison oak above 3500 feet on the northern section of the trail, though it fills in again near Strawberry Camp. Bring a walking stick to counteract the slope and navigate slippery sections.

Santa Lucia fir, a rare species endemic to the Santa Lucia Mountains, inhabits the steep, rocky slopes along the Black Cone Trail.

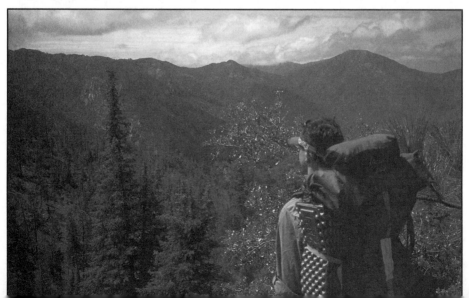

In summer, temperatures can reach the upper 90s Fahrenheit along this exposed 8.6-mile trail, and coastal fog obscures your views. In spring, ticks are a nuisance, but onshore winds promise far-reaching views east to the Arroyo Seco and west to the Big Sur watershed and broad Pacific. Fragrant wildflowers blanket the ridgelines, gullies, and steep ravines. In winter the possibility of snow keeps nighttime temps below freezing as howling winds funnel up the canyons. The fog rolls well offshore in fall, ushering in wonderful views, comfortable temps, and diminished tick, fly, and mosquito populations. However, water can be scarce along much of the route. Fill up at Mosquito Springs, White Cone Springs (0.4–0.8 mile past Venturi Camp), the headwaters of the North Fork Big Sur (not reliable by late summer), Black Cone Camp, and Strawberry Creek.

This trail serves as an important link between the northern and southern Ventana Wilderness, connecting the trails of the Carmel, Little Sur, and Big Sur watersheds with those of the Arroyo Seco watershed. The route from China Camp offers at least three point-to-point trips. If you can arrange a shuttle vehicle, destinations include: (1) Arroyo Seco Campground (26.2 miles); (2) Church Creek Trailhead (24.1 miles); and (3) Horse Pasture Trailhead (27.6 miles). The latter two trips can also be loop trips if you're willing to hike several steep miles up Tassajara Road (5.4 miles from the Church Creek Trailhead and 5.2 miles from the Horse Pasture Trailhead). Or your loop can begin and end at the Church Creek Trailhead via the Church Creek, Pine Ridge, Black Cone, Marble Peak, and Horse Pasture Trails (see TRIP 54 Church Creek to Pine Valley Camp, page 221). The Black Cone Trail descends (albeit gently) more than 1700 feet in the 7.8 miles between Pine Ridge and Strawberry Camp—if you're willing to return along the trail and regain this elevation, several point-to-point trips lead through the heart of the wilderness.

Out-and-back destinations from China Camp include: (1) Mosquito Springs Camp (17.2 miles round-trip); (2) South Fork Camp (36 miles round-trip); (3) Strawberry Camp (30.2 miles round-trip); and (4) Willow Springs Camp (38.4 miles round-trip).

Trip Description

See TRIP 52 Pine Ridge, Sykes Hot Springs, & Big Sur (page 207) for the first 7.3 miles of this route to the **Black Cone Trail junction** atop **Pine Ridge** (4540').

If you're in desperate need of water, you can either descend 0.3 mile farther along the **Pine Ridge Trail** to **Pine Ridge Camp** (a spring runs year-round in all but the driest years) or hike 0.8 mile along the **Black Cone Trail** to the **Mosquito Springs Trail junction** (a half-mile spur leads to year-round water at **Mosquito Springs Camp**).

At the Black Cone Trail junction, a metal plaque nailed to a charred snag points the way. Veer left and head south along the western flanks of 4965-foot **South Ventana Cone.**

Over 0.8 mile the loose-packed trail passes low-lying thickets of manzanita, scrub oak, ceanothus, yerba santa, and a few yuccas. The first prominent saddle marks the **Mosquito Springs Camp Trail junction** (8.1 miles, 4470').

SIDE TRIP ■

Mosquito Springs Camp Trail leads east, dropping 500 feet in half a mile. This can be a slippery descent over loose tread obscured by overgrowth. Fortunately, someone has placed yellow flagging at the major switchbacks. As the trail levels off, you'll reach **Mosquito Springs Camp** (8.6 miles, 3940'), which offers a few flat tent sites nestled between granite talus and aggressive growth stemming from the 1999 Kirk Complex Fires. Be aware that the one or two decent sites lie along the runoff path for winter storms. True to the camp name, mosquitoes thrive here in spring and early summer, diminishing again by fall. While water is available before camp during the wet season (November through April), it's reliable year-round at camp in all but the driest years.

■ ■

From the junction, the Black Cone Trail contours just west of the ridgelines that separate the **Big Sur** and **Arroyo Seco** drainages. You'll meander on and off the spine, eventually arriving at a saddle atop a steep, narrow canyon that holds the western headwaters of **Tassajara Creek,** just below point 4135 feet on the USFS map. The saddle hosts **Venturi Camp** (10.7 miles, 4100'), littered by such random artifacts as a pair of pliers and a rusty rake. There's enough room for two tents, but the nearest water is 0.4 mile farther along the trail at **White Cone Springs.** The sheer topography exposes the camp to strong, cold winds that funnel up from the canyon.

Beyond camp the trail skirts the western flanks of an enormous white granite peak known locally as **White Cone.** Over the next 0.3 mile you'll pass two impressive peaks marked as 4721 feet and 4719 feet on the USFS map (the trail doesn't thread the peaks as drawn on the USFS map, but remains well below them on the contour). You'll soon reach the first of three reliable springs (11.1 miles, 4240'), though this one may run dry in drought years. White Cone Springs is 0.1 mile farther, gushing over moss-covered white granite cliffs. Head east 0.4 mile toward a massive granite face to find the **third spring** (11.5 miles, 4100').

Beyond the springs, the trail descends toward a prominent forked **ridge** (12.1 miles, 4100'), offering views northwest to the Big Sur watershed and Pacific. From this vantage point, you can see most of the remaining 3 miles of the Black Cone Trail as it winds past the western flanks of **Black Cone** before dropping into **Strawberry Valley.**

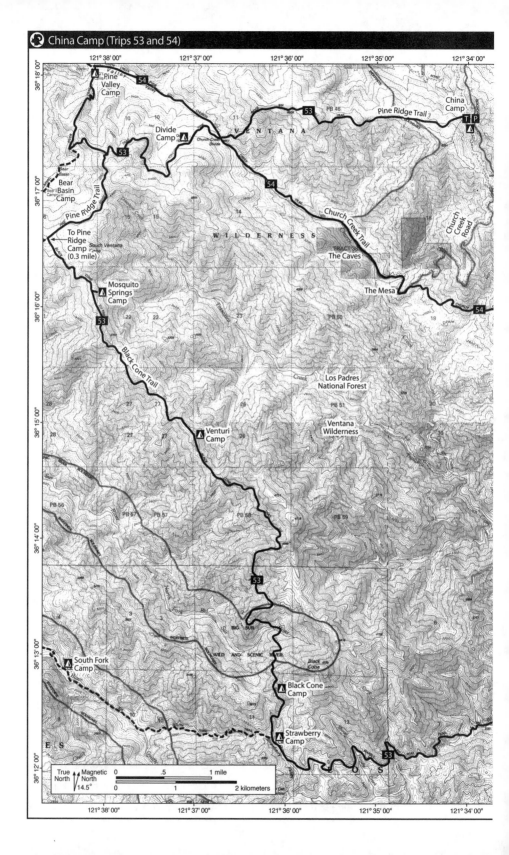

121° 38' 00"   121° 37' 00"   121° 36' 00"   121° 35' 00"   121° 34' 00"

36° 18' 00"

Pine Valley Camp

54

53

Pine Ridge Trail

China Camp

T P

V E N T A N A

Divide Camp

PB 46

53

54

Church Creek Divide

Bear Basin Camp

36° 17' 00"

Pine Ridge Trail

Church Creek Trail

Church Creek Road

To Pine Ridge Camp (0.3 mile)

South Ventana Cone

W I L D E R N E S S

TRACT 38
The Caves

Mosquito Springs Camp

36° 16' 00"

53

The Mesa

PB 50

Black Cone Trail

Creek

Los Padres National Forest

PB 51

36° 15' 00"

Venturi Camp

Ventana Wilderness

PB 56

PB 57   PB 57

PB 58

PB 59

36° 14' 00"

53

36° 13' 00"

BIG   SUR

South Fork Camp

WILD AND SCENIC RIVER

Black Cone

Black Cone Camp

E   S

Strawberry Camp

53

36° 12' 00"

True North   Magnetic North   0   .5   1 mile
14.5°   0   1   2 kilometers

121° 38' 00"   121° 37' 00"   121° 36' 00"   121° 35' 00"   121° 34' 00"

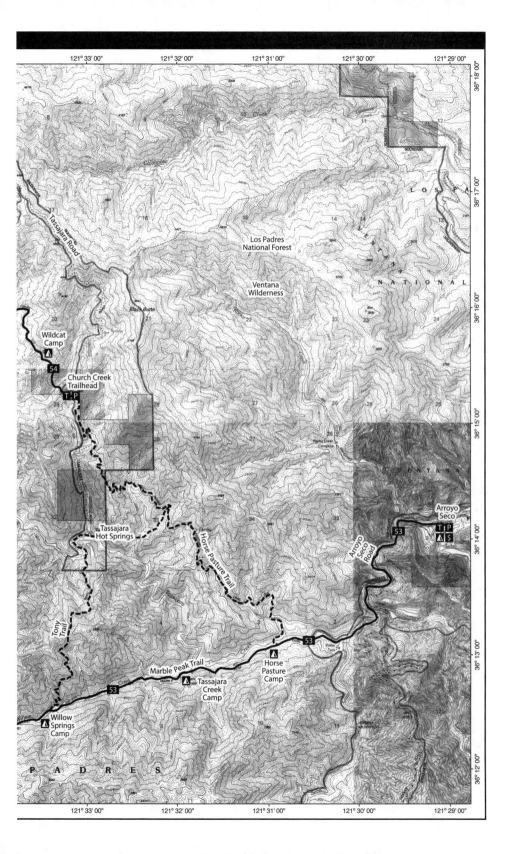

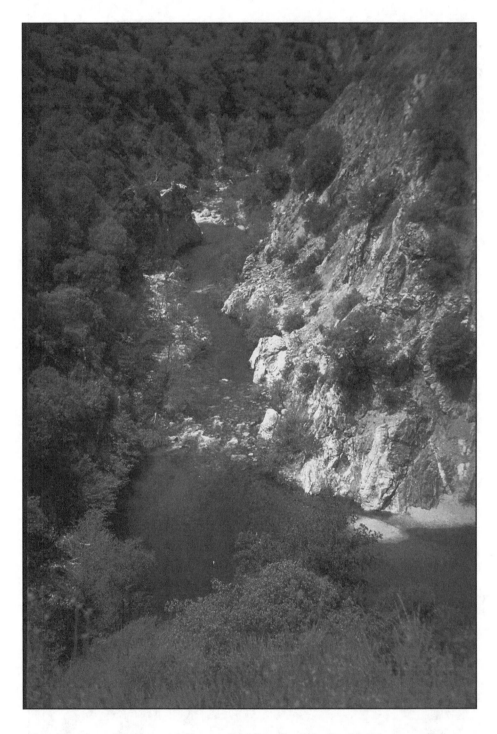

After a strenuous 25 miles, reward yourself with a refreshing dip along the Arroyo Seco.

Onward, the trail dips through a small canyon that channels a headwater of the **North Fork Big Sur River** (12.6 miles, 3670'). Across the canyon, the trail ascends to **Shotgun Ridge** (12.9 miles, 3700'), which overlooks the dozens of creeks, creeklets, springs, ravines, gullies, and broad valleys of the Big Sur drainage below. The ridge was named for a rusty 20-gauge shotgun that was left in the brush with other debris by the crew that forged this trail in the 1960s.

Beyond the ridge, the mostly waterless route reaches another small seep trickling from the mountainside (13.3 miles, 3610'). Fifty yards farther you'll reach the 200-yard spur down to comfortable **Black Cone Camp**. A year-round spring issues forth from the hillside in camp, which can accommodate up to four tents with room to spare. Nearby, look for an ice-mold stove that the Forest Service installed when the camp was established in the 1960s.

Beyond the spur, the trail leads 0.3 mile toward a large reliable **creek** (13.6 miles, 3600'), another headwater of the North Fork Big Sur. The creek lies along the northeastern flanks of Black Cone, which dominates the eastern skyline less than half a mile from the trail. From here you'll contour past three minor ridges to the divide (14.3 miles, 3690') between **Strawberry Creek,** the **Salinas River** headwaters, and the North Fork Big Sur. The trail gradually descends an old bulldozed firebreak. Although the trail widens, poison oak makes a comeback along the remaining 0.8 mile to **Strawberry Camp.**

As you descend into Strawberry Valley, you'll cross two small seasonal creeklets (usually dry by midsummer), following the second creeklet 0.1 mile to **Strawberry Camp**. The Black Cone Trail ends here at the **South Fork Trail junction** (15.1 miles, 2840'). Though perched in a small valley, the camp lies on sloping ground. The site can accommodate up to four tents in the shade of a sprawling oak. While the creek may run dry by late summer, a 0.3-mile jaunt downslope to the **Marble Peak Trail junction** will lead to water.

For a description of the remaining 12.1 miles to **Arroyo Seco Campground,** refer to TRIP 56 Willow Springs & Strawberry Camps (page 234) and follow that trail description in reverse.

Trip 54

CHURCH CREEK TO PINE VALLEY CAMP

LENGTH AND TYPE: 17-mile out-and-back, 34.2-mile loop, 22.3-mile point-to-point (Los Padres Dam), or 32.5-mile point-to-point (Arroyo Seco)

RATING: Strenuous to challenging

TRAIL CONDITION: Passable to difficult, poison oak

HIGHLIGHTS: This route leads past ancient sandstone formations deep within Church Creek canyon, highlighted by vast oaks and ponderosa pines amid grassy slopes and spring wildflowers.

TO REACH THE TRAILHEAD: To reach the Church Creek Trailhead, drive 5.4 miles past the China Camp entrance along Tassajara Road. At 5.2 miles you'll pass the Horse Pasture Trailhead on your left. Continue 0.2 mile farther to a sharp left bend through a conspicuous gully. Park in the small lot on your right and walk 50 feet back up the road to the crossing at the Church Creek Trailhead. There are no facilities or water at the trailhead.

If you miss the trailhead and continue down Tassajara Road, you'll reach another parking area in 1.1 miles. There, 17.2 miles from the Carmel Valley Road junction, a dirt road leads to a Zen Buddhist monastery that contains Tassajara Hot Springs.

TRIP SUMMARY: From the Church Creek Trailhead, hikers can choose from at least four route options, each featuring a stay at beautiful Pine Valley. Destinations include: (1) Pine Valley (17 miles out-and-back) via the Church Creek and Carmel River Trails; (2) Los Padres Dam Trailhead (22.3 miles point-to-point) via Pine Valley, Hiding Canyon, and the Carmel River; (3) Arroyo Seco Campground (32.5 miles point-to-point) through Church Creek with a detour to Pine Valley via the Pine Ridge, Carmel River, Black Cone, and Marble Peak Trails; or (4) the Church Creek Trailhead (34.2 miles out-and-back) with a detour to Pine Valley via the Pine Ridge, Black Cone, Marble Peak, and Horse Pasture Trails and Tassajara Road. While the last two routes could bypass the detour to Pine Valley, that 1.7-mile trail leads to one of Ventana's premier camps. As is the case with most wilderness trails, these routes suffer from overgrown brush and poison oak, faint tread, fallen snags, and other obstacles.

The out-and-back route along the Church Creek Trail ascends 2070 feet in 6.8 miles to Church Creek Divide, at the junction with the Carmel River Trail to Pine Valley. Though this route to the divide is 3.2 miles longer and gains 670 feet more elevation than the Pine Ridge Trail, it offers your only chance to take in Church Creek canyon's incredible sandstone formations. Remnants of a seafloor formed millions of years ago, these ancient beds jut from the canyon walls along the downthrown side of the Church Creek Fault. Native Esselen tribes once used these outcrops as shelters. Many of their pictographs remain on cave walls.

Trip Description

A sign at the trailhead (2180') states that Pine Ridge Trail is 7 miles away and Pine Valley 8 miles. You'll quickly cross a small stream and enter the **Ventana Wilderness**. The trail parallels the creek in the shade of bigleaf maples, live oaks, Coulter pines, and ceanothus thickets. For the next half mile the well-defined yet slightly overgrown trail recrosses the creek three times and ascends minor ridges and gullies to the **first of seven divides** (0.8 mile, 2770').

Pause at the saddle to take in views southwest to the **Church Creek** and **Tassajara Creek** confluence, northwest to massive sandstone beds along the canyon bottom, and west along

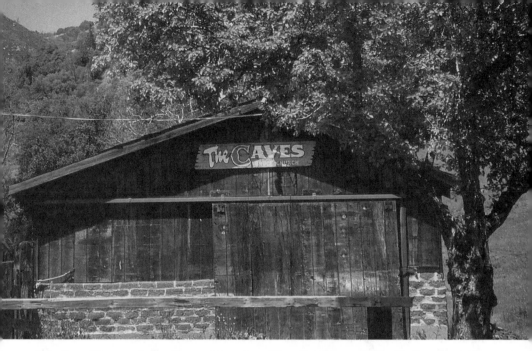

"The Caves" is named after the sandstone formations that form primitive shelters along the ancient canyon walls above Church Creek.

the spine of the ridge that separates the **Big Sur** and **Arroyo Seco** watersheds. The **Black Cone Trail** closely follows this distant ridge.

Beyond the saddle, you'll meander past tilted sandstone layers and descend into **Wildcat Camp** (1.1 miles, 2750'). This small camp is limited to one tent site along a narrow bench shaded by bays, elderberries, alders, and sycamores. The reliable creek dwindles to a trickle in summer and fall.

Past camp, you'll cross the creek and begin a moderate climb past chaparral, chamise, sage, and bush poppies. Over the next 0.6 mile the trail wriggles across two divides, crosses a seasonal creek (dry by late summer), and reaches the **third divide** (1.7 miles, 3240'), offering a view southeast toward **Junipero Serra Peak,** which lords 5862 feet over the **Santa Lucia Range.**

You'll continue between sandstone outcrops featuring smooth overhanging rims and convex floors and walls. A honeycomb pattern along the sandstone faces is the result of weathering, which forms deep cavities known as **tafoni**. Archaeological evidence proves the Esselen used larger tafoni caves for shelter from the sun, wind, and rain.

The trail briefly strays from the formations and descends half a mile past brushy slopes, crossing a small reliable **creek** (2.2 miles, 2760'). Past the gully, the trail steepens for a 0.2-mile descent to a large arroyo, or dry boulder-strewn creek bed, lined with yuccas, Coulter pines, sycamores, sage, and poison oak. Onward, the trail climbs 200 feet to the fourth divide along broad grassy slopes, radiant in spring with blooming owl's clover, lupines, poppies, and popcorn flowers. From this divide, you can see the trail along the east canyon wall past the fifth divide to **Church Ranch Road.**

At points over the next 0.3 mile the tread grows faint and confusing, particularly where a large fallen live oak blocks the trail. Clear deer trails lead down to the creek, while the less distinct main trail contours northwest above the creek. You'll cross a shallow gully and small seasonal creek, then ascend a minor ridge past oak- and pine-clad slopes to the fifth divide.

Labeled THE MESA on the USFS map, this broad, flat-topped divide lies just below the junction with Church Ranch Road. Climb the steep, oak-studded grassy slopes past a dilapidated sign a few feet from the junction (3.4 miles, 2690'). The trail joins this private road and contours past **The Mesa** 0.8 mile to **Church Ranch Bridge.** Cross the bridge for views across the canyon of sprawling black oaks, Coulter pines and their massive cones, and recently charred Santa Lucia firs.

You'll soon enter **Bruce Church Ranch** through an open wooden gate posted PRIVATE PROPERTY (4.2 miles, 2580'). For the next 1.5 miles the trail crosses the ranch past grazing horses, wooden barns, and fences. From the entrance gate, the road abruptly turns after 0.2 mile, crosses the creek, and leads to private homes. At this turn, the Church Creek Trail continues straight along a vague trail (4.4 miles, 2590').

Beyond the ranch, the trail closely follows Church Creek for the next 0.3 mile before beginning a moderate ascent of the east bank toward a minor ridge. Pause here for views of the sloping sandstone beds that parallel **Church Creek Fault,** as well as the open ridges and oak savannas back along the trail. Past an often-dry creek bed (4.7 miles, 2630'), the trail reenters the Ventana Wilderness and climbs 0.2 mile, skirting prime wildlife habitat. These oak savannas teem with grazing deer, moles, rabbits, mice, stealthy bobcats, and scavenging coyotes. Acorn woodpeckers hammer away noisily at the thick bark of oaks and pines, building caches for their favorite nut.

As the trail again strays from the creek, it climbs past scattered oaks to the **sixth divide** (5.3 miles, 3130'). Notice the striking differences in plant communities amid the sandstone outcrops, with chaparral on higher slopes, small clusters of Santa Lucia firs and ponderosa pines nestled along the canyon, and open oak woodlands below. Past two small seasonal creeks, the trail wraps along steep slopes through dense thickets of ceanothus, manzanita, scrub oak, and poison oak.

Fire-scarred madrones, ponderosas, black oaks, and manzanitas have made an impressive comeback since the 1999 Kirk Complex Fires ravaged these slopes. Unfortunately, these aggressive, fire-adapted species are quickly overtaking the trail. Someone has managed to slash back much of the encroaching vegetation, but regular maintenance is needed to keep the trail clear. Beyond these densely overgrown sections, the trail crosses several gullies past the often-dry headwaters of Church Creek to the seventh and final divide, **Church Creek Divide** (6.8 miles, 3651').

PICTURES FROM THE PAST ■ ■ ■ ■ ■ ■ ■ ■ ■ ■ ■ ■ ■ ■ ■ ■ ■

On Bruce Church Ranch, amid arching overhangs and rock shelters labeled THE CAVES on the USFS map, visitors will find a series of ancient pictographs. The many handprints on these rock walls offer proof of the practically vanished Esselen people, whose homeland once encompassed the Ventana Wilderness. A 1972 excavation of the rock shelters along Church Creek recovered artifacts that prove the Esselen survived in this canyon for many years following the arrival of Spanish missionaries in 1770, perhaps remaining in remote areas of the Santa Lucia Range through the mid-1800s.

Hostility toward American Indians was commonplace in California during this period. Most Esselen either assimilated, succumbed to disease, or were killed in warfare. Tragically, much of their culture, trading systems, religion, and language were also lost. No one knows why the Esselen left this rock art, but in 1929, poet Robinson Jeffers wrote the following verse to commemorate the pictographs:

Hands

Inside a cave in a narrow canyon near Tassajara
The vault of rock is painted with hands,
A multitude of hands in the twilight, a cloud of men's palms, no more,
No other picture, There's no one to say
Whether the brown shy quiet people who are dead intended
Religion or magic, or made their tracings
In the idleness of art; but over the division of years these careful
Signs-manual are now like a sealed message
Saying "Look: we also were human; we had hands, not paws. All hail
You people with the cleverer hands, our supplanters
In the beautiful country; enjoy her a season, her beauty, and come down
And be supplanted; for you also are human."

— *Reprinted by permission of Jeffers Literary Properties*

■ ■

The divide marks the junction with the **Pine Ridge** and **Carmel River Trails.** If you're bound for **Pine Valley**, see TRIP 49 Pine Valley (page 199) for a description of camp and the 1.7-mile route into the valley via the Carmel River Trail. If you're bound for **Arroyo Seco Campground** or a grand wilderness loop along the **Black Cone Trail,** see TRIP 53 Black Cone Trail to Arroyo Seco (page 215) for details.

CHAPTER seventeen

Arroyo Seco

■ ■ ■ ■ ■ ■ ■ ■ ■ ■ ■ ■ ■

N EAR ITS SOURCE, the Arroyo Seco is anything but a dry wash, as its Spanish name might suggest. Only as it approaches the Salinas River does it dwindle into a desiccated sandy riverbed. This relatively unknown river originates in the eastern Ventana Wilderness amid some of Big Sur's most spectacular backcountry. Its fanlike drainage encompasses numerous tributaries. The Arroyo Seco is fed from the north by Paloma and Piney Creeks; from the west by Tassajara, Church, and Willow Creeks; and from the southwest by Lost Valley Creek. To the south its headwaters descend off the east face of Coast Ridge and the north face of Cone Peak, and to the southeast it flows from Junipero Serra Peak into Roosevelt and Santa Lucia Creeks. Together these tributaries slice through diverse mountainous terrain, carving narrow gorges that shelter deep emerald pools.

As with most of the Ventana Wilderness, the best time to visit the Arroyo Seco is in spring or fall. Be aware that ticks and mosquitoes flourish in spring and summer, and in fall many small tributaries run dry. During heavy winter storms, the small creeklets, creeks, and rivers swell rapidly and can be difficult or dangerous to cross. Summer is an excellent time to enjoy the river's numerous swimming holes, though air temperatures are often uncomfortably hot, and flies can be a nuisance.

The narrow, winding 18-mile Arroyo Seco Road—or Arroyo Seco–Indians Road, as labeled on the USFS map—threads through the wilderness, connecting Santa Lucia Memorial Park Campground near Jolon with the Arroyo Seco resort area, west of the Salinas Valley town of Greenfield. The road has been permanently closed to public vehicles since its seasonal closure in late fall 1994. The stretch between the Arroyo Seco Campground and Escondido Campground remains closed to all vehicles, due to landslides. The road is open to hikers, equestrians, and bicyclists year-round, if they can get past the landslides. The stretch between Escondido and Memorial Park campgrounds is closed seasonally, starting with the first rains of the season through approximately April. Contact Monterey County Public Works for current road conditions: (831) 755-4800, www.co.monterey.ca.us/publicworks.

The road's fate is uncertain. Los Padres National Forest officials proposed to remove landslide debris and perform road maintenance to reopen the road. Opposition from

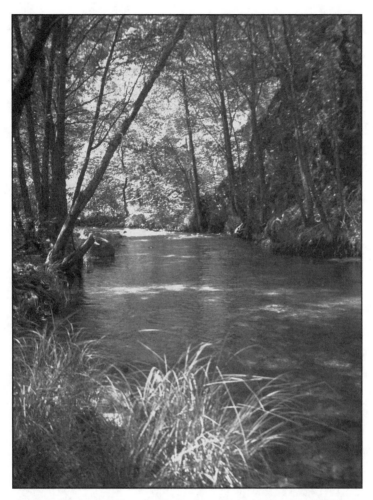

Calm pools along Willow Creek are densely shaded by alders above Tassajara Camp.

environmental organizations, including the Ventana Wilderness Alliance and the Center for Biological Diversity, sought to have the problematic road either closed to vehicle traffic entirely or restored with less impact to the Arroyo Seco watershed.

DIRECTIONS: From the north, drive south on U.S. Highway 101 to Salinas and exit at Arroyo Seco Road/Mission la Soledad in the town of Soledad. Drive 1.1 miles west on Arroyo Seco Road to a sharp bend left, where it meets Fort Romie Road (County Road G17). From this junction, Arroyo Seco Road merges with County Road G17 for 8.5 miles south to a junction with Elm Avenue (County Road G16). Turn right on Elm and drive 5.8 miles southwest to the junction with Arroyo Seco. Bear left (west) on Arroyo Seco.

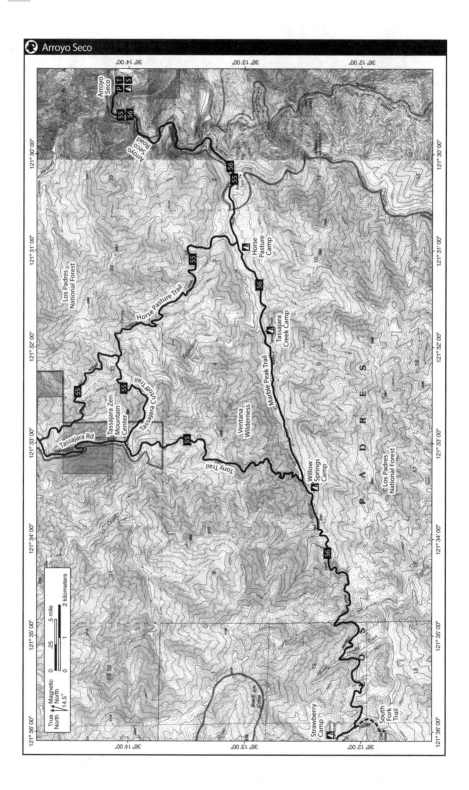

From the south, drive north on U.S. Highway 101 and take the Route 101 Business exit in Greenfield, 15 miles north of King City. Half a mile from the exit, you'll reach Elm Avenue. Turn left on Elm and drive 5.8 miles southwest to the junction with Arroyo Seco Road. Bear left (west) on Arroyo Seco.

Arroyo Seco Road merges with Carmel Valley Road (County Road G16) for 6.5 miles until you reach a fork. Bear left along Arroyo Seco Road, which leads 4.4 miles to a bridge over the Arroyo Seco. Onward half a mile, the road enters the self-service pay station at popular Arroyo Seco Campground (see below for campground details).

If you're not camping, continue along the road 0.4 mile beyond the entrance to a large parking lot and a gate where the pavement ends. From here you must traverse the narrow, winding road on foot, bike, or horse. The Marble Peak Trailhead lies 2.4 miles farther along Arroyo Seco Road.

VISITOR CENTER: Big Sur Station: (831) 667-2315. The station is on Highway 1, 4.2 miles south of Andrew Molera State Park and just south of Pfeiffer Big Sur State Park. Open daily 8 a.m.–6 p.m. Memorial Day through Labor Day, 8 a.m.–4:30 p.m. the rest of the year. USFS Monterey District Headquarters, King City: (831) 385-5434.

NEAREST CAMPGROUND: The northern section of Arroyo Seco Road ends at Arroyo Seco Campground (39 sites, $15–30/night for primitive sites and $20–40/night for car camping), along the lower Arroyo Seco. Facilities at the year-round campground include flush toilets, hot showers, and RV sites.

INFORMATION: There's a $5/night parking fee at the campground. Fire permits are required for all stoves in the backcountry. Dogs are permitted and allowed off leash, except in designated campgrounds, where a 6-foot or shorter leash is required.

WEBSITE: www.fs.usda.gov/lpnf

PHONE: Los Padres National Forest Headquarters: (805) 968-6640

Trip 55

TASSAJARA HOT SPRINGS

LENGTH AND TYPE: 19.2-mile out-and-back, 15.3-mile loop, or 11.5-mile point-to-point

RATING: Moderate to strenuous

TRAIL CONDITION: Passable to difficult, poison oak

HIGHLIGHTS: Hikers follow Tassajara Creek through narrow gorges that shelter hidden pools, while guests of the Tassajara Zen Mountain Center can enjoy the mineral-rich hot springs.

TO REACH THE TRAILHEAD: This hike begins where the pavement ends on Arroyo Seco Road.

TRIP SUMMARY: This route along Arroyo Seco Road and the Marble Peak Trail to the Tony Trail or the Horse Pasture and Tassajara Cutoff Trails accesses rugged, steep-walled Tassajara Creek canyon and its invigorating hot springs and swimming holes.

Only take this route when the Tassajara Zen Mountain Center is open. The center is open only to guests with reservations from late April to early September: (831) 659-2229 or (415) 865-1899 for reservations, sfzc.org/tassajara. From late September to early April, Tassajara is closed to the public while the resident community immerses itself in Zen training. The public does have right-of-way through the grounds year-round, but the monks would prefer not to have unregistered guests. Without reservations you cannot use the hot springs or bathhouses.

The climb from Willow Creek canyon to Tassajara can be arduous. The trail is overgrown, and along steeper sections the narrow tread suffers from slides and washouts. Expect flies, ticks, and lots of poison oak. Nevertheless, these routes via the Tony, Horse Pasture, and Tassajara Cutoff Trails lead into one of Ventana's most beautiful canyons.

The route from Arroyo Seco offers several out-and-back, loop, and point-to-point options, including: (1) Arroyo Seco to Tassajara Zen Mountain Center to the Church Creek Trailhead via the Tony Trail and Tassajara Road (11.5 miles point-to-point, if you can arrange a shuttle vehicle); (2) Arroyo Seco to Tassajara Zen Mountain Center via the Horse Pasture and Tassajara Cutoff Trails, returning via the Tony Trail (15.3-mile loop); and (3) Arroyo Seco to Tassajara Zen Mountain Center via the Tony Trail (out-and-back 19.2 miles). Choose this last route if you're unable to arrange a shuttle vehicle. The Horse Pasture Trail is overgrown with waistdeep poison oak, ruling it out for those highly allergic to this plant. The Tony Trail is steeper and considered abandoned by the US Forest Service, though as of this writing it was passable.

PROTECTING THE STEELHEAD ■ ■ ■ ■ ■ ■ ■ ■ ■ ■ ■ ■ ■ ■

Steelhead trout have thrived in coastal waters and freshwater rivers for millions of years. Now these fish are endangered. The Arroyo Seco is one of the few tributaries of the Salinas River that supports a small population of the threatened trout. Unfortunately, loss and damage of their freshwater habitat is a leading reason for their population decline.

Fortunately, wilderness advocates have launched a campaign to permanently preserve the wild and free Arroyo Seco from dams, diversions, and new development by adding it to the National Wild & Scenic River System. This designation is part of the Wild & Scenic Rivers Act of 1968. As of 2010, a bill was introduced to protect about 19 miles of the Arroyo Seco.

Wilderness advocates urge the public to voice support for permanent protection of the Arroyo Seco. For more information contact the Ventana Wilderness Alliance: (831) 423-3191 or ventanawild.org.

■ ■

Trip Description

Arroyo Seco Road continues from a locked gate directly above the parking lot (1540'). The road beyond winds high above the **Arroyo Seco**. Listen for the swift river below as it cascades past smooth outcrops and plunges into deep pools. You'll be tempted to take one of the many short spurs to the banks of these refreshing pools to escape the heat and sun along the exposed road.

After 2.4 exposed miles, the road widens at a turnout where cars once parked for the **Marble Peak Trailhead** (1340'). Set out from the signed junction on your right, descending narrow, steep **Marble Peak Trail.** You'll brush past manzanita brush and poison oak in the shade of sprawling coast live and black oaks. The steep trail drops to a sturdy **bridge** (2.7 miles, 960') across a narrow stretch of the Arroyo Seco, 150 yards above the river's confluence with **Willow Creek,** fed by **Tassajara** and **Church Creeks.** You'll find a refreshing swimming hole just below the bridge.

Beyond the bridge, you'll follow an old roadbed, then veer west on a broad path to a steep bluff. This bluff overlooks the Arroyo Seco, Willow Creek, and the **Horse Pasture Trail,** which slices through dry chaparral along Tassajara Creek canyon. Onward, the trail parallels Willow Creek Fault and ducks through two gullies to the **Horse Pasture Trail junction** (3.6 miles, 1070').

To reach Tassajara Creek canyon, you'll either take the Horse Pasture Trail 2.1 miles to the **Tassajara Cutoff Trail,** which leads a mile to the monastery, or continue on the Marble Peak Trail to the **Tony Trail,** which climbs 3.1 miles of steep switchbacks to the monastery. Both routes are laborious and suffer from encroaching brush. Though it offers an easier grade through the canyon, the Horse Pasture Trail is overgrown with waist-high poison oak, and there are no campsites along the trail. Neither route is suitable if you're toting a heavy pack.

Although the Forest Service doesn't make trail maintenance or construction a priority, it would be valuable to build a trail along Tassajara Creek to the Tassajara Cutoff Trail. This new route would connect to Tassajara Road and eliminate the need to maintain the Horse Pasture and Tony Trails, not to mention lead through one of the backcountry's most spectacular canyons.

In the meantime, you're better off staying at one of the camps along **Willow Creek** (**Willow Springs** is a favorite) and dayhiking to the hot springs. Remember, reservations are required at the **Tassajara Zen Mountain Center,** and it's closed to the public between late September and early April.

SIDE TRIP ■

The 4.8-mile **Horse Pasture Trail** (3.6 miles, 1070') crosses brush-choked slopes high above Tassajara Creek on its 1300-foot ascent to **Tassajara Road.** It's a hot, exposed route in summer and a tick-infested trek in spring. Regardless, it's useful if you're headed to the **Church Creek Trailhead,** Tassajara Cutoff Trail, or the Zen Mountain Center.

After 2.1 miles, you'll reach the **Tassajara Cutoff Trail junction.** This trail leads a mile to Tassajara Creek and 0.3 mile farther to the monastery. Gorgeous pools line the narrow canyon, offering welcome opportunities to swim and lounge about on smooth, sun-warmed rocks.

The Horse Pasture Trail continues another 2.1 miles to Tassajara Road, where a left turn leads 0.2 mile to the Church Creek Trailhead and 1.3 miles to the monastery.

■ ■

A few feet past the Horse Pasture Trail junction, amid open stands of oaks and pines, a 70-foot spur leads from the Marble Peak Trail to the well-established though unofficial **Horse Pasture Camp** (3.7 miles, 1070'). Equestrians frequent this idyllic camp amid a small rock-studded meadow, which in spring is blanketed in colorful wildflowers. Camp can accommodate

A refreshing swimming hole entices backpackers just below Horse Bridge.

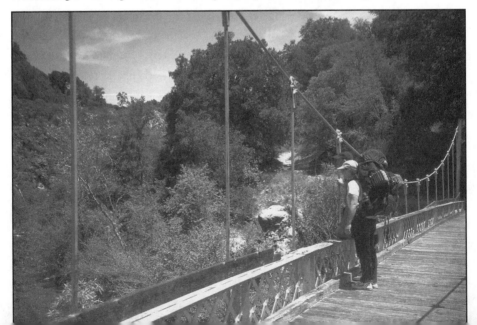

up to two tents in the shade of live oaks and maples. Two small cascades gurgle away not 50 feet from camp, but the route to Willow Creek is heavily overgrown with poison oak.

Beyond the spur to camp, the Marble Peak Trail widens along an abandoned road. You'll climb high above the creek past two small gullies with reliable springs, enter a side canyon lined with poison oak, then descend to **Tassajara Creek Camp** (4.7 miles, 1150'). Two sites lie along the south bank. To reach the first site, descend from the main trail to a flat bench downstream from the confluence of Willow and Tassajara Creeks. Overlooking the confluence a minute farther along the main trail, the second site can accommodate up to three tents in the shade of maples and live and valley oaks. Campers can also take a dip in small pools along the alder-lined creek.

A few hundred yards past camp, you'll reach the first of 15 boulder-hops across Willow Creek. The first 11 occur in fairly rapid succession over the next mile as the trail closely follows the river's course. The 12th crossing is 0.2 mile farther, the next 0.4 mile farther, and the 14th a half mile beyond that. From late spring until the first winter rains, you should make it without wetting a toe. Along the south bank 150 feet past the last crossing, you'll reach the **Tony Trail junction** (6.5 miles, 1800').

Here you'll find an unofficial primitive camp with two small sites, each with a fire ring and room for up to two tents. The camp lies under a dense canopy of alders, maples, and sycamores with a lush understory of ferns, poison oak, and thimbleberries, which produce edible berries in early summer.

The Tony Trail leads 3.1 miles to Tassajara Creek and the Zen Mountain Center. The public has legal right-of-way across the monastery grounds to Tassajara Road, though the monks prefer to not have unannounced guests (reservations must be made in advance). The monastery is closed to visitors from fall to spring. In summer, visitors with reservations may enjoy the creekside hot springs, waterfalls, and swimming holes. Visitors may stay overnight in private or communal rooms. Day-use fees ($30/adults, $12/children) include soaks in the bathhouses. A vegetarian lunch is also available by reservation and costs $13/adults and $9/children.

From the Tony Trail junction, you'll cross Willow Creek and an adjacent **creeklet** (your only source of water until Tassajara Creek) and ascend a steep, unstable slope on a moderately overgrown trail. Though the trail is marked ABANDONED on USFS maps, it shows signs of recent maintenance, unlike many "maintained" trails within the wilderness. Check for hitchhiking ticks in spring. You'll ascend 16 switchbacks to precarious slopes above Willow Creek, climbing 1150-foot ridge in 1.5 miles. Pause atop this ridge for views of the Willow Creek drainage to the south and Tassajara Creek drainage to the north.

From this point, the trail is virtually all downhill the 1.6 miles to Tassajara Creek and the monastery. A small unofficial trail leads half a mile upstream to a **waterfall**—impressive in winter, though a mere trickle by late summer. The trail crosses the creek and leads 0.4 mile downstream past meditation grounds, bathhouses, small rooms, and residences to the parking lot and Tassajara Road. The steep, unpaved road continues 1.5 miles farther to the Church Creek Trailhead (11.5 miles, 2180'). Heavy rains may close this stretch.

PARADISE FOUND ■

The Tassajara Zen Mountain Center is nestled in rugged, mineral-rich Tassajara Creek canyon. Humans have used these healing grounds for centuries. The native Esselen people used the hot springs as traditional ceremonial grounds, as depicted in surviving pictographs on cave walls in Church Creek canyon.

In the 1860s, crews forged Tassajara Road and built the original resort cabins and pools along the banks of Tassajara Creek. Today the site is home to *Zenshin-ji* (Zen Mind Temple), a Soto Zen Buddhist monastery established in 1966. From May through August, Tassajara welcomes guests to workshops, retreats, and work-study programs in this remote wilderness valley. For more information visit sfzc.org/tassajara.

■ ■

Trip 56

WILLOW SPRINGS & STRAWBERRY CAMPS

LENGTH AND TYPE: 24.2-mile out-and-back, loop, or point-to-point

RATING: Strenuous

TRAIL CONDITION: Passable to Willow Springs; dense poison oak, brush, and faint tread to Strawberry Camp

HIGHLIGHTS: Wind your way through narrow gorges and verdant canyon bottoms past crystal-clear tributaries and cool, dark pools.

TO REACH THE TRAILHEAD: This hike begins where the pavement ends on Arroyo Seco Road.

TRIP SUMMARY: This route from Arroyo Seco Road along the Marble Peak and South Fork Trails to Strawberry Camp and beyond offers multiple out-and-back and point-to-point destinations, including: (1) Willow Springs Camp (13.8 miles out-and-back); (2) Pine Ridge Trail junction via Black Cone Trail (14.6 miles one way, with option to continue 15.8 miles to Pfeiffer Big Sur State Park or 5.4 miles to Pine Valley); (3) Tassajara Hot Springs (11.5 miles point-to-point to the Church Creek Trailhead); and (4) Tassajara Hot Springs via Tony Trail (19.2 miles out-and-back).

From Arroyo Seco Campground, you'll climb steep Arroyo Seco Road for 2.4 miles above the lower Arroyo Seco. Short spurs from the road drop to the banks of the river, where you can roam the canyon floor, swimming, sunning, climbing, and boulder-hopping around each bend.

Trip Description

See TRIP 55 Tassajara Hot Springs (page 229) for the first 6.5 miles of this route to the **Tony Trail junction.**

Past the Tony Trail junction (1800') on the **Marble Peak Trail,** you'll make three boulder-hops across **Willow Creek** in fairly rapid succession over the next 0.4 mile, emerging at **Willow Springs Camp** (6.9 miles, 1970') amid a magnificent grove of live oaks. One of the most charming camps along the Marble Peak Trail, Willow Springs is large enough to accommodate up to 12 tents, depending on one's willingness to camp on slightly sloping ground. In early morning, even the soundest sleepers will wake to the chorus of numerous birds marking their territories and finding mates along the fertile canyon ripe with insects, acorns, seeds, and fruit.

Past camp the trail ascends through shaded gullies, then climbs a series of switchbacks more than 800 feet in 1.3 miles to the first of two saddles. Pause for views down Willow Creek canyon and beyond to the **Salinas Valley.** From here you'll head south 0.1 mile to the second, more prominent saddle (8.2 miles, 2770') at the head of Willow Creek canyon, overlooking the headwaters of Willow and **Zigzag Creeks.**

Ahead, the Marble Peak Trail descends one of the most level, well-graded routes in the Ventana's chaparral landscape. The trail traverses two major side canyons and contours past numerous smaller gullies before crossing reliable **Camp Creek** (10.4 miles, 2760'). You'll climb from this canyon to the fourth saddle, then descend to less reliable **Shovel Handle Creek** (11.3 miles, 2720'). After a steep climb 200 feet across a minor ridge, you'll pass a fairly reliable small spring and reach the second saddle. From here the trail descends 0.2 mile to the **South Fork Trail junction** (11.8 miles, 2750').

At the junction, turn right onto the 5.2-mile **South Fork Trail,** which quickly crosses **Strawberry Creek** and climbs gently upstream 0.3 mile into **Strawberry Valley** and **Strawberry Camp** (12.1 miles, 2840'). The sole site lies on slightly sloping ground and is big enough for up to three tents. This is a popular camp among equestrians due to the small open valley and it's proximity to water through late summer. In fall the creek may seem more like a seep, though you can usually find water a few feet downstream.

Directly above camp lies the **Black Cone Trail junction** (12.1 miles, 2840'). This incredibly scenic 7.8-mile route traverses some of Ventana's highest ridges and mountains, connecting the trails of the Arroyo Seco drainage with the trails of the **Big Sur River** and **Carmel River** drainages. If you're bound for the coast, the Black Cone Trail links up with the **Pine Ridge Trail** at **Pine Ridge** (see TRIP 53 Black Cone Trail to Arroyo Seco, page 215). For a broader wilderness tour, the Pine Ridge Trail leads west 15.8 miles to **Pfeiffer Big Sur State Park** and east 5.4 miles to **Pine Valley** (see TRIP 52 Pine Ridge, Sykes Hot Springs, & Big Sur, page 207).

Trip 57

JUNIPERO SERRA PEAK

LENGTH AND TYPE: 12.4-mile out-and-back

RATING: Strenuous to challenging

TRAIL CONDITION: Passable to difficult, poison oak

HIGHLIGHTS: Epic panoramas from the highest peak in the Santa Lucia Range

TO REACH THE TRAILHEAD: If you're driving north or south on Highway 101, take the Jolon Road exit, 10 miles south of Greenfield and a mile north of the Salinas River crossing. Take Jolon Road (County Road G14) 17.8 miles south to the Mission Road junction. Turn onto Mission Road and drive 0.2 mile to the Hunter Liggett Military Reservation gate (expect to show your driver's license and vehicle registration to enter). In 4.9 miles you'll reach a four-way junction with Del Ventura Road. Turn left and in 0.8 mile bear right along the paved road. Del Ventura turns into Milpitas Road at an unspecified spot. Travel 12 miles from the intersection, cross Rattlesnake Creek, and enter US Forest Service land. Just 5 miles farther you'll reach a spur road on your right, which leads 250 feet to the gated trailhead for Junipero Serra Peak via the Santa Lucia Trail. Just before the gate you'll find a turnout that can accommodate 10 cars.

If you're bound for Memorial Park and the Arroyo Seco Trailhead, continue on Milpitas Road 0.1 mile past a spur road on your left that leads to the USFS Indian Station. A tenth of a mile past this spur, you'll reach Santa Lucia Memorial Park Campground on the right. Here the pavement ends and the road continues 0.1 mile to the end of Milpitas Road. At this junction, take the left fork and travel a few yards, then fork left again. The road dead-ends at the gated trailhead. Park on the shoulder without blocking the gate.

If you're bound for the Lost Valley Trailhead at Escondido Camp, take the right fork from the end of Milpitas Road and drive along Arroyo Seco Road 2.6 miles to Escondido. This road closes from the first heavy rains until spring, when weather and road conditions

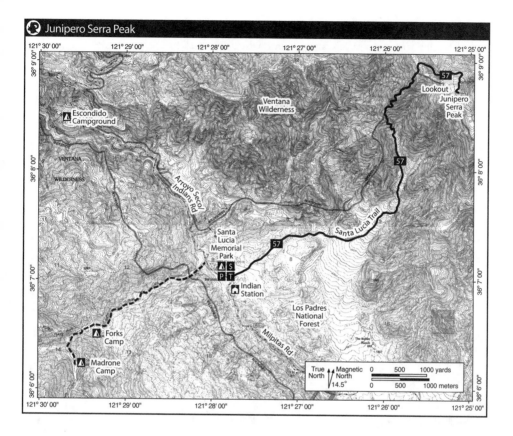

improve. Contact Los Padres National Forest Headquarters for current road conditions: (805) 968-6640, www.fs.usda.gov/lpnf.

TRIP SUMMARY: This strenuous hike climbs nearly 4000 vertical feet in 6.2 miles across boulder-strewn hillsides, pine groves, and blue and valley oak woodlands to the summit. During the wet season, new growth highlights ancient exposed sandstone along the valleys, knolls, cliffs, and ridges. Vibrant wildflower displays progress upslope as spring advances. On clear days from the summit you'll catch glimpses of the Sierra Nevada across the Salinas and San Joaquin Valleys.

The best time to summit is during the wet season (November through April), when air quality is best and temperatures are moderate along this exposed route. Snow blankets the mountain at higher elevations after winter storms. Ticks thrive as temperatures rise, while summer brings an onslaught of flies, soaring temperatures, and blankets of fog that obscure coastal views.

Forged by the Forest Service in the early 1900s, the Santa Lucia Trail historically linked Indian Station to Arroyo Seco Campground with a detour to Junipero Serra Peak, formerly known as Sta'yokale among local American Indians.

The trail served as the only access through the eastern section of the Ventana Wilderness until Arroyo Seco Road was completed in 1939. Though its northern and southern trailheads remain open today, they are not regularly maintained. In places, the tread is faint and head-high brush aggressively encroaches on the trail.

Our Lord's candle, a semiarid yucca, thrives on rocky, open slopes where it blooms a candle-like stalk of creamy white flowers in late spring.

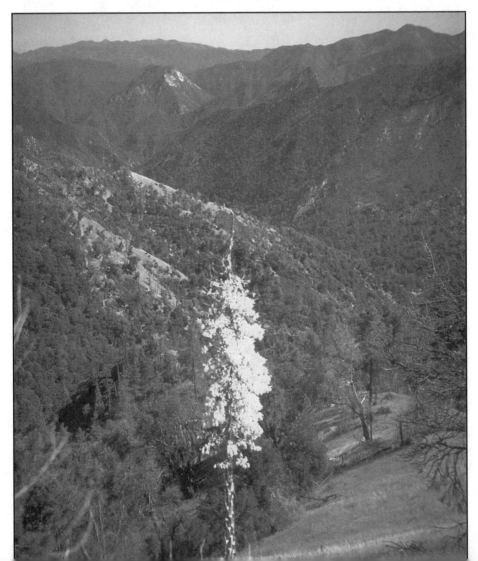

Trip Description

From the gated trailhead at road's end (2090'), the broad **Santa Lucia Trail** leads through open grassland to the east end of **Santa Lucia Memorial Park,** adjacent to steep sandstone cliffs. You'll ascend a minor ridge, climb briefly northeast, and arrive at a minor gap. Onward, the trail leads northeast past live oaks and open terrain. If you're not bound for the summit but would like to take in some of the scenery, end your climb atop the next ridge, which offers outstanding views.

Along the way you may notice the anomalous prickly pear cacti. Although **Junipero Serra Peak** does boast unusual and rare plant species, this cacti is not endemic to the **Santa Lucia Range.** Spanish missionaries brought the drought-tolerant species from Mexico as early as 1769. Modern-day specimens probably derive from stock planted by early settlers.

From the scenic ridge, you'll turn east and climb to a **saddle** (1 mile, 2350'). From this saddle, the route continues along an abandoned road to a dry creek bed lined with willows and sycamores, the latter featuring bark that resembles a jigsaw puzzle. In a few minutes you should pass a rusty **abandoned tractor** (1.4 miles, 2320'). Onward, the path narrows and gradually climbs to a junction with a **southbound trail** (1.6 miles, 2430'). Beyond this junction the trail climbs an unrelenting steep grade.

Dense brush encroaches on the trail as you enter a steep-walled arroyo canyon. In winter and spring, a small stream meanders through the wash. Lining the channel are large granite boulders, transported here during heavy floods that reshape this landscape about once every 100 years. You'll continue along a faint trail between two parallel washes before crossing the west wash (2.6 miles, 3170').

The steep route crosses a small meadow past heavy chaparral thickets to a second sloping meadow. From here you'll switchback through head-high brush to a prominent saddle and a junction with the north-trending abandoned section of the **Santa Lucia Trail** (3.7 miles, 4170'), marked by a dilapidated sign that claims you're 2 miles from the summit. You'll notice a faint trail leading east up the ridge. Fortunately, your route switchbacks toward the ridge along a more moderate grade. From this point, you're more than halfway to the summit.

Over the next 0.8 mile the trail tops a ridge, veers left past oak-clad slopes, and crosses through dense manzanita thickets to a notable saddle. Turning east, you'll skirt the north slopes and pass a junction with the heavily overgrown, abandoned **Junipero Serra Camp Trail,** which drops 600 feet in 0.4 mile to the site of the former camp. Beyond the junction you'll pass enormous Coulter and sugar pines as you climb toward a saddle between a ridge and the summit. Below the saddle, the trail leads a quarter mile to a minor ridge, where it turns south and climbs to more open terrain. The trail wanders up the western flank, then climbs south to an abandoned 40-foot **lookout tower** (6.2 miles, 5862') at the summit.

From this vantage point atop the highest peak in the Santa Lucia Range, you'll take in virtually the entire northern range, including the **Ventana and Silver Peak wildernesses, Hunter Liggett Military Reservation,** and the **Big Sur** coast. To the northwest, conspicuously flat-topped **Uncle Sam Mountain** (4766') and notched, barren **Ventana Double Cone** (4853') rise behind **Tassajara Creek** and **Church Creek** canyons. Sixty miles of visible coastline spread out beyond the **Coast Ridge.** To the west, 5155-foot **Cone Peak** rises less than 3 miles from the glistening blue **Pacific** (or perhaps engulfing fog bank). **Piñon Peak** (5264') caps a prominent ridge that extends east, masking most of the Salinas Valley, while beyond it lies the **Diablo Range,** 35 miles to the south. On extremely clear days, usually between winter storms, you may spot the high crests of the **Sierra Nevada** across the **Salinas and San Joaquin Valleys.** About 165 miles east, any visible peaks are most likely those along the east edge of Kings Canyon National Park. When ready, return the way you came.

STA'YOKALE, SACRED PEAK ■ ■ ■ ■ ■ ■ ■ ■ ■ ■ ■ ■ ■ ■ ■

Formerly known as Sta'yokale, Pimkolam, and Santa Lucia Peak, Junipero Serra Peak has long been of great spiritual importance to Salinian American Indians. The Salinian people continue to gather here for ceremony and prayer, trusting in the healing wisdom of this sacred mountain.

The following traditional Salinian creation story, retold by the Salinian Nation Cultural Preservation Association, explains the peak's significance:

A long time ago, waters from the ocean rose and flooded the entire world, except for the very top of Sta'yokale. Those First People who survived the deluge gathered on top with Eagle (Sa'yyo). Sa'yyo asked Kingfisher to dive down and get some mud from the bottom of the water. Kingfisher did so, but when he returned to the surface, he died. Sa'yyo scraped mud from beneath Kingfisher's nails, which he rolled into four balls. He threw one of the balls to each of the four directions. The waters receded, and the world became as it is today. And the First People who had died were brought back to life.

■ ■

CHAPTER eighteen

Big Sur

■ ■   ■   ■   ■   ■   ■   ■   ■   ■   ■   ■

N ESTLED ALONG THE BASE of the rugged Santa Lucia Range, Big Sur shelters a wealth of natural treasures. From steep, redwood-lined canyons to headlands that tumble precipitously into the sea, this land is more than a string of towns or stretch of coastline. Though its attributes are many, Big Sur's beauty will elude halfhearted travelers not wanting to venture far from Highway 1.

This chapter varies from Chapter 10: Pfeiffer Big Sur State Park. While trails in that park are limited to day-use access, trails described in this chapter offer overnight treks into Los Padres National Forest and the vast Ventana Wilderness, and backcountry camps are mentioned in each route. Except for the Manuel Peak Trail, these routes do not begin at Pfeiffer Big Sur State Park, but near the town of Big Sur.

You'll hike past wildflower-strewn golden hillsides, oak woodlands, fragrant coastal scrub, and pine-studded ridges. The higher you climb, the more rewarding the views become, with glimpses east into the sheer Santa Lucias and west to the rugged coast. Hikers can access the Pine Ridge Trail at Big Sur Station, a half mile south of Pfeiffer Big Sur State Park. This is unquestionably the most popular route into the Ventana Wilderness. It leads from high above the Big Sur River to the canyon floor, linking spacious riverside camps, refreshing swimming holes, and thermal pools, including the often-crowded Sykes Camp. Other routes access portions of Big Sur from Coast Ridge Road (closed to vehicles).

DIRECTIONS: Pfeiffer Big Sur State Park is on the east side of Highway 1, 26 miles south of the Carmel Valley Road (County Road G16) junction in Carmel and 28 miles north of the Nacimiento-Fergusson Road junction near Kirk Creek Campground. Big Sur Station is also on the east side of Highway 1, a half mile south of the state park entrance. The complex serves the US Forest Service, CalTrans, and California State Parks.

VISITOR CENTER: Big Sur Station: (831) 667-2315. The station is a half mile south of the park entrance. Open daily 8 a.m.–6 p.m. Memorial Day through Labor Day, 8 a.m.–4:30 p.m. the rest of the year.

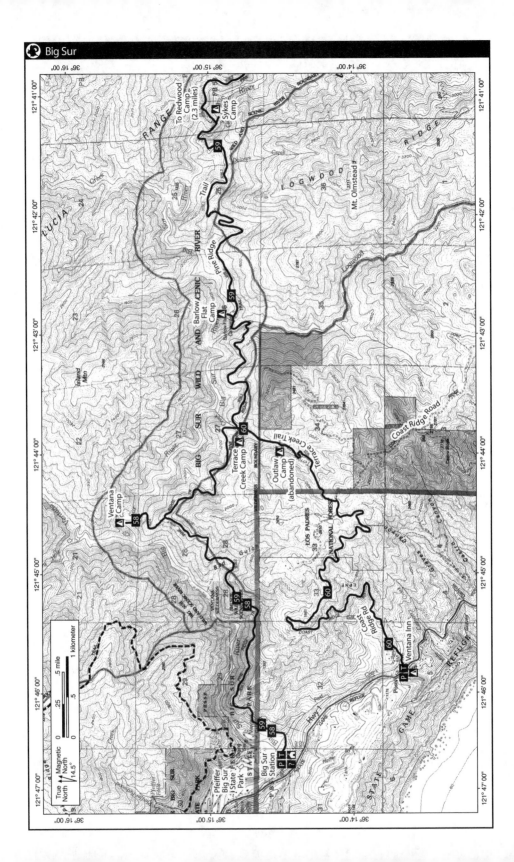

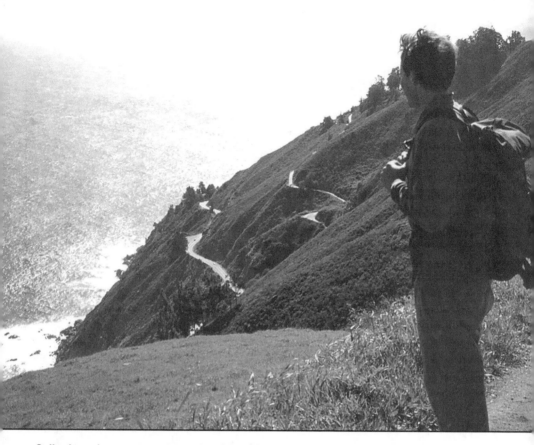

Solitude seekers must venture only a few miles from Highway 1 before being continuously rewarded the farther they climb.

NEAREST CAMPGROUND: Pfeiffer Big Sur State Park (218 sites, $35/standard site, $45/river site, $150/group site; reservations recommended). Along the Big Sur River, this 1006-acre park offers showers, Wi-Fi, and swimming. For more information call (800) 444-7275 or visit parks.ca.gov.

INFORMATION: Pfeiffer Big Sur State Park charges a day-use fee of $10. No dogs allowed on park trails. Fire permits required for all stoves and/or campfires (free and available at Big Sur Station). Campfires permitted from late November through April (fire season posted at trailhead). No wilderness permits are required in Ventana Wilderness.

WEBSITE: parks.ca.gov or www.fs.usda.gov/lpnf

PHONE: Big Sur Station: (831) 667-2315; Los Padres National Forest Headquarters: (805) 968-6640

Trip 58

VENTANA CAMP

LENGTH AND TYPE: 10.2-mile out-and-back

RATING: Moderate

TRAIL CONDITION: Well maintained to clear, poison oak

HIGHLIGHTS: Follow the Big Sur River as it cascades through steep, narrow canyon walls that shelter deep swimming holes.

TO REACH THE TRAILHEAD: At Big Sur Station the Pine Ridge Trailhead is at the end of the parking lot beyond the visitor center. Self-pay parking is $4/night for overnight guests. You'll find water, flush toilets, and maps at the visitor center.

TRIP SUMMARY: Pine Ridge is the most heavily used trail in the wilderness, as most hikers set their sights on Sykes Camp and the 100°F hot springs. Barely 4 miles into that 10-mile trek is the junction to Ventana Camp, which boasts one of Ventana's finest swimming holes. Though far from a hidden treasure, it makes a wonderful weekend trip. If you go in spring or fall, when summer crowds have diminished and temperatures are still pleasant, you'll likely have the brisk pool all to yourself.

Trip Description

The well-marked and heavily used **Pine Ridge Trail** starts from the end of the parking lot (370'). You'll briefly skirt a fenced-in pasture, then enter the cool, damp redwood- and fern-lined gullies high above **Pfeiffer Big Sur State Park Campground**. After a gradual descent and crossing of perennial **Post Creek** (0.7 mile, 280'), the trail climbs steady switchbacks to a steep ridge (0.8 mile, 850'). Pause to take in the view down canyon, where the **Big Sur River** abruptly turns from southwest to northwest on its final stretch to **Molera Beach**. Also notice the flats where the river meets the major fault of the Big Sur drainage, the **Sur Thrust Fault,** which steadily slips, compresses, and erodes rocks in its path. The river closely follows this swath of destruction to the **Pacific.**

Onward, the tread turns to loose gravel along sunny slopes with scattered views into the steep-walled river gorge. Although you'll hear cascading falls directly below, the only way to access this section of the river is along the **Gorge Trail** (see TRIP 21 Gorge Trail, page 107). Across the canyon are the exposed south-facing slopes of **Manuel Peak,** clearly marked by the **Manuel Peak Trail,** which slices through dense chaparral thickets (see TRIP 20 Manuel Peak Trail, page 105). This vegetation stands in stark contrast to this trail's forested north-facing slopes.

The trail continues through shady redwood gullies and tanoak groves devastated by sudden oak death (see sidebar, page 165, for details). Soon you'll reach a sign that marks the state park boundary and your entry into the **Ventana Wilderness** (2.3 miles, 900').

You'll climb north nearly 300 feet in the next 0.3 mile to the trail's high point, then turn east for a quick descent through two gullies. The second gully (3.3 miles, 1240') boasts a seasonal 40-foot waterfall that cascades from trailside cliffs in winter and spring, though by summer barely a trickle is heard. Onward, the trail climbs half a mile past several overlooks, then descends to a nearby ridge and the **Ventana Camp Trail junction** (3.9 miles, 1500'), marked by a dilapidated sign.

Ventana Camp Trail is a strenuous 1.2-mile spur that drops 840 feet down a series of short switchbacks to the river. From the junction, turn left down the trail and you'll quickly reach an unofficial campsite. Though waterless and not as scenic as Ventana Camp, this is where those unwilling to slog heavy gear down the steep grade choose to camp. It can hold up two tents on sloping ground. After a series of 14 switchbacks, the trail emerges at **Ventana Camp** (5.1 miles, 660'), perched atop a broad terrace on the upper Big Sur.

Shaded by oaks, madrones, and redwoods, the camp can accommodate large groups at 10 sites that flank the river. In summer, a large swimming hole in the river bend offers respite from the heat. Just past this bend, the river turns south-southwest through a steep-walled gorge, where the collective flow of the watershed's tributaries and runoff funnel through a notch less than 10 feet wide and plunge into one of Ventana's most alluring swimming holes.

If you're eastbound on the Pine Ridge Trail, refer to the following trip description for the remaining 1580-foot gain and 970-foot loss in elevation over the next 5.7 miles to **Sykes Camp**. The strenuous 900-foot vertical toil back to the Pine Ridge Trail is best done in early morning or late afternoon.

JUST WHAT THE DOCTOR ORDERED ■ ■ ■ ■ ■ ■ ■ ■ ■ ■ ■ ■

While artifacts found in the Santa Lucia Range date back 10,000 years to the Esselen, Salinian, and Ohlone-Rumsen people, Big Sur remained largely unexplored through the early 20th century. A flood of settlement and industry at the end of the 19th century emphasized the need for a direct trading route in and out of the region.

Frustrated with the time it took to reach his Big Sur patients from Monterey, Dr. John Roberts dreamed of an efficient, safe road, and even conducted early surveys. Entering the political arena as county supervisor, then state legislator, he lobbied for the construction of what would become America's most scenic roadway. Construction began in 1919, and Highway 1 opened to the public in 1938.

Trip 59

SYKES & REDWOOD CAMPS

LENGTH AND TYPE: 23.8-mile out-and-back

RATING: Moderate to strenuous

TRAIL CONDITION: Well maintained to clear, poison oak

HIGHLIGHTS: Stroll the free-flowing Big Sur past sheltered swimming holes, mineral-rich hot springs, and redwood forests to these idyllic camps.

TO REACH THE TRAILHEAD: At Big Sur Station the Pine Ridge Trailhead is at the end of the parking lot beyond the visitor center. Self-pay parking is $4/night for overnight guests. You'll find water, flush toilets, and maps at the visitor center.

TRIP SUMMARY: Winding deep into the heart of the Big Sur River drainage, the lower Pine Ridge Trail from Big Sur Station to Sykes Camp is the most popular route into the Ventana Wilderness. The total elevation gain and loss along this stretch are 2380 feet and 1490 feet, respectively. The well-maintained trail winds past three other camps in the 10 miles to Sykes Camp. Expect plenty of foot traffic in summer, while spring break brings hordes of hikers to Sykes to cluster about the 100°F hot springs, which can get crowded and, at times, rowdy.

Despite the crowds, pesky flies, and mosquitoes, summer is the best time to visit for a brisk swim (mid- to high 50s Fahrenheit) or to lounge atop the Big Sur's sunny banks and boulders. Swimming is also tolerable on warmer spring and fall days. In spring wild irises emerge from the damp forest floor, while lupines, poppies, hound's-tongues, and starflowers bloom in natural riverside bouquets, highlighted by the occasional delicate tiger lily. Temperatures remain pleasant in fall, as breezes scatter colorful autumn leaves across the canyon floor. From winter through early summer, ticks thrive amid the trailside brush. Fortunately, vegetation rarely encroaches on this well-maintained trail. If you crave solitude, hike the trail in winter. Be aware, however, that the river can rise swiftly during winter storms, making crossings deep and treacherous. The only ford along this trail is at Sykes Camp, and you can avoid this crossing to reach the hot springs.

From Sykes Camp, the Pine Ridge Trail leads 2.4 miles east to Redwood Camp, where you'll find peace beneath the trees even in busy summer months.

Trip Description

See TRIP 58 Ventana Camp (page 244) for the first 3.9 miles of this route to the **Ventana Camp Trail junction** (1500').

From this junction, the **Pine Ridge Trail** ascends 70 feet and descends 260 feet over the next 1.4 miles to **Terrace Creek Camp.** *Ventana* (Spanish for window) holds true to its name along this trail, which offers framed glimpses down the **Big Sur** drainage to the sheer peaks and ridges of the **Ventana Wilderness** and distant **Pacific**. Notched and barren **Ventana Double Cone** lords over the northeastern skyline. Legends claim a rock bridge once connected its twin peaks, framing a window-like summit nearly 5000 feet above the ocean. Whether or not that's true, the double summit served as a prominent landmark for Spanish vessels in the late 18th and 19th centuries.

Enjoy the views, as the trail soon enters shady gullies laced with ferns and moss-covered boulders amid seasonal springs. After a brief climb to a nearby ridge, you'll descend south into steep, redwood-lined **Terrace Creek** canyon. Here you'll find **Terrace Creek Camp** and the **Terrace Creek Trail junction** (5.3 miles, 1320').

The small camp flanks the creek just upstream from the junction. Don't expect solitude, as hikers stream past en route to **Sykes Camp** or back to **Big Sur Station**. You'll find one large main site for up to three tents along the east bank a few yards from the junction, just below a pit toilet. Three smaller sites lie upstream, two downstream. The steep canyon remains cool even in summer heat. In spring, carpets of redwood sorrel, mats of ferns and mosses, and delicate fairy bells line the babbling creek to its confluence with the Big Sur. If you're bound for **Coast Ridge Road** via the **Terrace Creek Trail,** see TRIP 60 Highway 1 to Terrace Creek Camp (page 251) for the trail description.

Beyond the signed camp junction, the Pine Ridge Trail ascends 510 feet and descends 210 feet in the next 1.4 miles to **Barlow Flat Camp** (see side trip on the following page). You'll skirt a ridge and head east along its marble slopes to two seasonal springs. Past the second spring, the trail enters a damp redwood glen. Microclimates vary dramatically as the trail climbs to more arid slopes and sun-drenched ridges. Across the canyon, sheer granite walls reflect the sound of roaring rapids far below in the steep canyon.

Past a second ridge, the trail switchbacks and descends into **Logwood Creek** canyon (6.5 miles, 970'). The creek is an easy boulder-hop in all but the wettest months. After crossing, you'll ascend 0.1 mile to a saddle, from which a short, steep spur climbs 200 feet in 0.1 mile to a 1290-foot summit. Detour here for far-reaching views south along the canyon. Past the spur, the trail descends 0.1 mile to the signed **Barlow Flat Camp Trail junction** (6.7 miles, 1040').

Beyond the signed camp junction, the Pine Ridge Trail ascends 900 feet and descends 690 feet in the next 2.9 miles to Sykes Camp. The trail starts out on a moderate 500-foot climb past a wall of fragile ferns, fed in wet season by a 40-foot waterfall above the trail. You may miss it entirely in summer. You'll climb through two increasingly larger redwood gullies and emerge amid arid slopes cloaked with fragile wild iris beneath oaks, madrones, and a few pine saplings. As you crest a minor ridge (8.2 miles, 1640'), the vegetation changes to a chaparral community of chamise, ceanothus, and poison oak.

SIDE TRIP ■

The **Barlow Flat Camp Trail** descends steep switchbacks 150 feet in 0.2 mile to the outskirts of **Barlow Flat Camp** (6.9 miles, 890'). This is the most spacious camp along the Pine Ridge Trail, often welcoming large groups in summer. The first three sites sit atop a flat, redwood-shaded bench above the south bank of the Big Sur. Three more open sites are nestled amid fragrant bays, maples, alders, and sycamores closer to the water's edge. Five more sites lie beneath redwoods, tanoaks, and peeling madrones along the north bank. The crossing is often wet until summer and may be impassable during or after heavy winter rains. A narrow trail leads upstream past the fifth site to an 80-foot-long swimming hole and sandy beach.

The swimming opportunities at Barlow Flat are excellent. Its sun-drenched rocky outcrops are perfect for basking in the sun and diving into some of the deeper pools. Expect water temps in the low 50s Fahrenheit in spring and fall and the low 60s on warm summer days. Temps may rise 10°F on a hot summer day.

A cross-country route leads to more alluring swimming holes downstream, though passage can be treacherous in rainy season. The first pool is adjacent to the site farthest downstream along the south bank. Onward, 150 yards downstream, cascades plunge through the narrow gorge into deep, hidden pools. From late spring through fall, it's best to wade rather than scale the sheer canyon walls. Don't even attempt passage in winter, as the frigid river can be swift and dangerous. Beyond an Olympic-sized pool, a gossamer 80-foot fall plunges from a small tributary into the Big Sur. If you're willing to swim and wade a minute farther downstream, you'll reach another emerald pool.

■ ■

Beyond this exposed ridge, you'll descend 200 feet to a cool, damp redwood gully cloaked with six-fingered ferns, which bear delicate palmate fronds. Beyond the gully, the route contours 0.2 mile along **Dolores Creek** canyon to a small knoll and dips directly above hidden **Sykes Hot Springs**. You'll continue your descent southeast, switchback northwest, then descend 150 feet to the Big Sur. The trail emerges at **Sykes Camp** and the **Sykes Hot Springs Trail junction** (9.6 miles, 1080').

Most hikers end their trek at Sykes, as the Pine Ridge Trail ascends 1760 feet and descends 1130 feet in the next 2.3 miles to **Redwood Camp**. This less-traveled stretch is predictably ill maintained. Encroaching brush poses a nuisance in wet season when hitchhiking ticks are abundant.

SIDE TRIP ■

Sprawled along a 0.1-mile stretch of the Big Sur, **Sykes Camp** offers campers their choice of 10 sites. The best lie upstream from the Pine Ridge Trail.

From the trail junction, cross the river and head upstream to a sandy beach and adjacent emerald pool. This wet ford can be swift and treacherous in winter as the river swells. You'll soon reach the first of six sites, with room for up to two tents beneath live oaks and madrones. Fifty feet farther upstream, you'll reach a pit toilet amid three large redwoods. The second and third sites lie nearby along a narrow gravel bench. Each can accommodate up to three tents.

A larger fourth site is perched above the rocky bank in the shade of fragrant bays, madrones, and live oaks, whose roots grasp riverside boulders. Secluded pools below this site are often less crowded than pools closer to the hot springs. Perch atop the sun-baked boulders and watch small trout dart between the white water cascades and calm pools.

Beyond the fourth site, the camp trail leads 60 feet upstream, crosses the river, and emerges on a sandy beach beside another attractive pool. Just above this pool lies the fifth site, which can accommodate up to two tents. Onward, 80 feet past a bend, is the similarly small sixth site, atop a sandy flat bordered by a smooth rock face and alders.

Downstream, the unmarked 0.4-mile spur to **Sykes Hot Springs** is heavily used and easy to follow—ignore erroneous descriptions of bushwhacking from camp. Those who want to keep their feet dry will have to navigate sheer rock faces laced with poison oak. The preferred route requires a few boulder-hops or wades that may be difficult or impassable in rainy season.

From where the Pine Ridge Trail crosses the Big Sur, head downstream along the south bank 25 feet to the first crossing. Onward, you'll pass a small single-tent site, recross the river, and reach two more sites, equipped with a pit toilet. Beyond the third site, the trail crosses the river twice in 100 feet and arrives at a fourth site. A third of a mile downstream, you'll catch a whiff of sulfur from the first of several small hot seeps.

The trail ascends 60 feet to the first of three small pools, each large enough for up to four adults. Directly below the pool lies a stone- and sandbag-lined hot tub, 6 feet across and 2 to 3 feet deep. Perched beside the clear, bracing waters of the Big Sur, these mineral-rich 100°F pools are among Ventana's most popular destinations. Don't expect a private soak in summer or on weekends and holidays in spring and fall.

■ ■

From Sykes Camp, you'll cross the Big Sur and climb 0.3 mile to a long, narrow saddle. Passing a rocky ledge, the trail crosses a gully and small seasonal creek. Leaving the canyon, switchbacks climb to a south-trending ridge (10.6 miles, 1680'), offering impressive views down the Big Sur's steep **North Fork** and **South Fork** drainages. The terrain and temperatures vary widely as the brushy route leads to a second exposed ridge, ducks through a small redwood-fringed gully, then returns to the dry slopes of chamise, manzanita, scrub oak, live oak, black sage, and scattered pines and yuccas. Just as suddenly, you'll reenter shady groves along Redwood Creek.

Descending 0.1 mile, you'll reach an unmarked spur on the right (11.9 miles, 1780') to Redwood Camp's larger sites. If you miss this narrow spur, just continue 150 yards farther past two small sites and cross the river. The larger sites now lie a minute downstream.

The first site on the east bank sits amid large boulders and old-growth redwoods. Seventy feet downstream past a small seep, the trail leads to the biggest site, which can accommodate up to 10 tents. This site is perched atop a flat bench carpeted in wild strawberries, starflowers and sorrel in the shade of redwoods, tanoaks, and madrones.

If you continue eastbound on the Pine Ridge Trail, expect conditions to worsen. Overgrown brush, loose tread, and exposed slopes make the 2770-foot climb over the next 3.9 miles to **Pine Ridge** a strenuous adventure.

Sykes Hot Springs is one of Big Sur's most popular backcountry destinations.

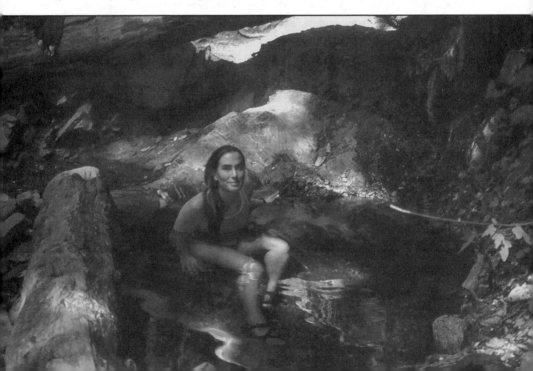

From Pine Ridge, the **Black Cone Trail** leads into the heart of the wilderness, skirting some of Ventana's highest peaks and ridges (see TRIP 53 Black Cone Trail to Arroyo Seco, page 215). If you intend to hike the entire 23.1 miles of the Pine Ridge Trail, Redwood Camp is an excellent place to rest before beginning the long climb. Better yet, start your hike from **China Camp** to avoid excessive elevation gain (see TRIP 52 Pine Ridge, Sykes Hot Springs, & Big Sur, page 207).

Trip 60

HIGHWAY 1 TO TERRACE CREEK CAMP

LENGTH AND TYPE: 11.6-mile out-and-back or 12.9-mile loop

RATING: Moderate

TRAIL CONDITION: Clear, poison oak

HIGHLIGHTS: Take in dramatic views of the furrowed Santa Lucia Range above steep coastal canyons that shelter redwood-flanked creeks.

TO REACH THE TRAILHEAD: The trailhead is on Highway 1 at gated Coast Ridge Road (North Coast Ridge Road on the USFS map) beside the Ventana Inn. The inn is on the east side of Highway 1, 2.2 miles south of Pfeiffer Big Sur State Park and 10 miles north of Julia Pfeiffer Burns State Park. Drive 0.1 mile along the inn entrance road to the public parking area on your left, for day use only. If you're planning to camp, you must park at one of the turnouts along Highway 1 adjacent to the entrance road. From the parking area, walk up the entrance road till it forks. The left branch climbs past the restaurant, while the right branch leads to the gated trailhead.

TRIP SUMMARY: This 5.8-mile route along Coast Ridge Road and Terrace Creek Trail to Terrace Creek Camp can be approached as either an out-and-back or loop trip. You could continue east along the Pine Ridge Trail to swimming holes at the riverside Barlow Flat, Sykes, and Redwood Camps or return 5.3 miles to Big Sur Station via the westbound Pine Ridge Trail (see TRIP 59 Sykes & Redwood Camps, page 246). The latter route finishes with a 1.7-mile stroll south on Highway 1 to the inn. Though a strenuous day hike, the loop makes a pleasant weekend trip. To avoid excessive elevation gain and end on a moderate downhill gradient, consider starting from Big Sur Station.

From Coast Ridge Road, you'll climb more than 1500 feet and traverse a spectacular ridge crest. The Terrace Creek Trail closely follows its namesake's banks as the creek builds to support a narrow strip of redwoods. Temperatures drop as you descend the lush canyon through an oasis of ferns, fungi, and mosses to redwood-shaded Terrace Creek Camp.

The best times to hike this route are in winter and spring, when the swollen creek cascades past verdant new growth. Spring paints the flanks of Coast Ridge with abundant poppies, lupines, baby blue eyes, and myriad other emerging wildflowers. In summer, cool Terrace Creek canyon offers respite from the sweltering heat, though views along Coast Ridge Road disappear beneath a thick blanket of fog.

Trip Description

This hike begins along the first 4.2 miles of **Coast Ridge Road,** which offers convenient mile markers. From the gate (1040'), the road skirts the prestigious **Ventana Inn** and its short guest trails. In a few minutes, you'll pass several private driveways and cross a shallow redwood-fringed gully (1 mile, 1420').

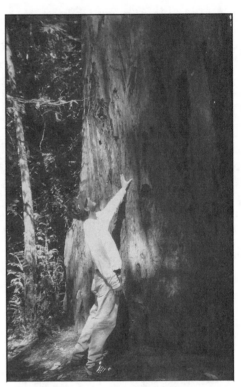

Ancient 1000-year-old redwoods form a narrow band winding through the Big Sur River canyon.

Past this creeklet, the trail crosses a smaller gully, where a creek cascades 40 feet down a sugary white **marble stalagmite** (1.2 miles, 1460'). This formation developed as marble deposits flowed downstream and accumulated at the base of the gully. Marble is one of the oldest rocks in the youthful **Santa Lucia Range,** stretching back hundreds of millions of years to a mountain range in what is now Mexico. The ancient rocks migrated north along the numerous northwest-trending faults to create some of the region's most dramatic features.

Beyond the gully, you'll continue to climb exposed **Coast Ridge.** Briefly returning to shade, the route passes through a second **locked gate** (1.5 miles, 1635'). After half a mile, the trail switchbacks and leads to impressive views northwest along the **Big Sur River** canyon to the **Pacific.** Continue 0.3 mile to a saddle, where dramatic inland views feature 4853-foot **Ventana Double Cone,** whose barren notched peak dominates the skyline just 5 miles northeast.

The road veers right from the saddle to a minor **gully** (3 miles, 2100'), passing a steep, gated private driveway on your left. Onward, the vegetation changes to rolling grasslands, highlighted in spring by spectacular wildflowers. You'll steadily climb four minor ridges, then crest a fifth, which offers the best views thus far.

From the saddle, you'll cross to an adjacent ridge and head north toward a prominent saddle. At mile 4, the road turns east past a spur road on your left. A hundred yards farther, you'll reach a second saddle and the signed **Terrace Creek Trail junction** (4.2 miles, 2590'), also on your left.

From this junction, you'll descend 1270 vertical feet along the steep 1.6-mile trail. Start out past encroaching brush that rebounded aggressively following a fire years back. Keep watch for abundant poison oak. After 0.3 mile, the trail crosses the typically dry head-waters of Terrace Creek and switchbacks down oak- and madrone-clad slopes.

You'll follow the east bank for the next quarter mile before crossing the creek to continue your descent of the steep canyon. The creek holds true to its name, as it cascades past terraces of lush ferns, emerging mushroom caps, and delicate redwood sorrel. Follow the switchbacks another mile through the primeval redwood forest to **Terrace Creek Camp** and the **Pine Ridge Trail junction** (5.8 miles, 1320').

Nestled along the creek beneath a narrow belt of redwoods, the camp offers three small sites above the trail junction (with a pit toilet) and three below the junction. The largest site, with room for up to three tents, lies along the east bank above the **Pine Ridge Trail.**

If you're continuing east or west along the Pine Ridge Trail, refer to TRIP 59 Sykes & Redwood Camps (page 246).

Trip 61

HIGHWAY 1 TO COAST RIDGE ROAD

LENGTH AND TYPE: 7-mile out-and-back

RATING: Challenging

TRAIL CONDITION: Difficult, poison oak

HIGHLIGHTS: Clear days along Coast Ridge Road reveal 50 miles of coastal views. If fog shrouds the coast, gaze east to marvel at Ventana's nearly mile-high peaks.

TO REACH THE TRAILHEAD: This route begins along a private road on the east side of Highway 1, 7.9 miles south of Pfeiffer Big Sur State Park and 3 miles north of Julia Pfeiffer Burns State Park. Turn east off Highway 1 and park along the road without blocking access. The road continues as a private driveway, restricted to vehicles but open to hikers. After 1.1 miles, the road curves right to the signed, gated DeAngulo Trailhead.

TRIP SUMMARY: The lightly used DeAngulo (day-an-GOO-low) Trail climbs to dramatic views along Coast Ridge. Be prepared to face diminished tread, fallen debris, overgrown brush, and minor slides that challenge even the most experienced backcountry hiker.

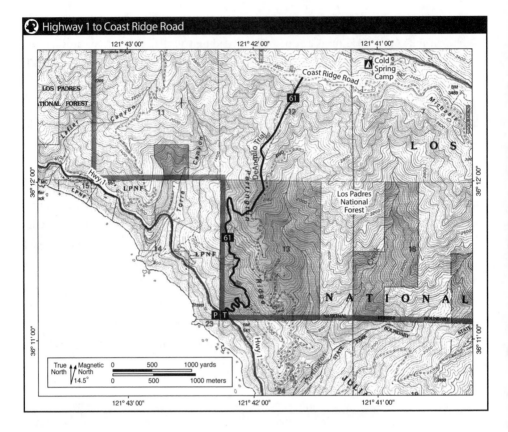

Highway 1 to Coast Ridge Road

Trip Description

Although the **DeAngulo Trail** does not officially begin along the private road, the trail description and mileage is measured from **Highway 1** (600').

The road crosses through an open gate and ascends wide switchbacks past two private driveways. You'll climb past fragrant, invasive eucalypti and dense thickets of sage, lupine, poison oak, golden yarrow, and coyote brush to dense oak woodlands, where the **road forks** (0.6 mile, 1410'). The right fork switchbacks up a private driveway 0.1 mile to a locked gate. You'll veer left through a second open gate (0.7 mile, 1450') and pass a dilapidated sign assuring hikers that the trail does eventually begin. After a few minutes, the road passes another private residence, then switchbacks past three more private driveways. Continue climbing through a hairpin right turn to the signed **DeAngulo Trail junction** (1.8 miles, 1600'), a thousand feet above Highway 1.

Fringed with poison oak, the trail heads north through open grasslands, skirting just east of a private residence. After 100 yards, you'll cross a small shady gully past scrapped cars and make your way around a large fallen tanoak. The trail crosses a second shallow

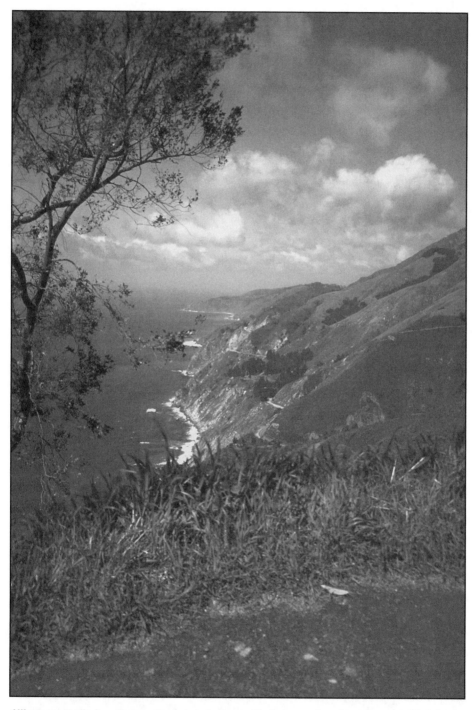

Hikers must climb a steep yet scenic private road before meeting the remote and lightly traveled DeAngulo Trail.

redwood-lined gully, briefly follows an abandoned roadbed, and skirts around a downed bay tree in another shallow gully. You'll cross several more gullies, slippery with leaves from numerous dead or dying tanoaks afflicted by sudden oak death, which has killed these trees by the thousands (see sidebar, page 165). Flags may hang from dead limbs and branches, marking the vanishing trail.

Continue climbing the steep, shady canyon to more open slopes and cross a junction with a dirt road. The trail switchbacks up a grassy ravine, climbing toward a large ponderosa pine draped with vine-like poison oak (2.3 miles, 2080'). Follow a trail sign left past a private road and stroll beneath a canopy of madrones, live oaks, bays, tanoaks, and pines to a **junction** (2.4 miles, 2170') marked by a conspicuous pine.

Avoid the abandoned road, which leads to a gully lined in poison oak. Instead, switchback right into a small grove of young pines. A minute farther the trail turns left and merges with an **old tractor path** (2.5 miles, 2240'). Head north 60 yards, then follow the next trail sign uphill to the right.

Leaving the roadbed, you'll climb past arid yuccas, which sport brilliant cream flowers on large stalks in early summer, and toyons, which produce vibrant red berries in winter. In spring, lupines, poppies, owl's clover, and baby blue eyes blanket these steep slopes. The trail climbs steadily along switchbacks to an oak-clad knoll (3 miles, 279') between **Torre** and **Partington Canyons**. Take a break and enjoy the views, as the trail continues on an extremely steep grade (about 30%) along bulldozer tracks forged during the 1985 Rat Creek Fire.

On loose rubble, you'll climb a dry wash straight up **Partington Ridge** past drought-tolerant ceanothus, scrub oaks, and yuccas. The trail passes an abandoned road (3.2 miles, 3140') on your left and continues a minute farther to a trail junction. Turn left here for a moderate, quarter-mile climb along grasslands past scattered pine and oak woodlands to **Coast Ridge Road** (3.5 miles, 3520'). If you miss the spur trail, the bulldozed wash also reaches the road along a shorter albeit more strenuous route.

From here you can either head back the way you came or continue along the road. If you turn right and hike 0.7 mile to **Cold Spring Road**, then turn left and hike 0.6 mile, you'll reach **Cold Spring Camp**. If you turn left, the road leads 8.8 miles to the **Ventana Inn** on Highway 1 (see TRIP 60 Highway 1 to Terrace Creek Camp, page 251). Whatever you decide, enjoy the solitude and spectacular views along this lonely ridgetop.

CHAPTER nineteen

Cone Peak

■　■　■　■　■　■　■　■　■　■　■　■　■

TOPPING OUT BELOW 6000 FEET, the Santa Lucia Range by no means approaches the lofty reaches of the Sierra Nevada, which soars more than 14,000 feet above the San Joaquin and Sacramento Valleys. But the rugged Santa Lucias certainly surpass any of the Lower 48 coastal ranges in terms of topographical relief. These peaks drop so precipitously to the rocky coves and pounding Pacific, their vertical canyon walls appear to fold in upon themselves.

No mountain illustrates this better than Cone Peak. Within 3 miles of the coast, Cone rises nearly a mile. The astonishing grade from the beach at Limekiln to the summit is the most extreme coastal slope in the contiguous United States. This abrupt change in elevation, along with a variety of soil types, supports impressive ecological diversity, including old-growth redwoods, ancient oak woodlands, endemic stands of Santa Lucia firs, and an isolated grove of sugar pines.

Despite the rugged terrain, Cone Peak and its flanks are accessible via many trails and roads. When it opens in spring, Cone Peak Road (aka Central Coast Ridge Road) enables hikers to reach the summit in less than two hours. Four trailheads start along this road: the Cone Peak Summit Trail, Vicente Flat Trail, Coast Ridge Trail, and San Antonio Trail. A network of trails also wind through Limekiln and Hare Canyons, while other trails lead to upper San Antonio Creek and Devils Canyon.

> **DIRECTIONS:** The first four trail descriptions in this chapter start along Cone Peak Road (driving directions follow). Directions for TRIP 66 Highway 1 to Vicente Flat are listed in that route's summary information.
>
> From the north, drive 54 miles south of Carmel on Highway 1 to the Nacimiento-Fergusson Road junction, on the east side of the highway. From the south, drive 44 miles north of Cambria and 36 miles north of San Simeon on Highway 1 to the junction. Kirk Creek Campground is on the west side of the highway, 0.1 mile north of the junction.
>
> Head east on Nacimiento-Fergusson Road and climb 7.3 very windy miles to the signed junction with Central Coast Ridge Road (better known as Cone Peak Road). Turn left and drive north on Cone Peak Road.

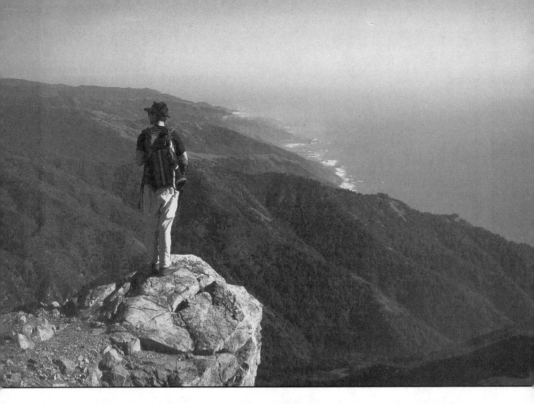

Peace and solitude atop Cone Peak, the most extreme coastal slope in the lower 48

If you're driving north or south on Highway 101, take the Jolon Road exit, 10 miles south of Greenfield and a mile north of the Salinas River crossing. Take Jolon Road (County Road G14) 17.8 miles south to the Mission Road junction. Turn onto Mission Road and drive 0.2 mile to the Hunter Liggett Military Reservation gate (expect to show your driver's license and vehicle registration to enter). In 2.9 miles turn left onto paved Nacimiento-Fergusson Road, which winds 17.9 miles to the signed junction with Central Coast Ridge Road (Cone Peak Road), 300 yards past the USFS Nacimiento Station. Turn right and drive north on Cone Peak Road.

As you drive north on 6.6-mile Cone Peak Road, a saddle at Mile 3.7 marks the Vicente Flat Trailhead, while the San Antonio Trailhead is at Mile 3.9, and the Cone Peak Trailhead at Mile 5.2.

Cone Peak Road is closed from roughly November through May (specific dates vary depending on weather and road conditions). Contact Los Padres National Forest Headquarters or Big Sur Station for details (see below).

VISITOR CENTER: Pacific Valley Station: (805) 927-4211. Open daily 8 a.m.– 5 p.m. The station is on the east side of Highway 1, 3 miles north of the Sand Dollar Beach Day-Use Area, 60 miles south of Carmel, and 30 miles north of Hearst San Simeon State Historical Monument (Hearst Castle).

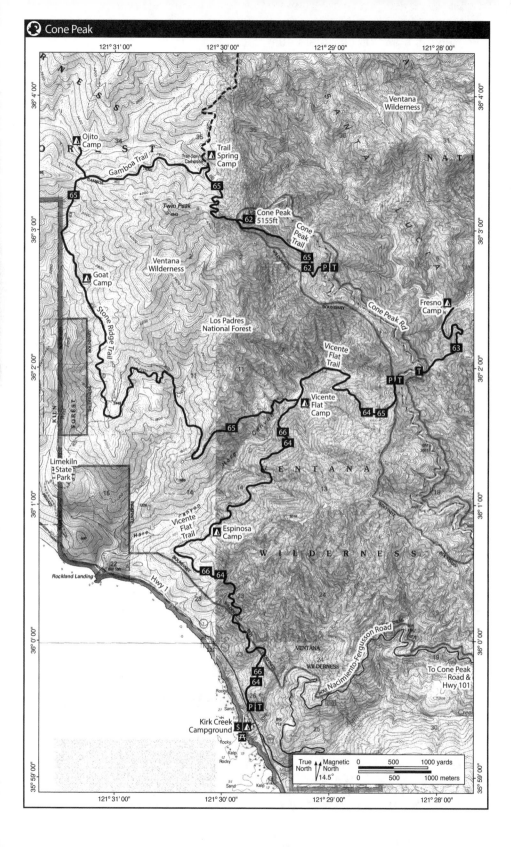

NEAREST CAMPGROUND: Kirk Creek Campground (34 sites, $22/night; reservations recommended) is on the west side of Highway 1, 0.1 mile north of the Nacimiento-Fergusson Road junction. Kirk Creek campsites are available on a first-come, first-serve basis or by reservation. You can make reservations online at recreation.gov or by calling (877) 444-6777. This campground offers magnificent views of the Big Sur coast and a short trail to the beach.

INFORMATION: Fire permits required for all stoves. Dogs permitted and allowed off leash, except in designated campgrounds, where a 6-foot or shorter leash is required. No horses or bikes allowed on trails.

WEBSITE: www.fs.usda.gov/lpnf

PHONE: Los Padres National Forest Headquarters: (805) 968-6640; Big Sur Station: (831) 667-2315

Trip 62

CONE PEAK TRAIL

LENGTH AND TYPE: 6.4-mile out-and-back

RATING: Moderate

TRAIL CONDITION: Clear

HIGHLIGHTS: The fast track to epic views from 5155-foot Cone Peak

TO REACH THE TRAILHEAD: The signed trailhead is on the west side of Cone Peak Road at Mile 5.2 beside a small turnout for up to four cars. There are no facilities or water at the trailhead.

TRIP SUMMARY: This is the shortest trail to one of the highest peaks in the Santa Lucia Range. Trails to 5862-foot Junipero Serra, 4853-foot Ventana Double Cone, and 4417-foot Mt. Carmel require significantly more elevation gain and mileage to summit. If you're bound for this summit

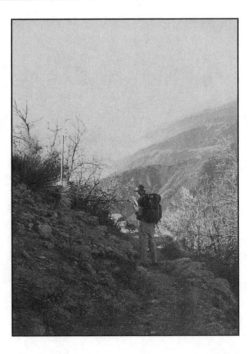

Fire-adapted species such as chamise and manzanita inhabit the flanks of Cone Peak and encroach on the trail as they vigorously grow back following a fire.

when Cone Peak Road is closed (November through May), tack on the additional 5.2 miles each way between the trailhead and junction with Nacimiento-Fergusson Road.

Lording over the southern Ventana Wilderness, Cone Peak offers boundless views along the rugged flanks of the Santa Lucias to the rocky Pacific. The hike is best enjoyed in spring and fall, when fog banks roll well offshore. In winter, snow may fall on the summit, and temperatures can drop below freezing. Bring plenty of water and extra clothing along this exposed trail, and be prepared for rapidly changing conditions.

THE HIGH ROAD ■

In 1542, Juan Cabrillo sailed past the forbidding Santa Lucia Range and wrote, "There are mountains which seem to reach the heavens, and the sea beats on them." Spanning 200,000 acres of raw wilderness, these granite and marble peaks rise more than 5000 feet above the Salinas Valley to the east and plunge west to the rugged Pacific shoreline.

If you're looking for an easy hike or drive into these mountains, think again. Few roads cross the wilderness, making it one of the largest roadless coastal tracts in the Lower 48. Fortunately, if you're reluctant to brave overgrown trails with loose tread and steep grades, there is Nacimiento–Fergusson Road, which connects the "Salad Bowl" to the surf in little more than an hour's drive.

From the east, the road crosses the oak-fringed San Antonio Valley and Hunter Liggett Military Reservation before climbing into the Santa Lucias. Three miles past the divide, you'll reach the US Forest Service's Nacimiento Station, the only structure along the route. A quarter mile farther, the road passes Old Coast Road to the south and Cone Peak Road to the north, which access most trailheads in this chapter. Where the road plummets to the Pacific, fog often engulfs the river canyons, replenishing redwoods that line these deep gullies.

■ ■

Trip Description

From the signed trailhead on the west side of **Cone Peak Road** (4000'), you'll climb past dense thickets of manzanita, wartleaf, and tree poppies, which bloom brilliant yellow by late spring. These fire-adapted species are thriving in the wake of the 1999 Kirk Complex Fires, California's 10th largest recorded wildfire, which scorched more than 90,000 acres of wilderness.

The trail climbs to a nearby saddle for your first stunning overlook of the southern **Santa Lucia Range.** Approaching a ridge, you'll turn north to a second saddle (0.5 mile,

4030'). As the trail steepens, the views encourage you onward. Watch your footing as you pass two rubble-lined gullies that continually erode onto the trail.

Skirting past a downed tree, you may notice the first instance of encroaching poison oak, a rarity at this altitude. Aggressive brush makes steady inroads, but dedicated Ventana hikers and wilderness advocates bring pruning sheers and machetes with them to keep it in check.

PRODIGIOUS CONE PEAK ■ ■ ■ ■ ■ ■ ■ ■ ■ ■ ■ ■ ■ ■ ■

Remarkable in many aspects, Cone Peak has intrigued people for millennia with its varied topography, geology, botany, and cultural history. Its western slopes form the steepest coastal grade in the continental United States. Its bedrock comprises metamorphic rocks of the Salinian block, among the oldest rocks in the Santa Lucia Range. Its spectacular cliffs boast marble from an ancient seafloor that was transported here from Mexico along northwest-trending faults.

In the late 1800s, entrepreneurs found an overwhelmingly rugged peak that sheltered a wealth of natural resources. They would extract lumber, lime, tanbark, and even gold from these slopes and clefts. One company erected four enormous kilns along Limekiln Creek to purify some of the largest limestone deposits along the central California coast. The kilns still stand amid the redwoods at Limekiln State Park, along Cone Peak's western flanks.

Intrigued by the abrupt, distinct climatic zones from sea level to 5155', botanists came in search of new plant species. Habitats vary from cool, damp redwood forests to rolling oak savannas and sun-scorched chaparral, each zone hosting dramatically different flora and fauna. In the 1830s, botanists first described the area's Coulter and sugar pines and Santa Lucia firs. The latter form an extensive stand on the peak's northwest slopes. Isolated from Sierra Nevada stands, secluded stands of sugar pines are limited to the highest peaks of the Santa Lucias.

■ ■

Onward, you'll reach an unmarked junction (1.2 miles, 4380'), where a spur on your left leads 100 feet south along the ridge for encompassing views of the Santa Lucias. To your right, the main route switchbacks down a ridge with scattered views through the remains of charred trees. The trail veers northwest to the **Cone Peak Summit Trail junction** (2 miles, 4830'), atop a narrow ridge. If you're bound for **Trail Spring Camp** and the **Gamboa Trail junction,** refer to TRIP 65 Cone Peak Loop (page 266) and follow that trail description in reverse.

Cone Peak Summit Trail climbs the remaining 325 feet in 0.3 mile. Start out southeast past drought-tolerant scrub oaks, manzanitas, sticky monkeyflowers, and yuccas, which shoot forth stalks of densely clustered, edible white flowers. As the trail switchbacks to cooler north-facing slopes, the vegetation shifts to a cluster of endemic Santa Lucia firs and an isolated stand of sugar pines. The switchbacks soon lead to a dramatic **ledge** (2.2 miles, 4760') above a sheer rock face inhabited by cliff swallows, which dart skyward in search of tasty insects.

From the ledge, a final series of short switchbacks leads to the **summit** (5155'). Climb the lookout tower for more encompassing views. Breathe deeply, relax, and enjoy. Clockwise from the north are the barren peaks of 4853-foot **Ventana Double Cone** and 3709-foot **Pico Blanco.** To the northeast rises 5862-foot **Junipero Serra,** the highest peak in the Santa Lucia Range. The ancient oak savannas of the **San Antonio and Nacimiento Valleys** stretch south and southeast. From the summit, a 3.2-mile ridge drops west to the **Pacific,** comprising the steepest coastal slope in the Lower 48—even steeper than the drop from 14,494-foot Mt. Whitney to Owens Valley. On the clearest days, often after winter storms, you can see the **Sierra Nevada** peaks east across the **Salinas and San Joaquin Valleys.**

Trip 63

FRESNO CAMP

LENGTH AND TYPE: 3-mile out-and-back

RATING: Challenging

TRAIL CONDITION: Difficult to impassable, poison oak

HIGHLIGHTS: Find solitude at this camp amid the vast, remote wilderness.

Fresno Camp is primitive and difficult to access, but the solitude is worth the trek.

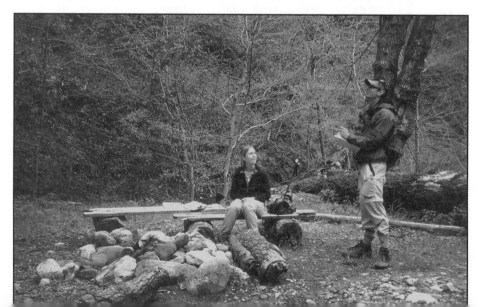

TO REACH THE TRAILHEAD: The trailhead is on the east side of Cone Peak Road at Mile 3.9. Trailhead parking is at Mile 3.7, just above the Vicente Flat Trailhead.

TRIP SUMMARY: You can approach this as either a 3-mile round-trip day hike or an overnight out-and-back trip with a stay at Fresno Camp, one of Ventana's largest camps. Thick brush encroaches on this lightly traveled trail.

Trip Description

From the turnout at Mile 3.7, you'll hike 0.2 mile farther along **Cone Peak Road** to the trailhead at Mile 3.9—factor this out-and-back stretch into your overall mileage. The unmarked trailhead (3290') is at an abandoned roadbed on the right-hand side of the road. Hike 200 yards along the heavily overgrown trail past chamise, broom, and wartleaf to a LOS PADRES NATIONAL FOREST sign at the **Ventana Wilderness** boundary. To the southeast lie the headwaters of the **Nacimiento River**.

After 0.2 mile, you'll reach a saddle that offers sweeping views of the **San Antonio River** canyon. Along a series of switchbacks, the trail makes an easily missed hairpin turn from east to west through head-high brush intermixed with poison oak, then veers east to north through a dry **gully** (0.8 mile, 2710'). From here you'll leave the roadbed and descend the fire-scarred slopes past thriving thickets of tanoak, madrone, and live oak.

The trail soon arrives at the usually reliable headwaters of the **San Antonio River** (1.3 miles, 2590'). You'll briefly parallel the drainage past a large fallen oak, then switchback southwest to the lush canyon floor at **Fresno Camp** (1.5 miles, 2320'). The first site sits atop a boulder-strewn flat just past the confluence of the river and the small creek your route paralleled. There's room for up to five tents in the shade of large maples and sycamores. The second site lies 120 yards upstream atop two large shady terraces.

Despite its proximity to Cone Peak Road, Fresno Camp remains one of Ventana's least-visited camps, likely due to the overgrown trail and unmarked trailhead. Judging from animal prints found along the flood plain, bears, bobcats, and cougars visit camp more often than humans. Be aware that severe winter storms may flood the camp.

Trip 64

VICENTE FLAT TRAIL

LENGTH AND TYPE: 4.8-mile out-and-back or 7.7-mile point-to-point

RATING: Moderate

TRAIL CONDITION: Clear to passable, poison oak

HIGHLIGHTS: Follow a narrow band of old-growth redwoods along sheer Hare Canyon.

TO REACH THE TRAILHEAD: The marked trailhead is on the west side of Cone Peak Road at mile 3.7 near a small turnout for up to five cars. There are no facilities or water at the trailhead.

TRIP SUMMARY: The Vicente Flat Trail descends 7.7 miles from Cone Peak Road to Highway 1. You can approach the trail as either an out-and-back or point-to-point hike. If you can arrange a shuttle vehicle, start from Cone Peak Road. This downhill route offers tremendous views of the coast, the sheer canyon, redwoods, and rolling golden savannas. The 4.8-mile out-and-back to Vicente Flat Camp is an excellent day hike or weekend trip.

Although you can hike the trail year-round, it can get quite cool and damp in the shady canyon in winter. Spring brings colorful wildflowers and new growth to the open slopes. Summer fog often obscures coastal views, while moderate fall temperatures keep fog banks well offshore.

Trip Description

From a saddle (3190') on the west side of **Cone Peak Road,** the **Vicente Flat Trail** climbs southwest toward a nearby ridge. From the ridge, you'll descend to another saddle and begin a series of short switchbacks that overlook **Hare Canyon**'s sheer north wall, composed of banded gneiss and other Salinian metamorphic rocks. Barely 3 miles long, the gorge rises from sea level to more than 3000 feet, making it one of the world's deepest canyons.

The trail descends past healthy, fire-regenerated thickets of yerba santa, chamise, and scrub oak to a small **ridge** (0.7 mile, 2500'). From here a more moderate gradient descends pine-clad slopes past the charred remains of Coulter pines that still bare their enormous cones. Onward, you'll pass large redwoods that succumbed to the 1999 Kirk Complex Fires. Some of these fire-scorched giants along upper **Hare Creek** have sprouted vibrant new shoots from their trunks, calling to mind bristled pipe cleaners.

Farther along the shady trail, gurgling water heralds your arrival on the banks of Hare Creek (1.1 miles, 2500'). You'll follow the intermittent creek for a quarter mile beneath more fire-ravaged redwoods before crossing it and a side gully. In another quarter mile, the steep trail recrosses the creek. Over the next 0.3 mile, you'll head southwest into the lush canyon, crossing the creek seven more times.

Past the fifth crossing, you'll reach **Vicente Flat Camp** (2.2 miles, 1700'). The first site is perched amid redwoods atop a flat creekside bench, with room for up to three tents. The second, more spacious site sits along the north bank and includes a table and fire ring. The third and fourth sites lie just downstream past old-growth redwoods at the extreme southern limit of their range.

Onward, the trail leads to **Vicente Flat** itself, a small meadow that hosts **two small sites** (2.4 miles, 1650'). Along the edge of the flat, two parallel paths skirt west. The upper

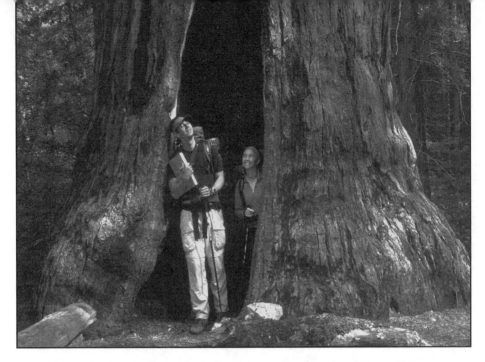

Ancient fire scars from large cavities inside old-growth redwoods at Vicente Flat.

trail, the main Vicente Flat Trail, climbs 0.1 mile through poison oak thickets to the **Stone Ridge Trail**. Avoid the poison oak in favor of the lower spur, which detours 70 feet to two creekside sites and rejoins the main trail only yards from the **Stone Ridge Trail junction** (2.5 miles, 1620').

If you're continuing on the scenic westbound Stone Ridge Trail, refer to TRIP 65 Cone Peak Loop. If you're bound for the coast, refer to TRIP 66 Highway 1 to Vicente Flat (page 271) and follow that trail description in reverse.

Trip 65

CONE PEAK LOOP

LENGTH AND TYPE: 15-mile out-and-back, loop, or point-to-point

RATING: Challenging

TRAIL CONDITION: Passable, poison oak

HIGHLIGHTS: Climb through coastal oak woodlands, pastoral hillsides, and thriving chaparral for tremendous views from 5155-foot Cone Peak.

TO REACH THE TRAILHEAD: The marked trailhead is on the west side of Cone Peak Road at Mile 3.7 near a small turnout for up to five cars. There are no facilities or water at the trailhead.

TRIP SUMMARY: You can approach this 15-mile loop as either an extremely strenuous day hike or a more enjoyable yet still strenuous backpacking trip, staying at one or more of the four camps along the route. Most people hike the 2.2 miles to Vicente Flat Camp, spend the night, and get a fresh start the following day. The onward route is slow going, as sections of the Stone Ridge Trail are overgrown with brush with faint, steep tread. If you do opt for a multiday trek, stay a second or third night at Goat, Ojito, or Trail Spring Camps. Regardless of your route, don't miss the 0.3-mile spur to the summit.

Instead of hiking the entire loop, consider day hiking the scenic lower section of Stone Ridge Trail. This lightly used trail offers tremendous views of surrounding peaks in the Limekiln drainage. If you're willing to descend from the Hare/Limekiln Creek divide, the trail plunges into cool redwood- and fern-lined canyons amid Limekiln's remote headwaters.

This route is best enjoyed in spring, when grassy slopes are cloaked with colorful lupines, blue-eyed grass, and California poppies. You'll climb from 1500 feet to 5155 feet through lush redwood canyons, yucca-dotted slopes, open grasslands, arid chaparral, and oak woodlands. Use caution on steep, slippery trails along the oak-clad canyon walls, and watch for hitchhiking ticks amid the encroaching brush. In summer, temperatures can be brutal and fog usually obscures coastal views, while fall brings moderate temperatures and diminished fly, tick, and mosquito populations.

CLEARING THE TRAILS ■ ■ ■ ■ ■ ■ ■ ■ ■ ■ ■ ■ ■ ■ ■ ■ ■ ■

Over the past few decades, six major fires have swept through Los Padres National Forest: the 1977 Marble-Cone Fire, the 1985 Rat Creek Fire, the 1992 Cienega Fire, the 1993 Big Sur Gorge Fire, the 1999 Kirk Complex Fires, and the 2008 Basin Complex Fire. The latter scarred most of the Ventana Wilderness, burning 162,818 acres. In this era of fire suppression, enormous amounts of dead and downed trees build up, creating catastrophic damage when fires do sweep through.

Following a wildfire, charred trees and debris obscure trails and lay waste to camps. Free from the limiting shade of a forest canopy, the understory of shrubs such as ceanothus, poison oak, chamise, and manzanita aggressively sprouts new shoots, obscuring tread and sometimes choking the path altogether. Winter storms bring an onslaught of mudslides and washouts, which further erode trails, creating dangerous hiking conditions.

Fortunately, dedicated Ventana hikers and wilderness enthusiasts volunteer their time and efforts to help the US Forest Service maintain these scenic trails. If you'd like to get involved, visit the Ventana Wilderness Alliance at ventanawild.org or the Sierra Club's Ventana chapter at ventana.sierraclub.org.

■ ■

Trip Description

See TRIP 64 Vicente Flat Trail (page 264) for the first 2.4 miles of this route to **Vicente Flat** (1650').

Along the edge of the flat, two parallel paths skirt west. The upper trail, the main **Vicente Flat Trail,** climbs 0.1 mile through poison oak thickets to the **Stone Ridge Trail**. Avoid the poison oak in favor of the lower spur, which detours 70 feet to two creekside sites and rejoins the main trail only yards from the **Stone Ridge Trail junction** (2.5 miles, 1620'). If you're bound for the coast on the Vicente Flat Trail, refer to TRIP 66 Highway 1 to Vicente Flat (page 271) and follow that trail description in reverse.

From the signed junction, the Stone Ridge Trail climbs northwest through dense redwoods and tanoaks into sun-dappled oak woodlands. Beyond a minor gully lined with poison oak, you'll climb to a grassy knoll that offers views up sheer-sided **Hare Canyon** toward **Cone Peak**. The trail continues past oak savannas (2.8 miles, 1830') that harbor several picnic spots, ideal for day hikers from Vicente Flat. In spring this open terrain is carpeted in vibrant wildflowers.

As you skirt a ridge composed largely of marble, the narrow trail opens on spectacular coastal views. Watch your footing along a minor washout just before you reach the saddle that divides Hare Canyon and **Limekiln Canyon** (3.8 miles, 2030'). From the saddle, a 0.2-mile spur leads west atop a ridge for views thousands of feet down-canyon to the foamy surf.

The main trail descends from the saddle along the steep north-facing slopes of the Limekiln Creek drainage. Be on your guard for poison oak along this lightly used stretch. Increasingly steeper switchbacks lead past sprawling oaks to deep redwood-lined gullies. You'll have to clamber over and around large fallen oaks and redwoods in some sections, especially difficult if you're carrying a heavy pack. The trail leads north to the **creek** (4.6 miles, 1530'), where windstorms have toppled several large redwoods.

Across the reliable headwaters, the trail leads 10 yards downstream, climbs the canyon's steep west wall, switchbacks and leads north, skirting several large fallen tanoaks. Expect to find lots of debris from dead or dying oaks afflicted by sudden oak death (see sidebar, page 165). The trail continues across a minor ridge to a shallow canyon.

Following a seasonal stream west up the canyon, you'll climb first past shady redwoods then beneath live oaks and bays to two unofficial campsites. Perched beside the stream, each offers room for up to two tents. Beyond the second site, a curious trashcan sits alongside the trail. Regular garbage pickup service is not offered in the backcountry, so please pack out all your trash.

The trail beyond climbs southwest to an obvious oak-clad **saddle** (5.4 miles, 2030'), then northwest along a nearly level ridge. A hundred feet past a minor gully lined with

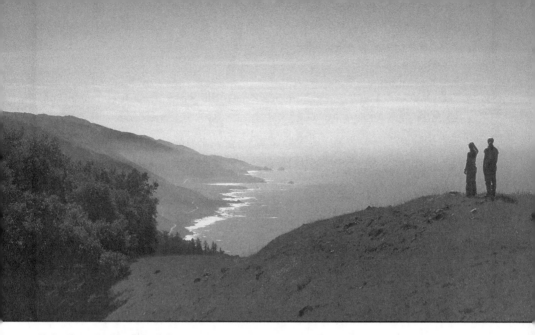

Enjoy breathtaking views from pastoral coastal oak woodlands.

madrones, oaks, and bays, the trail emerges in the open (5.9 miles, 2160'). For the next half mile, you'll enjoy sweeping views of the coast, Cone Peak, and sheer Hare and Lime-kiln Canyons. In spring, the otherwise golden hillsides are blanketed in lupines, poppies, buttercups, blue-eyed grass, mariposa lilies, shooting stars, and blue dicks. Watch the skies for common raptors, as well as the rare and endangered California condor, which boasts a massive 9-foot wingspan.

Onward, the trail follows a gentle contour and climbs a prominent ridge to a **minor gap** (6.4 miles, 2260') for filtered views through live oaks. Continue past a cluster of ponderosa pines to the headwaters of **West Fork Limekiln Creek.** Winding 0.8 mile through several shady gullies, the trail leads to a prominent **gully** (7.2 miles, 2170') of exposed, weathered marble. In all but the heaviest downpour, it's an easy hop across.

You'll soon enter the canyon's largest eastside gully along a boulder-strewn wash beneath a dense redwood canopy. The trail continues north across two more gullies, the second hosting a reliable creek. After veering 100 yards west to a grassy slope, you'll turn northwest to the **Goat Camp junction** (8.4 miles, 2500').

A short spur trail descends southwest to **Goat Camp,** nestled in the shade of oaks and sugar pines. Offering wonderful ocean views, this remote camp can accommodate up to four tents. During wet season, the nearest water source lies only a minute farther along the Stone Ridge Trail. In dry months, you'll need to return 0.6 mile to the large gully.

Fifty yards from the Goat Camp junction, the trail contours past Limekiln's north-ern headwaters, which in wet season supports a small creek that sustains a few staunch redwoods. Onward 0.1 mile, the trail begins a steep climb past the charred remains of a pre-1999 forest, now overgrown with ceanothus, broom, and yerba santa. Watch your footing on the loose tread, and be alert for hitchhiking ticks in spring. Switchbacks climb 500 feet to an obvious saddle and the three-way junction with the **Gamboa** and **Ojito Camp Trails** (9.3 miles, 3450').

SIDE TRIP ■

From the junction, the unmarked **Ojito Camp Trail** heads north, dropping 600 feet in the next 0.6 mile to Devils Canyon. On my last trip, encroaching brush and large fallen snags obstructed the route, though it was flagged and remained passable.

You'll descend a gentle grade to a nearby saddle, then plunge steeply to the south bank of **South Fork Devils Creek.** A faint overgrown trail leads 200 yards downstream along the swift creek to **Ojito Camp,** which has room for up to two tents. Those willing to venture cross-country will find myriad beautiful pools and cascades.

■ ■

Back at the saddle, the Gamboa Trail begins just left of a large pine snag, 50 feet before you reach a large fallen oak across the trail. The trail follows an ancient American Indian trading route past Coulter pines and Douglas and Santa Lucia firs. Filtered views overlook the South Fork's remote swimming holes and glistening **Pacific** beyond. Trail conditions along this stretch are dramatically better than on the Stone Ridge Trail. The route is well defined with no encroaching brush. Descend the gentle grade 1.6 miles to **Trail Spring Camp** and the **Coast Ridge Trail junction** (10.9 miles, 3800').

Trail Spring Camp offers one small site on sloping ground beside the unreliable headwaters of South Fork Devils Creek. To find water in dry months, anticipate a steep 300-foot descent 0.3 mile along the boulder wash. The **Coast Ridge Trail** continues 1.5 miles across the boulder-strewn gully to the end of **Cone Peak Road.** Twenty feet above camp is the signed **Cone Peak Trail junction** (10.9 miles, 3800').

Short switchbacks climb quickly to a broad, boulder-lined creek bed, only wet during heavy rains. Here enormous sugar pines tower above an open canopy of scorched manzanitas, tanoaks, scrub oaks, and ceanothus. As you climb longer switchbacks toward the isolated summit, you'll pass rare, endemic Santa Lucia firs, Santa Lucia bedstraw, and Santa Lucia lupines.

The trail reaches a narrow ridge between Devils and Limekiln Canyons that leads west to Cone Peak's neighbor, 4843-foot **Twin Peak**. Follow this ridge east to the **Cone Peak Summit Trail junction** (12.1 miles, 4830'). The 0.3-mile spur climbs short, steep switchbacks to the 5155-foot summit (see TRIP 62 Cone Peak Trail, page 260, for details).

From here it's 2 miles east along the Cone Peak Trail to Cone Peak Road. Again, refer to TRIP 62 Cone Peak Trail and follow that trail description in reverse. At Cone Peak Road, turn right and descend 530 feet in 1.5 miles to reach the **Vicente Flat Trailhead** at Mile 3.7. For directions to **Vicente Flat Camp**, see TRIP 64 Vicente Flat Trail (page 264).

Trip 66

HIGHWAY 1 TO VICENTE FLAT

LENGTH AND TYPE: 5.3-mile out-and-back or 7.7-mile point-to-point

RATING: Strenuous

TRAIL CONDITION: Clear, poison oak

HIGHLIGHTS: Climb from golden coastal bluffs to Vicente Flat Camp, nestled beneath ancient redwoods along Hare Creek.

TO REACH THE TRAILHEAD: The trailhead is on the east side of Highway 1, across the street from Kirk Creek Campground, 36 miles north of Hearst Castle, 41 miles north of Cambria, 38 miles south of Pfeiffer Big Sur State Park, and 54 miles south of Carmel. There are no facilities or water at the trailhead. If you're bound for Cone Peak Road and plan to use a shuttle vehicle, be aware that the road is closed during the wet season (November through April). See TRIP 64 Vicente Flat Trail (page 264) for more information.

TRIP SUMMARY: You can approach this primarily uphill route as either a scenic day hike or an out-and-back overnight. Or you can use Vicente Flat as a base camp for grander tours of the wilderness via the Stone Ridge, Gamboa, and Cone Peak Trails. If you can arrange a shuttle vehicle, consider the route from Cone Peak Road to Highway 1, which is virtually all downhill (see TRIP 64 Vicente Flat Trail).

From Highway 1, this route ascends nearly 2000 feet above the wave-swept coast. Bare golden terraces allow dramatic coastal and canyon vistas as the trail climbs pastoral hilltops into redwood-lined Hare Creek. Vicente Flat offers sites amid old-growth trees and atop a sun-drenched meadow.

Spring welcomes a profusion of wildflowers to the otherwise golden slopes. Watch for the rare and fragile orchid-like chocolate lily, which blooms along the lower portion of the trail. In wet months Hare Creek abounds with life. American dippers dive for food or bob along the banks, while California newts slither slowly to the water. Red, orange, yellow, and purple fungi emerge from the damp forest floor, and lush ferns, mosses, and horsetails thrive in the verdant canyon.

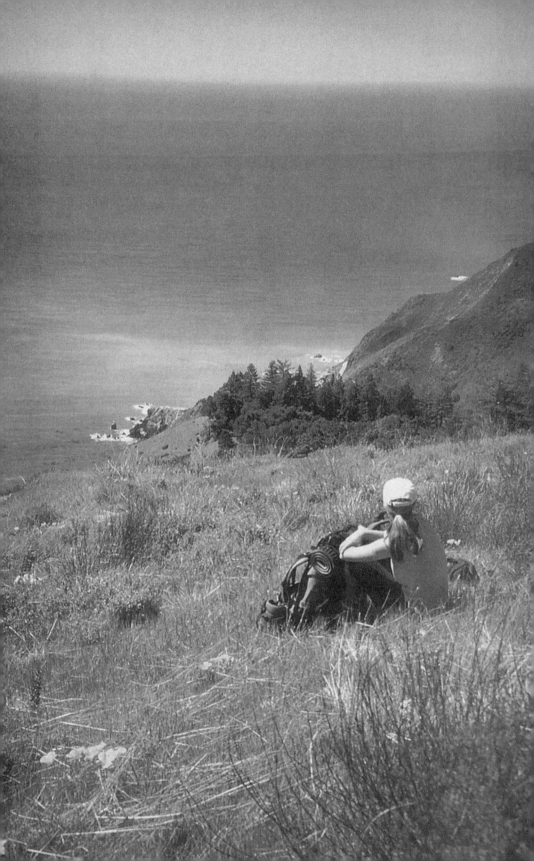

Trip Description

From its marked trailhead along **Highway 1** (190'), the **Vicente Flat Trail** quickly climbs a series of switchbacks north past coastal scrub, vibrant in spring with flowering lupines, poppies, sticky monkeyflowers, and sagebrush. In 0.3 mile you'll cross a minor gully, head toward a minor saddle, then turn north across rolling grasslands and sun-drenched coastal chaparral. Crossing a gully choked with invasive blackberry and broom species, you'll hear trickling from a nearby **spring** (0.9 mile, 700').

The grade steepens as the trail passes scattered yuccas, attesting to the aridity of these exposed slopes and switchbacks. You'll soon reach a **ridge** (1.4 miles, 1000') that offers spectacular views of the vast convergence of land and sea. This is a favorite day-hiking destination.

Onward, the trail enters the **Ventana Wilderness** and after 0.3 mile reaches shade beneath a canopy of oaks, madrones, and bays. Follow the ridgeline through four gullies past a dense band of redwoods. After a steep climb to a prominent ridge (2.9 miles, 1610'), pause to rest and enjoy the views. To the east is 5155-foot **Cone Peak** and its neighbor, double-notched **Twin Peak,** which loom over **Hare and Limekiln Creeks. Hare Canyon** is one of the world's deepest gorges, while **Limekiln Canyon** boasts the steepest coastal slope in the Lower 48 on its climb to Cone Peak.

The trail descends from the ridge, veering northeast through varied microclimates that support a wide range of drought-tolerant and moisture-loving plants. Yuccas dot the open, arid slopes, while redwoods cluster in the gullies. One hundred yards past a major gully along an unreliable creek, marked by a large fallen redwood, you'll reach a spur to **Espinosa Camp.**

The spur leads 100 feet to camp (3.4 miles, 1660'), which sits atop a minor ridge in the shade of live oaks, bays, redwoods, and rare, endemic Santa Lucia firs. Two small flats can accommodate up to four tents. Rock outcrops offer unobstructed views toward the coast. This is an excellent picnic spot, though the gully nearest camp is usually dry. Just 1.8 miles farther along the main trail, the roomier **Vicente Flat Camp** is adjacent to reliable Hare Creek.

Beyond the spur, you'll round a prominent ridge and skirt a large tanoak afflicted by sudden oak death, evidenced by its large cankerous wounds (see sidebar, page 165). On a contour 0.2 mile past camp, the trail reaches the first reliable water source, a creeklet that cascades past redwoods and lush ferns. Across the creeklet and through another gully, you'll emerge on open grassy slopes with ocean views. Here the trail veers east, tops out at 1860 feet, and begins a gentle descent to Vicente Flat.

Enjoy unsurpassed views during spring and fall, when typical summer fog and winter storm fronts have passed.

Soon you'll cross three typically dry rubble-strewn **gullies** (4.1 miles, 1800'), whose confluence lies 100 feet downslope. In winter, water plunges from adjacent marble faces, misting the surrounding greenery. Beyond the next dry redwood gully, the trail contours north and enters dense forest a quarter mile from Hare Creek. Several notably large redwoods mark your arrival at Vicente Flat.

A few feet past the creek, a spur cuts upstream to Vicente Flat Camp. Poison oak is less of a concern along this well-used stretch. The main trail continues a few yards to the **Stone Ridge Trail junction** (5.2 miles, 1620') and 0.1 mile beyond to the camp's lower reaches. See TRIP 64 Vicente Flat Trail (page 264) for a description of camp.

Silver Peak Wilderness

■　■　■　■　■　■　■　■　■　■　■　■　■

IN 1992, the Los Padres Condor Range & River Protection Act established the Silver Peak Wilderness. It originally protected 14,500 acres of this sheer region, where ridges plunge into deep V-shaped canyons and streams cascade past smooth boulders and deep pools on their way to the Pacific. An additional 17,055 acres are being added to these pristine lands within the Willow Creek and San Carpoforo drainages.

The wilderness encompasses a biologically rich landscape characterized by golden oak savannas, sun-drenched chaparral slopes, and lush riparian canyons. Northern and southern biogeographical regions converge here in a sharp dichotomy of vegetation. Redwoods push their southern limits amid verdant canyons carpeted in ferns and mosses. Watch for slithering salamanders and chatty winter wrens. Immediately adjacent, yet more typical of areas farther south, semiarid grasslands host yuccas, rufous-crowned sparrows, and scurrying alligator lizards. The wilderness also shelters such threatened and endangered species as the southern steelhead and the California condor.

Bounded on the west by the Pacific, the Silver Peak Wilderness rises thousands of feet to the crest of the Santa Lucia Range. Here, hikers can lose themselves amid river canyons, wildflower-strewn meadows, and high peaks that overlook the rugged coast.

DIRECTIONS: From San Simeon, head north on Highway 1, 1.5 miles past the Monterey County line. The Salmon Creek Trailhead is on the east side of the highway, at the heart of the Silver Peak Wilderness.

VISITOR CENTER: Pacific Valley Station: (805) 927-4211. The station is on the east side of Highway 1, a mile north of the Sand Dollar Beach Day-Use Area, 30 miles north of Hearst Castle, and 60 miles south of Carmel. Open daily 8 a.m.–5 p.m.

NEAREST CAMPGROUND: Plaskett Creek Campground (41 sites, $22/night; reservations recommended spring–fall and on holidays) is on the east side of Highway 1, 0.1 mile south of the entrance to the Sand Dollar Beach Day-Use Area, 40 miles south of Pfeiffer Big Sur State Park, and 35 miles north of San Simeon State

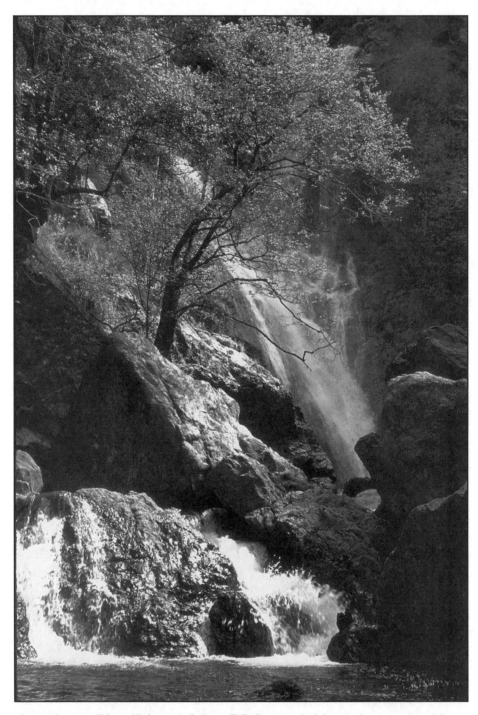

Just a short stroll from Highway 1, Salmon Falls is a wonderful stop along your coastal road trip.

Park. There's a maximum of eight people per site. Each site includes a picnic table, fire ring, and pedestal grill. Drinking water is available. For more information call Reserve America at (800) 444-7275 or visit ReserveAmerica.com.

INFORMATION: Fire permits required for all stoves. Dogs permitted and allowed off leash, except in designated campgrounds, where a 6-foot or shorter leash is required. Horses and livestock are allowed on the trail, but bikes are prohibited.

WEBSITE: www.fs.usda.gov/lpnf

PHONE: USFS Monterey District Headquarters: (831) 385-5434; USFS Pacific Valley Station: (805) 927-4211

Trip 67

PREWITT LOOP TRAIL

LENGTH AND TYPE: 12.8-mile out-and-back or loop

RATING: Strenuous

TRAIL CONDITION: Clear to difficult, poison oak

HIGHLIGHTS: Dramatic coastal views of sandy coves and jagged promontories from a remote canyon in the heart of Pacific Valley

TO REACH THE TRAILHEAD: The northern trailhead is on the east side of Highway 1, 30 miles south of Big Sur Station and 57 miles south of Carmel. The southern trailhead is on the east side of Highway 1, 0.8 mile north of the Pacific Valley Station, 2 miles north of Plaskett Creek Campground, and 17 miles north of Ragged Point. The following route description begins from the northern trailhead.

Parking for the northern trailhead is on the east side of Highway 1, at a turnout adjacent to the trailhead. There are no facilities or water at the trailhead. Parking for the southern trailhead is at the Pacific Valley Station. Parking is free at both trailheads.

TRIP SUMMARY: This hike leads past a diverse array of plant communities, from dense thickets of coastal scrub to cool redwood groves, oak and pine woodlands, and grassy savannas. The trail is best enjoyed in spring, when fields of delicate wildflowers boast profuse colors and aromas. For the best views, visit between October and April, when fog banks roll well offshore. On my last trip, the trail past Stag Camp was suffering from loose tread and active slides. Use caution.

Trip Description

From the turnout on **Highway 1,** stroll 50 feet down a single-lane dirt road to the signed **Prewitt Loop Trailhead.** According to the sign, the first backcountry camp, Stag Camp, is 4

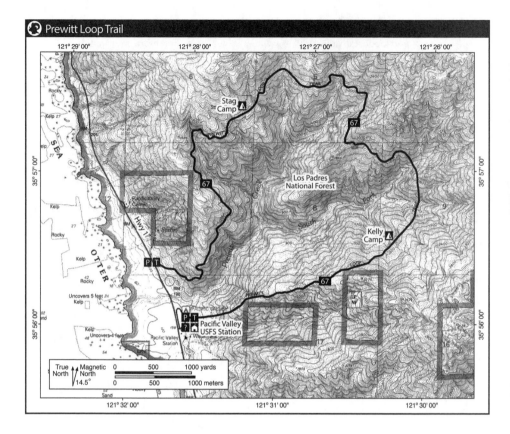

miles from the junction (actual mileage 4.1 miles) and the entire loop trail is 12 miles (actual mileage 12.8 miles).

From the junction, turn right onto the **Prewitt Loop Trail** and head southeast past ocean views through fragrant thickets of sagebrush, coyote brush, coffeeberry, and poison oak. In 0.1 mile you'll switchback north and climb past two small seeps amid chain ferns, horsetails, and a stand of willows. At the next switchback, the trail climbs southeast past two dry **gullies** (0.4 mile, 440').

Continue on a moderate grade past a dilapidated wooden gate marking the barbwire fence line of private property. Pause for views along the open coastal slope where **Prewitt Creek** meets the **Pacific** just north of **Sand Dollar Beach**. A few minutes past the gate, you'll reach a four-way junction (0.7 mile, 630') with an unmarked private trail that leads down to the small housing development in **Pacific Valley**.

Fifty yards farther southeast, the trail crosses an abandoned, overgrown roadbed and bends east for your first glimpse of the broad Prewitt Creek watershed. Narrow belts of redwoods stretch up canyon like veins, following the moisture-bearing gullies and ravines, while

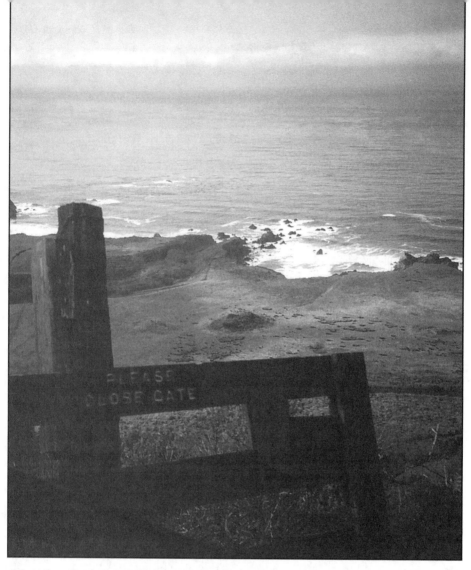

A broad marine terrace, which gave Pacific Valley its name, rises above the rocky shoreline and below the Prewitt Loop Trail.

more drought-tolerant oaks and pines stud the upper watershed. The trail contours past exposed south-facing slopes of arid chaparral and grasses, in dramatic contrast to the cooler, shadier north-facing slopes of mixed evergreens across the canyon.

The grade eases as you contour past three small dry gullies fringed with slender redwoods, live oaks, and bays. Climbing to grassy slopes studded with mature live oaks, the trail reaches the Prewitt Creek headwaters and crosses two small gullies 50 feet apart (2.6 miles, 1420'). Past the second gully, you'll switchback southeast to an easily missed spur **junction** (2.7 miles, 1530'). This spur doglegs left and climbs 150 yards to a dramatic overlook.

Past the spur, the main trail meanders through oak and pine woodlands populated by busy acorn woodpeckers, which store acorns to feed grubs they will later devour. Cross three prominent gullies (dry in all but heavy rain) to a stand of sycamores amid a fourth gully (3.8 miles, 1650'). Easily identified by mottled cream-and-white bark that resembles a jigsaw puzzle, the sycamores offer a place to picnic and enjoy canyon views. If you'd prefer a shadier spot with a picnic table, continue 0.3 mile to Stag Camp.

LUCKY COWS OR SPACE HOGS? ■ ■ ■ ■ ■ ■ ■ ■ ■ ■ ■ ■ ■

Gazing across the coastal terrace and lush grasslands at Pacific Valley, you may well wonder, "How lucky can a cow be?" Local cattle ranchers also feel pretty lucky, since they pay nearly a tenth of the market rate to graze each head of cattle on public vs. private lands. In 2004, the Forest Service charged allotment holders a measly $1.43 per AUM (animal unit month) for running cattle on the public land. Market rates on private land range from $12.50 to $15 per AUM. Cheap rent and a spectacular view—something to moo about.

However, all those happy hooves inflict a toll on the land. Cows graze native flora and fauna, trample delicate riparian zones, gouge and erode unstable slopes, and disperse seeds of invasive nonnative plants. They also disturb complex ecosystems by eating blooms that sustain butterflies, insects, and birds, in turn affecting predators further up the food chain.

Burger, anyone?

■ ■

A minute past the sycamore-lined gully, the trail passes a piped spring where water spills into a manmade trough. This is the most reliable water till you reach the **South Fork** headwaters, 6.8 miles from the trailhead. Many animals use this spring. Look for the tracks and scat of such species as coyotes, bobcats, gray foxes, and the occasional mountain lion.

Continue climbing past grassy slopes that in spring burst with decadent displays of lupines, shooting stars, and California poppies. The trail dips through a minor gully past ancient oaks nearly 4 feet in diameter, then bends south and leads straight to **Stag Camp** (4.1 miles, 1760'). In the shade of sprawling tanoaks and bays, the lone site offers room for up to three small tents and includes a table and fire ring. Although the trail leads through camp, you'll see few hikers along this little-used route.

Past this point, the trail is sketchy and not recommended. In spots, poison oak, rocks, brush, and large debris encroach on or obscure the tread. Although crews recently cleared much of the brush and slide debris from the trail, slopes along the creek's upper headwaters are prone to future slides. In fact, just past camp the trail crosses gullies past two major slides in an area known as **Big Slide** (4.9 miles, 1800').

Hardy hikers will continue along arid south-facing slopes where chaparral species such as coyote brush and chamise thrive. The revitalizing sound of water heralds your arrival at the South Fork (6.8 miles, 1880'). The trail crosses the rocky canyon on a fallen redwood and climbs a **ridge** (7.8 miles, 1950') between two of the headwater drainages. You'll veer north for the next 0.1 mile, switchback east 100 yards, then drop south into **Kelly Camp.**

Beyond the South Fork headwaters, the trail descends the remaining 3.5 miles to its southern trailhead at the **Pacific Valley Station.** If you parked your vehicle at the northern trailhead, you'll need to hike 0.8 mile north along Highway 1 to the turnout.

Trip 68

ALDER CREEK CAMP TO VILLA CREEK CAMP

LENGTH AND TYPE: 4.2-mile out-and-back, 4.7-mile point-to-point (Highway 1), or 8.4-mile point-to-point (Salmon Creek Station)

RATING: Strenuous

TRAIL CONDITION: Passable, poison oak

HIGHLIGHTS: Pause for unobstructed coastal views as you follow glassy creeks through peaceful groves of alders and redwoods.

TO REACH THE TRAILHEAD: Willow Creek Road is on the east side of Highway 1, 8 miles south of Nacimiento-Fergusson Road, 62 miles south of Carmel, a mile north of Gorda, and 8.4 miles north of the southern Buckeye Trailhead at the abandoned Salmon Creek Station.

Climb this rugged dirt road about 7 miles to an unmarked four-way junction and stay straight on the right fork, which makes a steep 1.5 mile descent into the Alder Creek drainage. The road ends at Alder Creek Camp, though it may be impassable during heavy winter rains. In summer it's a dry, dusty road. The signed northern Buckeye Trailhead lies on the north bank, 100 feet downstream from the main campsite.

TRIP SUMMARY: This route offers several day-hike or overnight options, including: (1) 4.2 miles round-trip to Villa Creek Camp; (2) 4.7 miles point-to-point from Alder Creek Camp to Highway 1 via the Buckeye and Cruikshank Trails; and (3) 8.4 miles point-to-point to Salmon Creek Station via the Buckeye Trail. If you can arrange a shuttle vehicle, consider the point-to-point treks, which offer unobstructed coastal views.

This hike is best enjoyed in spring and fall, when fog banks roll well offshore. Colorful spring wildflowers paint hillside oak savannas, while in fall, creekside alders and maples flash vibrant yellows, oranges, and reds. Seriously consider wearing pants on this hike to protect against ubiquitous poison oak and ticks.

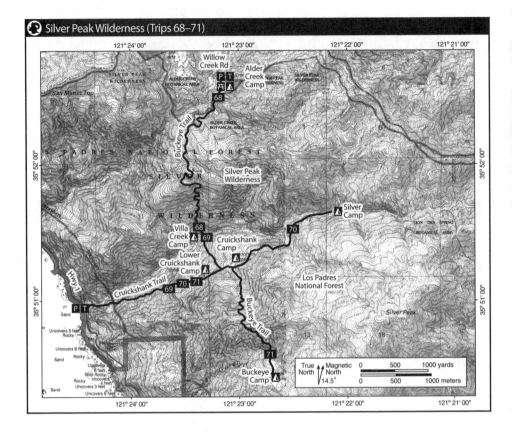

Trip Description

From its northern trailhead at **Alder Creek Camp** (2240'), the **Buckeye Trail** enters the creek's lush corridor, where poison oak is a common trailside companion. You'll quickly cross **Alder Creek** and begin climbing the canyon walls southwest through dense oak woodlands and encroaching ceanothus thickets.

Sections of this trail may be overgrown. (For the latest trail conditions, contact the Pacific Valley Station, (805) 927-4211, or the Ventana Wilderness Alliance, (831) 423-3191.)

After half a mile, the well-graded trail tops a grassy ridge between the **Villa Creek** and Alder Creek drainages. In spring, pause to picnic amid these wildflower-strewn slopes and watch as hawks kite over the tall grass in search of small prey. In 2003, flags marked the faint tread across the open slopes past stands of pines and oaks.

From the ridge, you'll veer right into the Villa Creek drainage, forging briefly through dense thickets of chaparral, primarily ceanothus. The trail abruptly switchbacks right and reenters the Alder Creek drainage, then heads toward a conspicuous serpentine outcrop at the divide.

From the divide, the trail skirts the western edge of open slopes 0.6 mile and drops past a seeping spring that supports thriving willows and exotic pampas grass. Onward, past a cluster of fragrant bays and a dry wash, the trail steepens on its final descent to the banks of Villa Creek. You'll emerge at **Villa Creek Camp** (2.1 miles, 1050), perched atop a small creekside bench.

There's room for up to three small tents in the shade of redwoods beside the year-round creek. You'll also find a table and a fire ring. In summer, the shade offers welcome respite from the sun-drenched upper canyon. During the wet season, colorful fungi sprout from the lush forest floor, though the camp may be damp and cold.

Trip 69

HIGHWAY 1 TO VILLA CREEK CAMP

LENGTH AND TYPE: 5.6-mile out-and-back

RATING: Moderate

TRAIL CONDITION: Clear, poison oak

HIGHLIGHTS: Gorgeous coastal views en route to a redwood-lined camp

TO REACH THE TRAILHEAD: The Cruikshank Trailhead is on the east side of Highway 1, 0.6 mile south of the Villa Creek bridge, 66 miles south of Carmel, and 4.5 miles north of the abandoned Salmon Creek Station. Park at the small turnout on Highway 1 adjacent to the trailhead. There are no facilities or water at the trailhead.

TRIP SUMMARY: From Highway 1, you'll climb the Cruikshank Trail east along Villa Creek's steep south canyon wall, then descend the Buckeye Trail north to cool, redwood-fringed Villa Creek Camp.

Trip Description

From the signed **Cruikshank Trailhead** on **Highway 1,** you'll quickly climb steep switchbacks through dense coastal scrub. Pause often to catch your breath and take in the dramatic coastal views. After a strenuous 600-foot ascent in less than a mile, the grade eases.

Continue along the south wall of deep, V-shaped **Villa Creek** canyon through shallow redwood-lined gullies. You'll cross a small creek fringed with redwood sorrel, starflowers, and ferns, then a minute later pass a few eucalyptus trees, probably planted here by early homesteaders. Two miles from the trailhead, you'll cross logs over a small creek and enter

Lower Cruikshank Camp (see TRIP 70 Cruikshank & Silver Camps, on the following page, for details). Just past camp lies the signed **Buckeye Trail junction** (2.2 miles, 1440').

At the junction, turn left onto the northbound **Buckeye Trail.** Past an open meadow that marks the **Cruikshank homestead,** you'll make a steep 450-foot descent in half a mile to **Villa Creek** (2.7 miles, 1070'), amid a narrow band of redwoods.

At the southern limit of their range, these redwoods are only able to find adequate moisture for survival along such small creeks. Drier conditions prevent the trees from obtaining the colossal size more commonly associated with old-growth stands farther north. Other than a few small patches of redwood sorrel, sword ferns, and seasonal wildflowers, the forest floor here is also comparatively bare.

Crossing to the north bank, you'll briefly follow the year-round creek downstream to a trail junction and seasonal side drainage. From this junction, the left fork descends to **Villa Creek Camp** (2.8 miles, 1050'), which offers a table, a fire ring, and room for up to three small tents.

The Buckeye Trail continues north along the right fork. If you're bound for **Alder Creek Camp,** refer to TRIP 68 Alder Creek Camp to Villa Creek Camp (page 281) and follow that trail description in reverse.

Fresh signs of mountain lion are commonly found along the Cruikshank Trail.

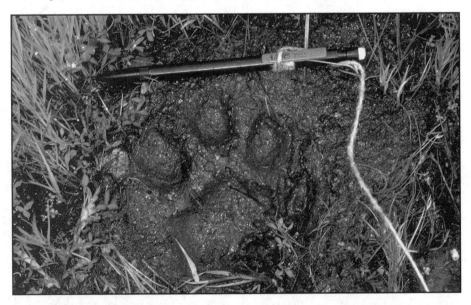

Trip 70

CRUIKSHANK & SILVER CAMPS

LENGTH AND TYPE: 6.2-mile out-and-back

RATING: Moderate to challenging

TRAIL CONDITION: Clear to difficult, poison oak

HIGHLIGHTS: This scenic trail climbs past fragrant coastal scrub and vibrant spring wildflowers to lush redwood forests.

TO REACH THE TRAILHEAD: The Cruikshank Trailhead is on the east side of Highway 1, 0.6 mile south of the Villa Creek bridge, 66 miles south of Carmel, and 4.5 miles north of the abandoned Salmon Creek Station. Park at the small turnout on Highway 1 adjacent to the trailhead. There are no facilities or water at the trailhead.

TRIP SUMMARY: The Cruikshank Trail climbs the Villa Creek drainage 6.5 miles to its headwaters below Coast Ridge Road. Due to poor trail conditions, including encroaching poison oak and fallen trees, it's best to avoid the trail beyond Silver Camp.

Depending on your stamina and susceptibility to poison oak, this route offers several day-hike or overnight options, including: (1) 4.4 miles round-trip to Cruikshank Camp (trails are clear and well maintained); (2) 6.2 miles round-trip to Silver Camp (trails passable with some poison oak); and (3) 9 miles round-trip to Buckeye Camp via the Cruikshank and Buckeye Trails (see TRIP 71 Highway 1 to Buckeye Camp, page 286). If you can arrange a shuttle vehicle, consider a point-to-point trip from the lower Cruikshank Trailhead to the abandoned Salmon Creek Station (refer to TRIP 72 Salmon Creek Station to Buckeye Camp, page 288), although sections of the lower Buckeye Trail may be overgrown.

Trip Description

From the signed **Cruikshank Trailhead** on **Highway 1**, you'll quickly climb steep switchbacks through dense coastal scrub. Pause often to catch your breath and appreciate the stunning coastal views. After a strenuous 600-foot ascent in less than a mile, the grade eases.

Continue along the south wall of deep, V-shaped **Villa Creek** canyon through shallow redwood-lined gullies. You'll cross a small creek fringed with redwood sorrel, starflowers, and ferns, then a minute later pass a few eucalyptus trees, likely planted here by early home-steaders. Two miles from the trailhead, you'll cross logs over a small creek and enter **Lower Cruikshank Camp** (1300').

In the shade of redwoods and bays, the first campsite is equipped with a fire ring. The trail continues 0.2 mile to a shady second campsite (2.2 miles, 1400'), equipped with a fire ring and a bench in the shade of sprawling oaks. Just past the second site, you'll reach the signed **Buckeye Trail junction** (2.2 miles, 1440').

From this junction, the northbound **Buckeye Trail** leads to **Villa Creek and Alder Creek Camps** (see TRIP 68 Alder Creek Camp to Villa Creek Camp, page 281), the eastbound **Cruikshank Trail** leads to **Silver** and **Lion Den Camps,** and the southbound Buckeye Trail leads first to **Buckeye Camp,** then 3.4 miles farther to the abandoned **Salmon Creek Station** (see TRIP 72 Salmon Creek Station to Buckeye Camp, page 288).

Continue east on the Cruikshank Trail to **Cruikshank Camp,** amid a small open meadow, site of the former **Cruikshank homestead** and an **American Indian midden** dating back to the Salinian Indians. Poison oak encroaches on the trail beyond this point.

Southeast of camp, the trail ascends 510 feet over the next 0.9 mile to **Silver Camp** (3.1 miles, 1950'), amid a picturesque grassland.

Past camp, poison oak and debris obstruct the narrow trail, which is hard to discern from the many deer paths that cross the route. If you're determined to hike farther, the trail leads 2.5 miles farther to **Silver Peak Road,** 2.9 miles to Lion Den Camp, and 3.4 miles to the junction of **Coast Ridge Road.**

Trip 71

HIGHWAY 1 TO BUCKEYE CAMP

LENGTH AND TYPE: 9-mile out-and-back or 7.9-mile point-to-point

RATING: Moderate to strenuous

TRAIL CONDITION: Clear to difficult, poison oak

HIGHLIGHTS: In spring, sprawling Buckeye Meadow boasts a carpet of colorful wildflowers.

TO REACH THE TRAILHEAD: The Cruikshank Trailhead is on the east side of Highway 1, 0.6 mile south of the Villa Creek bridge, 66 miles south of Carmel, and 4.5 miles north of the abandoned Salmon Creek Station. Park at the small turnout on Highway 1 adjacent to the trailhead. There are no facilities or water at the trailhead.

TRIP SUMMARY: This route to Buckeye Camp via the Cruikshank and Buckeye Trails is ideal in spring, when wildflowers and other budding plants blanket the open meadow. The trails are passable, though poison oak and washouts are common in places.

Other options include a 4.4-mile round-trip to Cruikshank Camp (trails are clear and well maintained) or, if you can arrange a shuttle vehicle, the 7.9-mile point-to-point trek from the abandoned Salmon Creek Station to the lower Cruikshank Trailhead (refer to TRIP 72 Salmon Creek Station to Buckeye Camp, page 288).

Trip Description

See TRIP 70 Cruikshank & Silver Camps (page 285) for the first 2.2 miles of this route to the signed **Buckeye Trail junction** (1440').

Turn right at the junction and head south on the **Buckeye Trail**. You'll climb the north slopes of **Villa Creek** canyon past oak and pine woodlands and across redwood-lined dry gullies. Unfortunately, trail conditions deteriorate, as encroaching plants obscure an already diminished tread.

In scattered shade, the trail climbs to an open saddle along **Redwood Gulch**. On my hike, red and pink flagging marked this indistinct stretch, which climbs south from the saddle toward a pine-rimmed minor ridge (3.1 miles, 2200'). Pause atop the ridge for far-reaching views.

From here the trail contours through dense coastal scrub past five gullies, dry in all but the heaviest rains. It's best to wear long pants along this stretch, as ticks are common during the wet season and poison oak is a year-round nuisance. Past the fifth gully, the route drops along poor tread to a small creek (4.1 miles, 1890') that's usually dry by summer. An easy hop across leads quickly to a second creek that also runs dry by summer. Onward, the trail leads north from the pleasant shade of maples and oaks to a large rocky outcrop, then southeast to the edge of **Buckeye Meadow**.

Entering the oak-rimmed meadow, you'll reach the smaller of **Buckeye Camp**'s two sites (4.5 miles, 2050'). Marked by a fire ring and a weathered table, this site offers room for up to

Sprawling oaks and buckeyes line the carpet of wildflowers each spring in Buckeye Meadow.

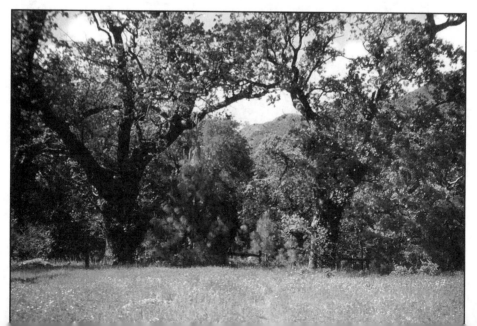

two tents. Onward, the trail threads between two large valley oaks and leads 100 yards farther to the large main site (2060'), which can accommodate several tents in the shade of a large fragrant bay. This is an ideal spot for a group outing, with plenty of room to play Frisbee or frolic in the broad meadow. A reliable spring-fed creek passes just south of camp, though in summer the shallow murky water may lose its appeal.

Scattered large ponderosa and Coulter pines and eucalyptus trees border the meadow, which in spring is painted with deep purple lupines. Enjoy the beautiful surroundings before returning to the trailhead. If you're after a grander tour of the wilderness, refer to the following trip and reverse the trail description.

A BLESSING & A CURSE ■ ■ ■ ■ ■ ■ ■ ■ ■ ■ ■ ■ ■ ■ ■ ■

While the dedication of Highway 1 in 1938 opened the Big Sur wilderness for all to enjoy, the construction project was also the source of devastating environmental damage, as crews dynamited and bulldozed coastal slopes to forge road cuts and bridges. Some of these scars remain, requiring continual maintenance and retrofitting. In stretches, heavy winter storms spawn landslides that can close the highway for extended periods. Invasive plant species compound the problem, as they choke out native flora, which loosens soil and boosts the potential for further slides.

Residents have long lobbied on behalf of the region, motivated by environmental concerns and fears that tourism might lead to rampant development and commercialism. Soon after the highway opened, residents lobbied the local board of supervisors and county planning commission to ban billboards and similar visual noise. As a result, visitors today can still enjoy stunning, uninterrupted vistas from the many turnouts along Highway 1.

■ ■

Trip 72

SALMON CREEK STATION TO BUCKEYE CAMP

LENGTH AND TYPE: 6.8-mile out-and-back, 7.9-mile point-to-point (Cruikshank Trailhead), or 8.4-mile point-to-point (Alder Creek Camp)

RATING: Strenuous

TRAIL CONDITION: Difficult, poison oak

HIGHLIGHTS: Another route to spectacular Buckeye Meadow, whose spacious grasslands burst forth with new life in spring

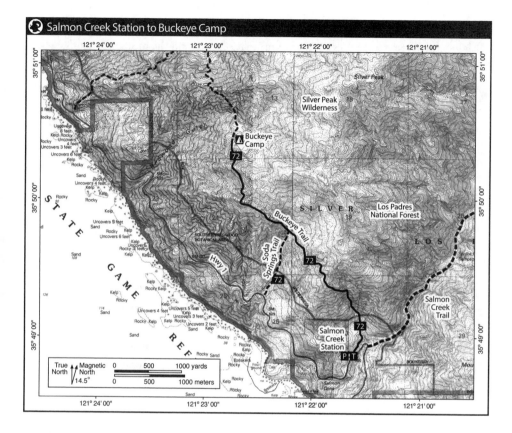

Salmon Creek Station to Buckeye Camp

TO REACH THE TRAILHEAD: The signed Buckeye Trailhead is at the abandoned Salmon Creek Station, 100 yards north of a tight bend in Highway 1, 8 miles south of Gorda, and 1.5 miles north of the posted San Luis Obispo County line. Park at the station. The trailhead is immediately west of the parking area. There are no facilities or water at the trailhead.

TRIP SUMMARY: The Buckeye Trail offers some of the best day-hike and overnight options in the Silver Peak Wilderness. If you can arrange a shuttle vehicle, point-to-point trips include: (1) 1.5 miles to Soda Springs Trailhead via the Buckeye and Soda Springs Trails; (2) 7.9 miles to the Cruikshank Trailhead via the Buckeye and Cruikshank Trails; and (3) 8.4 miles to Alder Creek Camp via the Buckeye Trail. Regardless of your itinerary, Buckeye Camp is a highlight. Perched amid an open meadow, the camp is roomy enough for a group outing.

Unfortunately, most of the trail beats through fast-growing coastal brush that each year aggressively overruns the trail. Those susceptible to poison oak should think twice, as this toxic plant is common along the coastal slopes.

The best time to hike the trail is between October and May, when fog banks roll well offshore, migrating gray whales spout within sight of land, and the meadows bloom anew. However, the wet months (November through April) also bring an onslaught of ticks, which wait alongside trails for unwary passersby. Wear light-colored pants and a long-sleeved shirt to help spot them. Though not breathable, rain pants or nylon pants may thwart these pesky hitchhikers altogether.

Summer is less desirable, as fog often obscures coastal views and warmer temperatures (usually above 70°F) bring an onslaught of nagging flies that persist through late fall.

Trip Description

The signed **Buckeye Trailhead** (230') lies just west of the abandoned ranger station's dilapidated garage. You'll cross a cattle guard and climb behind the station to a gated barbwire fence. Be sure to close the gate behind you.

After a steep, short climb past interwoven branches of poison oak and morning glory, the trail reaches a piped **spring** (0.2 mile, 410') that pours into large metal barrels. Continue climbing along a minor ridge to open slopes of fragrant coastal scrub, including sagebrush, yarrow, hedge nettle, and ceanothus. The ridge leads to a minor saddle (0.5 mile, 760') directly above Highway 1 for spectacular, unobstructed views of the coast.

Spring often brings windy, fogless days, exposing a dramatic convergence of land and sea.

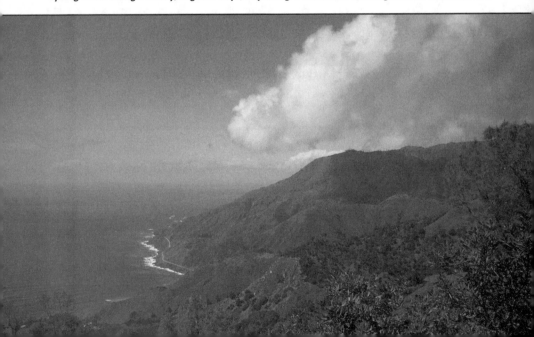

From the saddle, the trail crosses arid slopes flanked with open grasslands and scattered yuccas, climbing northwest past a barbwire fence to the **Soda Springs Trail junction** (1 mile, 860'). While the **Soda Springs Trail** leads a half mile to Highway 1, offering a shorter route to Buckeye Camp, the trail is steeper and often overgrown.

Past the junction, the trail crosses a bay-lined minor gully, which in wet season supports a small waterfall 30 feet northeast of the trail. You'll quickly cross three more gullies fringed with oaks, maples, bays, toyons, and buckeyes, offering shady respite from the exposed coastal slopes.

Just past a cascading creek, you'll reach an oak-clad minor ridge with impressive views. Cross another shady gully to a stand of ponderosa pines for views south toward **Piedras Blancas,** near Hearst Castle. Views open up to the north as you climb open oak and pine woodlands past a dry gully (3.3 miles, 2060'). From here the trail crosses a typically dry creek past a fence to the signed **Buckeye Camp** entrance at spacious **Buckeye Meadow.**

Skirting the oak-rimmed meadow, the trail reaches the main site (3.4 miles, 2060') in the shade of a large bay. This is an ideal spot for a group outing, with plenty of room for several tents. A reliable spring-fed creek passes just south of camp, though in summer the shallow murky water may lose its appeal. To reach the smaller second site, continue northwest, threading a pair of valley oaks at meadow's edge. The site lies just downslope, offering a fire ring, a weathered table, and room for up to two tents.

You can either return the way you came or loop north on the **Buckeye Trail** to the **Cruikshank Trailhead** along Highway 1 (refer to TRIP 71 Highway 1 to Buckeye Camp, page, 286 and follow that trail description in reverse). Be aware that this route may be overgrown and the tread obscured in places.

Trip 73

SALMON CREEK TRAIL TO SPRUCE CREEK & ESTRELLA CAMPS

LENGTH AND TYPE: 6.5-mile out-and-back or 6-mile point-to-point (Coast Ridge Road)

RATING: Moderate to strenuous

TRAIL CONDITION: Clear to difficult, poison oak, overgrown trail conditions past Spruce Creek Camp

HIGHLIGHTS: Follow mossy, forested Salmon Creek to impressive waterfalls, majestic oak woodlands, and vibrant spring wildflowers on the upper slopes.

TO REACH THE TRAILHEAD: The signed Salmon Creek Trailhead is at the tight bend in Highway 1, 8 miles south of Gorda, 27 miles south of Big Sur Station, 1.5 miles north of the posted San Luis Obispo County line, and 3.7 miles north of Ragged Point. Park at wide turnouts on either side of Highway 1. There are no facilities or water at the trailhead.

TRIP SUMMARY: This route offers several day-hike and overnight options. Don't miss the 0.2-mile round-trip day hike along Salmon Creek to Salmon Creek Falls. Though the falls are visible from the highway, be sure to brave the crowds on this popular trail. Another spectacular day-hike destination is Upper Salmon Creek Falls, 2.6 miles up the Salmon Creek Trail, between Spruce Creek and Estrella Camps. A short, steep unmarked spur leads down to the thundering falls, which cascade over large moss-covered boulders into an iridescent pool. Pause for an invigorating swim in spring and summer. Expect a quick dip, as water temperatures reach the high 50s Fahrenheit at best.

Backpackers can hike 2 miles to Spruce Creek Camp or 3.25 miles to Estrella Camp for year-round camping in the heart of the Salmon Creek drainage. Base yourself at either camp for day hikes farther into the wilderness. One favorite destination is Dutra Flat along the San Carpoforo Trail (see TRIP 74 Dutra Flat & San Carpoforo Camps, page 297).

Heavily overgrown trails and prevalent poison oak near Coast Ridge Road may limit your loop trip options. Trails descending from Coast Ridge Road are also in poor condition, as is the road itself in places. While the roadbed from the unmarked Willow Creek Road/Los Burros Road junction is sound, encroaching brush will scratch even the narrowest vehicles. Fallen trees, washouts, and heavy rains may make the road impassable. Check with the US Forest Service before attempting to drive the road (see Phone, page 277, for contact information).

Trip Description

From its trailhead on **Highway 1,** the **Salmon Creek Trail** climbs a moderate grade along the south bank of **Salmon Creek** toward the clearly audible falls. In 0.1 mile you'll reach the unmarked **Salmon Creek Falls Trail junction** (0.1 mile, 230'). No matter where you're headed, don't miss the 200-foot spur to the base of the falls, which winds past fragrant bays and large mossy boulders amid the cool mist.

After exploring the falls, carefully retrace your steps to this junction if you're bound for Spruce Creek Camp, the Spruce Creek Trail, or Estrella Camp. Don't be taken in by the heavily used, steep spur that continues up Salmon Creek to rocky promontories above the falls. Many hikers (perhaps misreading the USFS map that shows the trail following the river's course) mistake this spur for the Salmon Creek Trail, following it until it disappears into oblivion a mile upstream.

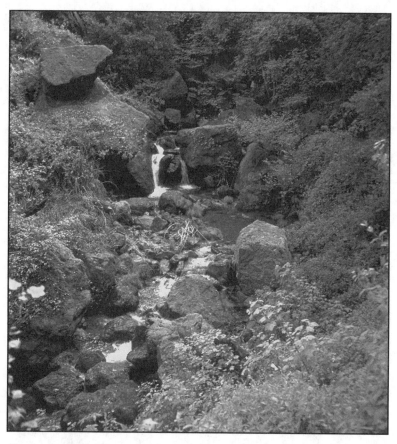

Spruce Creek flows past moss- and fern-covered boulders shaded by a lush riparian forest.

From the unmarked spur junction, you'll continue climbing a moderate grade up the south canyon wall. The trail soon switchbacks past a seasonal creek to a rocky viewpoint (0.3 mile, 760') that overlooks Salmon Creek's downstream passage to the **Pacific**. Fog may obscure the view in summer.

Notice the diverse plant life and dramatic vegetation shift in the canyon. A lush riparian forest of alders, maples, and bays along the canyon floor gives way to coastal scrub of fragrant sagebrush, sticky monkeyflowers, and coffeeberries, followed by a rocky, arid zone of succulents such as Our Lord's candle. The latter, a yucca, dies soon after sprouting a large stalk of cream-colored blossoms.

Onward, the trail switchbacks past a conspicuous mound of light-green, slippery **serpentine** (0.5 mile, 760'), California's state rock. Formed of basalt sediments from ancient seafloors, this stone slithered along fault lines to the surface. Many geologists believe this

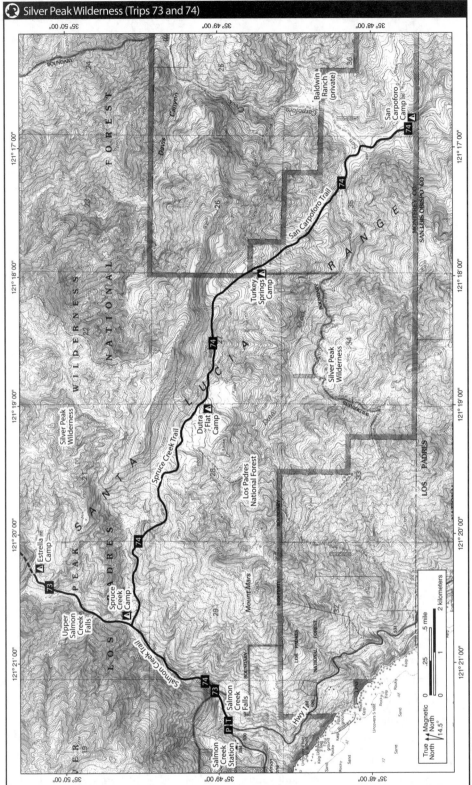

explains serpentine's slick appearance. Few plants can survive in shallow, nutrient-poor serpentine soils. A few "serpentine endemics" have adapted, including California poppies, yucca, and other tenacious succulents. Pause to enjoy unobstructed ocean vistas across Highway 1 and west down Salmon Creek's sheer V-shaped canyon.

The trail continues to climb the north-facing slopes through dense coastal shrub into the shade of sprawling live oaks and bays. Past a gradual turn east, you'll reach an easily overlooked **spur junction** (0.8 mile, 940'). This spur leads northeast 40 feet to two small unofficial camps. Each can accommodate up to two tents, though neither is as pleasant as Spruce Creek or Estrella Camps. The nearest reliable water is back down at Salmon Creek.

The main trail continues its moderate climb past fragrant black sage and sagebrush thickets and mats of hedge nettles, which boast deep lavender blossoms in spring. Just past an unreliable creek (dry in all but heavy rain), you'll reach a **crest** (1.5 miles, 1050'), then gradually descend past groves of Douglas firs, tanoaks, and bays amid dense huckleberry bushes. The trail contours along the south canyon wall, passing two more **seasonal creeks** (1.8 miles, 1010'). Even in winter, these crossings will be an easy hop.

Fifty feet past the last creek, you'll reach the signed **Spruce Creek Trail junction** (1020'). From here the **Spruce Creek Trail** leads southeast 2.5 miles to **Dutra Flat Camp,** 4 miles to **Turkey Springs Camp,** and 6 miles to **San Carpoforo Camp** (see TRIP 74 Dutra Flat & San Carpoforo Camps, page 297). The **Salmon Creek Trail** continues northeast a quarter mile to Spruce Creek Camp, 1.5 miles to Estrella Camp, and 4 miles to Coast Ridge Road. The trail past Estrella Camp may be overgrown with brush and impassable to Coast Ridge Road.

From the Y-junction, bear left and head steadily downslope past large old-growth Douglas firs and vine-like poison oak a quarter mile to **Spruce Creek Camp** (2 miles, 750'). This idyllic backcountry camp offers three sites at the confluence of **Salmon and Spruce Creeks**.

The trail leads directly to the first site, atop a flat on Spruce Creek's south bank. There's room enough for up to two tents, as well as a fire ring and a few large logs for seating. Do not use the abandoned pit toilet 100 feet downstream along Salmon Creek, as the steep topography and winter runoff pose a problem. Until the toilet is replaced, bring a shovel and dig a waste pit at least 6 inches deep and 100 feet from water. Watch where you sit, as poison oak is prolific.

The second site lies across Salmon Creek, just below the confluence. Though usually just a boulder-hop, this crossing may be wet or even impassable during heavy winter rains. Use a walking stick or handy branch to keep your balance. Once across, take a short spur north 20 feet past a rope swing to the site, which offers a table, a fire ring, a grill, and room for up to three tents.

The third site sprawls across adjoining flats along the Salmon Creek Trail, 40 feet upstream from the first site. There's a fire ring and room for up to three tents.

Beyond the third site, the trail begins a moderate climb of the north-facing slopes in the shade of young Douglas firs, bays, oaks, and ceanothus, whose blue blossoms fill the air with a lilac aroma in spring. You'll skirt high above the creek past small rapids and swirling emerald pools. While this stretch of the trail is clear of overgrown brush, a few small washouts between Spruce Creek and Estrella Camps require careful footing.

As you cross steep minor gullies, the sound of cascading water will lead you on. Just before a bend in the trail (2.6 miles, 1140'), a steep spur drops 150 feet to the base of **Upper Salmon Creek Falls**. More reminiscent of a deer trail, the precarious spur slides down loose rock past poison oak. Despite the challenging trail conditions, the alluring waterfall and swimming hole tempt many hikers down to the banks of Salmon Creek.

A few yards past the spur, you'll veer south 200 feet up a minor gully, cross its small seasonal stream, then switchback north up the Salmon Creek drainage (2.7 miles, 1150'). Skirting a few fallen trees, the trail opens on fine views of the canyon's forested slopes and the often-fogbound coast. Onward, the trail veers southeast away from the creek to a spur junction (3.1 miles, 1340'). This short spur leads to a grassy flat where deer commonly graze, an excellent place to stargaze a few paces from **Estrella Camp**.

Just past the junction, you'll arrive at the first two sites (3.25 miles, 1360'), perched on the west bank of Estrella Creek just above its confluence with Salmon Creek. The open first site has room for up to three tents, while the second site can accommodate up to four tents in the shade of a sprawling live oak. Both sites are equipped with a fire ring, and drinking water lies just downslope at year-round **Estrella Creek**.

Few people hike farther due to encroaching brush and poison oak a mile past camp to trail's end at **Coast Ridge Road**. For current trail conditions, call the Pacific Valley Station

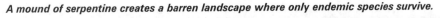

A mound of serpentine creates a barren landscape where only endemic species survive.

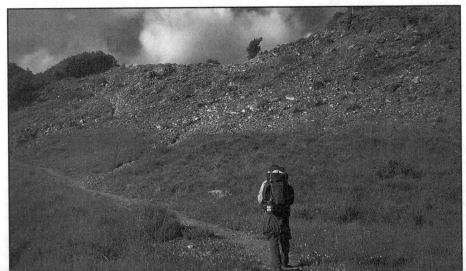

at (805) 927-4211. If you'd like join a volunteer maintenance crew, contact the Ventana Wilderness Alliance: (831) 423-3191, ventanawild.org. Though hard work, maintenance outings take in a spectacular loop trip up the Salmon Creek Trail to Coast Ridge Road and down the **Buckeye Trail.**

Trip 74

DUTRA FLAT & SAN CARPOFORO CAMPS

LENGTH AND TYPE: 15.6-mile out-and-back

RATING: Strenuous

TRAIL CONDITION: Passable to difficult, poison oak, cattle trails, faint tread

HIGHLIGHTS: Find solitude amid oak-studded golden hills, peaceful pine groves, and open meadows blanketed in fragrant spring wildflowers.

TO REACH THE TRAILHEAD: The signed Salmon Creek Trailhead is at the tight bend in Highway 1, 8 miles south of Gorda, 27 miles south of Big Sur Station, 1.5 miles north of the posted San Luis Obispo County line, and 3.7 miles north of Ragged Point. Park at wide turnouts on either side of Highway 1. There are no facilities or water at the trailhead.

TRIP SUMMARY: This route offers several out-and-back day hikes and overnight options, including: (1) 4 miles round-trip to Spruce Creek Camp, (2) 8.4 miles round-trip to Dutra Flat, (3) 12.2 miles round-trip to Turkey Springs Camp, and (4) 15.6 miles round-trip to San Carpoforo Camp. The Spruce Creek Trail becomes the San Carpoforo Trail at Dutra Flat.

The hike begins on a gentle ascent of the Salmon Creek drainage with views downcanyon to the often-fogbound coast. Onward, the trail climbs to the headwaters of the Spruce Creek drainage. Across the divide between the Spruce Creek and Dutra Creek watersheds, the San Carpoforo Trail winds past historic homestead sites and golden hills. You'll find a rich array of vegetation and terrain along the way, from riparian forests, to oak savannas, and wildflower-strewn open meadows.

Visit in spring to witness spectacular wildflower displays along the slopes of the San Carpoforo watershed. In winter, rain-saturated hillsides sprout vibrant green grasses and herbaceous plants. Year-round water sources are available at each camp in all but the driest years. Ticks are prolific during the wet season (November through April), flies and gnats are persistent in summer, and poison oak is unavoidable along the lower sections of the Spruce Creek Trail. On my hike, the last 100 yards to San Carpoforo Camp were overgrown with willow thickets and head-high stinging nettles.

Trip Description

See TRIP 73 Salmon Creek Trail to Spruce Creek & Estrella Camps (page 291) for the first 1.8 miles of this route to the **Spruce Creek Trail junction** (1.8 miles, 1020').

From the junction, turn right onto the less-traveled **Spruce Creek Trail,** which traces the slopes northeast of **Spruce Creek**. Unfortunately, poison oak is a common trailside companion along the overgrown trail.

Half a mile ahead, the trail breaks through the dense canopy of hardwoods and conifers to an open rocky barren (2.3 miles, 1200') and views north across the **Salmon Creek** drainage to 3590-foot **Silver Peak**. Past the barren, you'll turn south and follow year-round Spruce Creek past moss-covered boulders in the shade of bigleaf maples, sycamores, and oaks.

As you climb, notice how the vegetation changes from a riparian woodland to a mixed woodland of madrones, oaks, bays, and conifers. As you reach the divide between the Spruce Creek and **Dutra Creek** drainages (3.2 miles, 1950'), you enter a zone of brushy ceanothus, manzanita, and sage. The trail meets a gated barbwire fence at the saddle marking the divide. Be sure to close the gate behind you.

From here the vegetation and terrain shift dramatically from the steep, heavily forested canyons of Salmon and Spruce Creeks to rolling grasslands dotted with solitary oaks and stands of Coulter pines amid various seeps, springs, and meadows. The onward trail is virtually all downhill on a gentle to moderate grade.

Passing beneath a crimson canopy of tree-like manzanita, the trail descends to spacious meadows laced with small seasonal creeks and springs that are often dry by late spring. After 2.3 miles on the Spruce Creek Trail (called the **San Carpoforo Trail** from this point on), you'll arrive at **Dutra Flat Camp** (4.2 miles, 1930').

Once the site of an old homestead, this camp rests on a broad flat along a south-facing slope amid four large planted Monterey cypresses. With room enough for up to three tightly grouped tents, the site comes equipped with two fire rings and grills along with a table and bench. Rusty barbwire runs the perimeter, built to keep out cattle that feed on the grassy clearing above camp. In drier months, head uphill to find water at a spring-filled trough in the clearing.

A hundred feet south of camp is a marked junction with a spur that leads east 3 miles to **Coast Ridge Road**. Continue south on the San Carpoforo Trail. Ponderosa pines form small stands along these grassy slopes. In summer, go in search of several fruit trees on the south end of the flat. Reminders of the homestead that once occupied Dutra Flat, these trees still blossom and bear fruit.

Within sight of the dirt road from private **Baldwin Ranch,** which crosses the ridge to your west, you'll reach a minor gully. In wet months, water saturates the ground here, creating muddy seeps that preserve the tracks of visiting animals. Common visitors include bobcats, coyotes, gray foxes, and the occasional mountain lion.

Farther east the trail skirts a minor slide (4.7 miles, 1790'), so watch your footing. In spring this hillside supports decadent fields of purple lupine. Ahead, you'll veer southeast and descend a scenic ridge toward a notable lone oak on a small grassy knoll. Pause along the ridge for astounding views south across the **San Carpoforo drainage** and southern boundary of the **Silver Peak Wilderness.**

Before reaching the lone oak, you'll switchback south and descend to a minor gully (5.4 miles, 1560'), where several cattle paths cross the trail, headed north toward a creekside meadow. The trail contours to a minor ridge and the junction with another well-worn **cattle path** (5.8 miles, 1530') that hikers often mistake for the main trail. On my hike, pink flagging hung from a gray pine with a prominent forked top, marking this easily missed junction.

The cattle path leads straight past the gray pine, then plunges 0.7 mile down the southwest-facing walls of Dutra Creek canyon to **Baldwin Ranch Road.** From here, you could follow the less-scenic road 1.7 miles to the San Carpoforo Camp Trail.

If you prefer to continue on the main trail, turn left at the flagged junction just past the gray pine. In 0.3 mile, the trail crosses a small stream amid an open valley and arrives in **Turkey Springs Camp** (6.1 miles, 1410'). The peaceful site offers room for two tents in the shade of oaks and bays along a small spring-fed creek.

Beyond camp the trail meanders through the valley, crossing the creek four more times on its descent to Baldwin Ranch Road (7.3 miles, 740'). The trail merges with the well-graded road 0.3 mile farther to the signed **San Carpoforo Camp Trail junction.**

Turn right off the dirt road to cross a broad meadow to **San Carpoforo Creek.** This crossing is usually a knee-deep ford, though heavy winter rains may swell the creek, rendering it impassable. The trail continues downstream through dense willows and thickets of stinging nettles.

Brushing carefully past the nettles, you'll cross the creek once more to reach **San Carpoforo Camp** (7.8 miles, 650'), which offers room enough for up to five tents in the shade. In summer, swimming holes along the creek offer respite from the heat.

Note that the spelling of *San Carpoforo* on trail signs varies from "Carpoforo" to "Carpojo." USGS maps list it as Carpoforo, while locals pronounce it Carpojo.

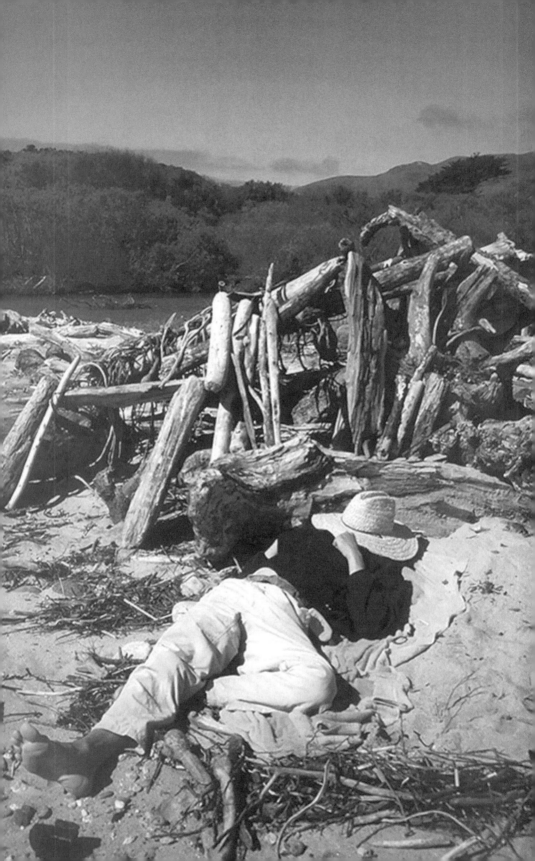

APPENDIX

Trips by Theme

Epic Views
Day Hikes
#2 Carmelo Meadow, Granite Point, & Moss Cove Trails

#3 Cypress Grove Trail

#4 South Shore, Bird Island, South Plateau, & Pine Ridge Trails

#6 Rocky Ridge Trail

#8 Soberanes Point Trails

#9 Point Sur State Historic Park

#10 Trail Camp & Headlands Trails

#12 East Molera Trail

#15 Bluffs, Spring, Panorama, & Ridge Trails

#16 Valley View Trail

#20 Manuel Peak Trail

#24 Tan Bark Trail & Fire Road Loop

#25 Ewoldsen Trail

#26 McWay Falls

#32 Ragged Point Nature Trail

#33 Piedras Blancas

#42 Manuel Peak & Pfeiffer Big Sur State Park

#57 Junipero Serra Peak

#62 Cone Peak Trail

Backpacking Trips
#37 Devils Peak & Mt. Carmel

#38 Ventana Double Cone via Ventana Trail

#47 Ventana Double Cone via Big Pines Trail

#51 Ventana Double Cone via Pine Valley

#53 Black Cone Trail to Arroyo Seco

#65 Cone Peak Loop

#66 Highway 1 to Vicente Flat

#67 Prewitt Loop Trail

#70 Cruikshank & Silver Camps

#72 Salmon Creek Station to Buckeye Camp

Waterfalls
Day Hikes
#17 Pfeiffer Falls Trail

#26 McWay Falls

#28 Limekiln Falls Trail

#32 Ragged Point Nature Trail

#73 Salmon Creek Trail to Spruce Creek & Estrella Camps

Backpacking Trips
#40 Coast Road to Pico Blanco Camp

#41 Pico Blanco

#45 Hiding Canyon & Round Rock Camps

#49 Pine Valley

#50 Hiding Canyon & Round Rock Camps

#73 Salmon Creek Trail to Spruce Creek & Estrella Camps

Wildflowers
Day Hikes
#25 Ewoldsen Trail

#30 Pacific Valley Trail

#36 San Simeon Nature Trail

Backpacking Trips

#40 Coast Road to Pico Blanco Camp
#44 Bluff & Carmel River Camps
#45 Hiding Canyon & Round Rock Camps
#56 Willow Springs & Strawberry Camps
#58 Ventana Camp
#59 Sykes & Redwood Camps
#74 Dutra Flat & San Carpoforo Camps

Swimming
Day Hikes

#1 Carmel River State Beach
#4 South Shore, Bird Island, South Plateau, & Pine Ridge Trails
#13 River Trail Loop
#21 Gorge Trail
#22 Pfeiffer Beach
#34 Hearst Memorial State Beach
#35 San Simeon State Beach

Backpacking Trips

#39 Little Sur & Jackson Camps
#40 Coast Road to Pico Blanco Camp
#41 Pico Blanco
#44 Bluff & Carmel River Camps
#45 Hiding Canyon & Round Rock Camps
#49 Pine Valley
#50 Hiding Canyon & Round Rock Camps
#55 Tassajara Hot Springs
#56 Willow Springs & Strawberry Camps
#58 Ventana Camp
#59 Sykes & Redwood Camps
#73 Salmon Creek Trail to Spruce Creek & Estrella Camps

Redwood Forest
Day Hikes

#7 Soberanes Canyon Trail
#17 Pfeiffer Falls Trail
#18 Nature Trail
#24 Tan Bark Trail & Fire Road Loop
#25 Ewoldsen Trail
Trips #27–29 (all trails)

Backpacking Trips

#39 Little Sur & Jackson Camps
#40 Coast Road to Pico Blanco Camp
#59 Sykes & Redwood Camps
#60 Highway 1 to Terrace Creek Camp
#64 Vicente Flat Trail
#69 Highway 1 to Villa Creek Camp

Oak Woodland
Day Hikes

#24 Tan Bark Trail & Fire Road Loop
#25 Ewoldsen Trail
#36 San Simeon Nature Trail
#60 Highway 1 to Terrace Creek Camp
#61 Highway 1 to Coast Ridge Road

Backpacking Trips

#37 Devils Peak & Mt. Carmel
#38 Ventana Double Cone via Ventana Trail
#54 Church Creek to Pine Valley Camp
#56 Willow Springs & Strawberry Camps
#65 Cone Peak Loop
#67 Prewitt Loop Trail
#72 Salmon Creek Station to Buckeye Camp

By the Ocean
Day Hikes

Trips #1–4 (all trails)
#5 Coastal Access Trails
#8 Soberanes Point Trails
#9 Point Sur State Historic Park
#10 Trail Camp & Headlands Trails
#11 Beach & Creamery Meadow Trails Loop
#15 Bluffs, Spring, Panorama, & Ridge Trails
#22 Pfeiffer Beach
#23 Partington Cove Trail
#26 McWay Falls
#30 Pacific Valley Trail
#31 Sand Dollar Beach & Jade Cove
#32 Ragged Point Nature Trail
#33 Piedras Blancas

By the Ocean *(continued)*
Day Hikes (continued)
#34 Hearst Memorial State Beach
#35 San Simeon State Beach

Backpacking Trips
Backcountry camping west of Highway 1 is not permitted except at Andrew Molera State Park's walk-in campground, a half mile from Molera Beach and 0.3 mile from the parking lot.

Surfing
#1 Carmel River State Beach
#11 Beach & Creamery Meadow Trails Loop
#22 Pfeiffer Beach
#30 Pacific Valley Trail
#31 Sand Dollar Beach & Jade Cove

Less-Traveled Destinations
Day Hikes
#12 East Molera Trail
#19 Buzzards Roost Trail
#24 Tan Bark Trail & Fire Road Loop
#61 Highway 1 to Coast Ridge Road

Remote Wilderness
Backpacking Trips
#38 Ventana Double Cone via Ventana Trail
#45 Hiding Canyon & Round Rock Camps
#47 Ventana Double Cone via Big Pines Trail
#48 Miller Canyon & Pine Valley Loop
#51 Ventana Double Cone via Pine Valley
#54 Church Creek to Pine Valley Camp
#74 Dutra Flat & San Carpoforo Camps

Accessible by Public Transportation
Day Hikes
Trips #1–4   (all trails)
Trips #5–9   (all trails)
Trips #10–15   (all trails)

Trips #16–21   (seasonal)
Trips #34–36   (all trails)

Backpacking Trips
Trips #58 & 59   (seasonal)

Author's Favorites
Day Hikes
Trips #1–4   (all trails)
#6 Rocky Ridge Trail
#8 Soberanes Point Trails
#9 Point Sur State Historic Park
#10 Trail Camp & Headlands Trails
#15 Bluffs, Spring, Panorama, & Ridge Trails
#16 Valley View Trail
#21 Gorge Trail
#22 Pfeiffer Beach
#23 Partington Cove Trail
#25 Ewoldsen Trail
#26 McWay Falls
#31 Sand Dollar Beach & Jade Cove
#61 Highway 1 to Coast Ridge Road

Backpacking Trips
#38 Ventana Double Cone via Ventana Trail
#40 Coast Road to Pico Blanco Camp
#41 Pico Blanco
#49 Pine Valley
#51 Ventana Double Cone via Pine Valley
#53 Black Cone Trail to Arroyo Seco
#55 Tassajara Hot Springs
#62 Cone Peak Trail
#64 Vicente Flat Trail
#65 Cone Peak Loop
#72 Salmon Creek Station to Buckeye Camp
#74 Dutra Flat & San Carpoforo Camps

Recommended Reading
Plant & Animal Identification

Evarts, John and Marjorie Popper (editors), *Coast Redwood: A Natural & Cultural History.* Los Olivos, CA: Cachuma Press, 2001.

Hensen, Paul and Donald Usner, *The Natural History of Big Sur.* Berkeley, CA: University of California Press, 1993.

Johnson, Sharon G., Pamela C. Muick, Bruce M. Pavlik, and Marjorie Popper, *Oaks of California.* Los Olivos, CA: Cachuma Press, 1991.

Johnston, Verna R., *California Forests & Woodlands.* Berkeley, CA: University of California Press, 1994.

Keator, Glenn, Ruth M. Heady, and Valerie R. Winemiller, *Pacific Coast Fern Finder.* Rochester, N.Y.: Nature Study Guild, 1981.

Lanner, Ronald M., *Conifers of California.* Los Olivos, CA: Cachuma Press, 1999.

Lyons, Kathleen, and Mary Beth Cooney-Lazaneo, *Plants of the Coast Redwood Region.* Boulder Creek, CA: Looking Press, 1988.

McMinn, Howard, and Evelyn Maino, *An Illustrated Manual of Pacific Coast Trees.* 2nd ed. Berkeley, CA: University of California Press, 1981.

Peterson, Roger Tory, A *Field Guide to Western Birds.* Boston: Houghton Mifflin, 1972.

Spellenberg, Richard, *National Audubon Society Field Guide to North American Wildflowers*, Western Region. New York: Alfred A. Knopf, 1998.

Stuart, John, and John Sawyer, *Trees & Shrubs of California.* Berkeley, CA: University of California Press, 2001.

Watts, Phoebe, *Redwood Region Flower Finder.* Berkeley, CA: Nature Study Guild, 1979.

Geology

Alt, David D., and Donald W. Hyndmand, *Roadside Geology of Northern & Central California.* Missoula, Mont.: Mountain Press Publishing Company, 2000.

Earnst, W.G. (editor), *The Geotectonic Development of California.* Englewood Cliffs, N.J.: Prentice Hall, 1981.

Howard, A.D., *Geologic History of Middle California.* Natural History Guide 43. Berkeley, CA: University of California Press, 1979.

Oakeshott, G.B., *Guide to the Geology of Pfeiffer Big Sur State Park,* Monterey County, California. California Division of Mines & Geology Special Report 11, 1951.

Page, B. M., *Migration of Salinian Composite Block in California & Disappearance of Fragments.* American Journal of Science, 282: 1694-1734. 1982.

Trask, P., *Geology of the Point Sur Quadrangle,* California. University of California Publications, Bulletin of the Department of Geological Sciences, 16(6): 119-186. 1926.

Van Andel, T.H., *New Views on an Old Planet: Continental Drift & the History of the Earth.* Cambridge, Mass.: Cambridge University Press. 1985.

Cultural History

Breschini, Gary S., *The Indians of Monterey County*. Carmel, CA: Monterey County Archaeological Society, 1972.

Breschini, Gary S., and Trudy Haversat, *An Overview of the Esselen Indians of Central Monterey County*. Salinas, CA: Coyote Press, 1993.

Brown, William S., *History of the Los Padres National Forest,* 1989-1945. San Francisco: US Forest Service, 1945.

Fink, Augusta, *Monterey County: The Dramatic Story of Its Past*. Santa Cruz, CA: Western Tanager, 1978.

Goodman, Judith (editor), *Big Sur Women*. Big Sur, CA: Big Sur Women's Press, 1983.

Kroeber, A.L., *Handbook of the Indians of California*. Berkeley, CA: Reprint. California Book Company, 1953.

Margolin, Malcolm, *The Ohlone Way: Indian Life in the San Francisco–Monterey Bay Area*. Berkeley, CA: Heyday Books, 1978.

Wall, Rosalind Sharp, *A Wild Coast & Lonely*. San Carlos, CA: Wide World/Tetra, 1992.

Regional Guides

Heid, Matt, *101 Hikes in Northern California 2nd edition*. Berkeley, CA: Wilderness Press, 2008.

Hensen, Paul and Donald Usner, *The Natural History of Big Sur*. Berkeley, CA: University of California Press, 1993.

Lorentzen, Bob, and Richard Nichols, *Hiking the California Coastal Trail: Volume 2*. Mendocino, CA: Bored Feet Publications, 1998.

Puterbaugh, Park and Alan Bisbort, *California Beaches*. San Francisco: Foghorn Press, 1996.

Ventana Chapter, Sierra Club (editors), *Trail Guide to Los Padres National Forest Northern Section*. Carmel, CA: PIP Printing, 1996.

INDEX

MAP INDEX

■ ■ ■ ■ ■ ■ ■ ■ ■ ■ ■ ■ ■

ABOUT THE AUTHOR

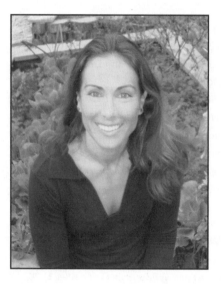

An avid hiker, backpacker, and naturalist, **Analise Elliot Heid** has pursued an outdoor lifestyle both professionally and recreationally. She currently works as an environmental educator, science teacher, and school garden program director along the California coast. Analise holds a B.S. in forestry from U.C. Berkeley, a M.A. in education from San Francisco State University, and works as a master teacher in the Cal State University Science Teacher and Researcher Program.